Study Guide
Cooper & Gosnell

Foundations of Nursing

Ninth Edition

Candice Kumagai

Formerly Instructor in Clinical Nursing
University of Texas at Austin
Austin, Texas

Martha Barry, MS, PN, CNM

Certified Nurse Midwife
OB Faculty Practice
Advocate Aurora Medical Group
Chicago, Illinois

ELSEVIER

ELSEVIER
3251 Riverport Lane
St. Louis, Missouri 63043

STUDY GUIDE FOR FOUNDATIONS OF NURSING, Ninth edition   ISBN: 978-0-323-81204-7

Notices

Knowledge and best practice in this field are constantly changing. As new research and experience broaden our understanding, changes in research methods, professional practices, or medical treatment may become necessary.

Practitioners and researchers must always rely on their own experience and knowledge in evaluating and using any information, methods, compounds, or experiments described herein. In using such information or methods they should be mindful of their own safety and the safety of others, including parties for whom they have a professional responsibility.

With respect to any drug or pharmaceutical products identified, readers are advised to check the most current information provided (i) on procedures featured or (ii) by the manufacturer of each product to be administered, to verify the recommended dose or formula, the method and duration of administration, and contraindications. It is the responsibility of practitioners, relying on their own experience and knowledge of their patients, to make diagnoses, to determine dosages and the best treatment for each individual patient, and to take all appropriate safety precautions.

To the fullest extent of the law, neither the Publisher nor the authors, contributors, or editors, assume any liability for any injury and/or damage to persons or property as a matter of products liability, negligence or otherwise, or from any use or operation of any methods, products, instructions, or ideas contained in the material herein.

Senior Content Strategist: Brandi Graham
Senior Content Development Specialist: Laura Goodrich

Printed in India

Last digit is the print number: 9 8 7 6 5 4

To the Student

Understanding fundamental concepts and principles of nursing will prepare you for patient care experiences. By mastering the content of your *Foundations of Nursing* textbook, you will have the necessary knowledge and skills for nursing practice. This Study Guide was created to help you achieve the objectives of each chapter in the textbook, establish a solid base of knowledge in the fundamentals of nursing, and evaluate your understanding of this critical information.

Each Study Guide chapter is organized into sections, each with its own topic and related objectives from the textbook. Different types of learning activities, including short answer, multiple choice, table activities, matching, figure labeling, and critical thinking activities assist you in meeting these content objectives. A new NextGen question has been added to each chapter. To maximize the benefits of this Study Guide and prepare for the learning activities:

1. Carefully read the chapter in the textbook and highlight, note, or outline important information.
2. Review the Key Points, access the Additional Learning Resources, and complete the Review Questions for the NCLEX® Examination at the end of each textbook chapter.
3. Complete the Study Guide exercises to the best of your ability.
4. Time and pace yourself during the completion of each exercise. You should spend approximately 1 minute for each multiple choice and matching question, and approximately 2 minutes for completion activities or short answer questions.
5. After completing an exercise, refer to the textbook page references as needed. You can then repeat any exercises for additional practice and review. A complete Answer Key is provided on the Evolve Resources website.

ADDITIONAL LEARNING RESOURCES

Additional Learning Resources are available on the Evolve website at http://evolve.elsevier.com/Cooper/foundations/.

Evolve

- Review Questions for the NCLEX® Examination (for each chapter)
- Answer Key for all Study Guide questions
- Calculators
- Fluids and Electrolytes Tutorial
- Immunization Schedule
- Spanish/English Glossary
- Additional Animations
- Additional Audio Clips
- Additional Video Clips
- Skills Performance Checklists
- Body Spectrum Electronic Anatomy Coloring Book

STUDY HINTS FOR ALL STUDENTS

- *Ask questions!* There are no bad questions. If you do not know something or are not sure, you need to find out. Other people may be wondering the same thing but may be too shy to ask. The answer could mean life or death to your patient, which certainly is more important than feeling embarrassed about asking a question..
- *Make use of chapter objectives.* At the beginning of each chapter in the textbook are objectives that you should have mastered when you finished studying that chapter. Write these objectives in your notebook, leaving a blank space after each. Fill in the answers as you find them while reading the

chapter. Review to make sure your answers are correct and complete, and use these answers when you study for tests. This should also be done for separate course objectives that your instructor has listed in your class syllabus.

- *Locate and understand key terms.* At the beginning of each chapter in the textbook are key terms that you will encounter as you read the chapter. Page numbers are provided for easy reference and review, and the key terms are in bold, blue font the first time they appear in the chapter. Phonetic pronunciations are provided for terms that might be difficult to pronounce.
- *Review Key Points.* Use the Key Points at the end of each chapter in the textbook to help you review for exams.
- *Get the most from your textbook.* When reading each chapter in the textbook, look at the subject headings to learn what each section is about. Read first for the general meaning, then reread parts you did not understand. It may help to read those parts aloud. Carefully read the information given in each table and study each figure and its caption.
- *Follow up on difficult concepts.* While studying, put difficult concepts into your own words to see if you understand them. Check this understanding with another student or the instructor. Write these in your notebook.
- *Take useful notes.* When taking lecture notes in class, leave a large margin on the left side of each notebook page and write only on right-hand pages, leaving all left-hand pages blank. Look over your lecture notes soon after each class, while your memory is fresh. Fill in missing words, complete sentences and ideas, and underline key phrases, definitions, and concepts. At the top of each page, write the topic of that page. In the left margin, write the key word for that part of your notes. On the opposite left-hand page, write a summary or outline that combines material from both the textbook and the lecture. These can be your study notes for review.
- *Join or form a study group.* Form a study group with some other students so you can help one another. Practice speaking and reading aloud, ask questions about material you are not sure about, and work together to find answers.
- *Improve your study skills.* Good study skills are essential for achieving your goals in nursing. Time management, efficient use of study time, and a consistent approach to studying are all beneficial.

ADDITIONAL STUDY HINTS FOR STUDENTS WHO USE ENGLISH AS A SECOND LANGUAGE (ESL)

- *Find a first-language buddy.* ESL students should find a first-language buddy—another student who is a native speaker of English and is willing to answer questions about word meanings, pronunciations, and culture. Maybe your buddy would like to learn about your language and culture. This could help in his or her nursing experience as well.
- *Expand your vocabulary.* If you find a nontechnical word you do not know (e.g., *drowsy*), try to guess its meaning from the sentence (e.g., *With electrolyte imbalance, the patient may feel fatigued and drowsy*). If you are not sure of the meaning, or if it seems particularly important, look it up in the dictionary.
- *Keep a vocabulary notebook.* Keep a small alphabetized notebook or address book in which you can write down new nontechnical words you read or hear along with their meanings and pronunciations. Write each word under its initial letter so you can find it easily, as in a dictionary. For words you do not know or for words that have a different meaning in nursing, write down how they are used and sound. Look up their meanings in a dictionary or ask your instructor or first-language buddy. Then write the different meanings or usages that you have found in your book, including the nursing meaning. Continue to add new words as you discover them. For example:
  - *Primary*—Of most importance; main (e.g., *the primary problem or disease*); The first one; elementary (e.g., *primary school*)
  - *Secondary*—Of less importance; resulting from another problem or disease (e.g., *a secondary symptom*); The second one (e.g., *secondary school* [*"high school" in the United States*])

Illustration Credits

Chapter 5
P. 29: Maslow A: *Motivation and personality,* ed 2, New York, 1970, Harper & Row.

Chapter 11
P. 75: Maslow A: *Motivation and personality,* ed 2, New York, 1970, Harper & Row.

Chapter 16
P. 113: Modified from Sheehy SB & Lombardi J: *Manual of emergency care,* ed 4, St. Louis, 1995, Mosby.

Chapter 17
P. 129: Clayton BD & Willihnganz M: *Basic pharmacology for nurses,* ed 17, St. Louis, 2017, Elsevier.

Chapter 23
P. 169: Elkin MK, Perry AG, Potter PA: Nursing interventions and clinical skills, ed 4, St. Louis, 2008, Mosby.

Chapter 31
P. 233: Hockenberry MJ, Wilson D: *Wong's essentials of pediatric nursing,* ed 8, St. Louis, 2009, Mosby.

Chapter 32
P. 242: Hockenberry MJ, Wilson D: *Wong's essentials of pediatric nursing,* ed 9, St. Louis, 2013, Mosby.

Contents

The Evolution of Nursing

Answer Key: A complete Answer Key is provided in your Additional Learning Resources on Evolve.

MATCHING

Directions: Match the nurse on the left with the contribution to nursing on the right.

Nurse	Contribution to Nursing
_____ 1. Dorothea Dix (1802-1887)	a. Credited with the development of the first nursing and hospital records
_____ 2. Clara Barton (1821-1912)	b. Pioneer crusader for elevation of standards of care for the mentally ill
_____ 3. Mary Ann Ball (1817-1901)	c. Worked for acceptance of African Americans in the nursing profession
_____ 4. Linda Richards (1841-1930)	d. Developed the American Red Cross in 1881
_____ 5. Isabel Hampton Robb (1860-1910)	e. Championed the rights and comforts of soldiers; organized diet kitchens, laundries, and ambulance service
_____ 6. Lavinia Dock (1858-1956)	f. Organized the first graded system of theory and practice in schools of nursing
_____ 7. Mary Eliza Mahoney (1845-1926)	g. Responsible for the development of public health nursing in the United States through the founding of the Henry Street Settlement in New York City
_____ 8. Lillian D. Wald (1867-1940)	h. Responsible, with Robb, for the organization of the American Society of Superintendents of Training Schools, which evolved into the National League for Nursing Education
_____ 9. Mary Adelaide Nutting (1858-1947)	i. Pioneer in nurse-midwifery
_____ 10. Mary Breckenridge (1881-1965)	j. Developed curriculum concepts and guidelines for student nurses

MULTIPLE CHOICE

Directions: Select the best answer(s) for each of the following questions.

11. For which circumstance is the nurse **most** likely to seek advice from the National Association for Practical Nurse Education and Service (NAPNES)?
    1. Being bullied and harassed by RN supervisor and coworkers
    2. Observing unprofessional behavior among nursing students
    3. Looking for a new job that provides opportunities to learn advanced skills
    4. Seeking to compare a facility policy to standards set for LPN/LVN practice

12. Which nursing action typifies the role of the LPN/LVN in case management nursing?
    1. Selects a clinical pathway to map time frames during hospitalization
    2. Coordinates and plans the care for a group of patients
    3. Cross-trains to assume duties that are usually performed by RNs
    4. Assists the RN in attaining desired patient outcomes of care

13. In which setting are most LPN/LVNs employed?
    1. Acute care hospital units
    2. Long-term care facilities
    3. Health care providers' (HCP) offices
    4. Home health agencies

14. Which nursing actions are appropriate to the roles/responsibilities of the LPN/LVN? **Select all that apply.**
    1. Uses active listening techniques when interacting with a depressed patient
    2. Reports changes in vital signs to the supervising RN and HCP in a timely fashion
    3. Takes initiative to create a comprehensive care plan for a newly admitted patient
    4. Ensures that the correct medication is given to the correct patient at the correct time
    5. Collects data from the patient, the family, and previous medical records

15. Which statement by a male nursing student is **most** likely to represent a factor associated with the high attrition rate of male students from nursing education programs?
    1. "The course of study is too prolonged and difficult."
    2. "I can make more money if I become a doctor."
    3. "The nursing instructors claim that I am not caring."
    4. "It's difficult for men to advance in the nursing profession."

16. A patient suddenly becomes unresponsive; therefore, he is unable to make decisions about health care options. What is the health care team **most** likely to do to determine the patient's wishes?
    1. Contact the patient's closest adult relative.
    2. Determine if the patient has a personal attorney.
    3. Seek opinions from the patient's primary HCP.
    4. Review the patient's advance directives.

17. One of the major problems of hospitals of the early nineteenth century has been addressed by which measure in contemporary health care?
    1. Focusing on women's health issues, such as heart disease
    2. Using Standard Precautions and improving hygienic practices
    3. Encouraging men to enter the nursing profession
    4. Reducing the nursing shortage during wartime

18. Which patient typifies the demographic changes of the population in the twenty-first century and represents an increased need for nursing care?
    1. A 3-month-old infant with developmental disabilities
    2. A 15-year-old homeless adolescent
    3. A 45-year-old man with diabetes
    4. A 78-year-old woman with chronic illness

19. Which nursing action reflects Florence Nightingale's vision of how to improve patient care?
    1. Includes the family in the patient education sessions
    2. Considers the patient's cultural and ethnic background
    3. Attends an in-service to learn about a new infusion pump
    4. Safeguards patient's privacy by maintaining confidentiality

20. Which situation includes the four major concepts that are the basis for nursing theories and models?
    1. The home health nurse assesses the patient's health and the home setting.
    2. The nurse studies nursing theory in an advanced-practice nursing curriculum.
    3. Nursing programs draw from several psychosocial and nursing theories.
    4. The patient is treated for hypertension, diabetes, and obesity.

21. Which patient is **most** at risk for being one of the "medically underserved" in the United States?
    1. A 30-year-old woman with newly diagnosed breast cancer
    2. An 86-year-old man who resides in a long-term care facility
    3. A 3-year-old whose parents recently emigrated for work
    4. A 60-year-old unemployed veteran who lives on the street

22. Using Maslow's hierarchy of needs, the nurse gives **priority** to which problem?
    1. Loneliness due to being away from family during hospitalization
    2. Inability to eat because of difficulty chewing and swallowing
    3. Anxiety due to recent diagnosis of cancer with poor prognosis
    4. Safety related to difficulty with balance during position change

23. A mother tells the nurse that her 17-year-old son, who has been wheelchair-bound for 1 year following an accident, is depressed because basketball season is starting and he was a star player for his high-school team. Using Maslow's hierarchy of needs, which intervention would address the adolescent's **priority** need?
    1. Advise the mother to check the wheelchair access ramps for safe access to the gym.
    2. Explore other interests and activities that would increase his self-esteem.
    3. Initiate a review of body systems to identify the cause of depression.
    4. Suggest the mother and son seek out a wheelchair basketball team.

24. The nurse has identified that a 56-year-old woman has an increased risk for heart problems because of family history. Which modifiable factors would be included in the teaching plan to promote health and self-help practices for wellness for this patient? **Select all that apply.**
    1. Smoking cessation and stress reduction
    2. Use of advanced technology and new medications
    3. Weight reduction and decreased alcohol consumption
    4. Cost of health insurance and specialist care
    5. Control over decision-making that affects the patient's own body and health

25. Which set of tasks would be assigned to an unlicensed assistive personnel (UAP) who has been cross-trained as a unit secretary?
    1. Direct visitors and give out patient information.
    2. Take vital signs and restock medications.
    3. Validate transcriptions and interpret vital signs.
    4. Ambulate patients and order unit supplies.

26. Which action **best** demonstrates the nurse's consistent effort to contribute to cost-containment?
    1. Obtains malpractice insurance
    2. Uses time and materials economically
    3. Questions excessive diagnostic testing
    4. Refers patients with no insurance to a sliding-scale clinic

27. The nurse is caring for a patient with immobility related to a chronic musculoskeletal disorder. Using Orem's theory of nursing, what would the nurse do?
    1. Monitor for self-care deficits.
    2. Arrange pillows to provide joint protection.
    3. Support existing coping mechanisms.
    4. Encourage ambulation down the hallway.

28. The nurse is caring for several patients on the medical-surgical unit. Which actions indicate that the nurse is providing care that adheres to the American Hospital Association's Patient Care Partnership? **Select all that apply.**
    1. Ensures that the housekeeping staff empties the trash receptacles in a timely fashion
    2. Assists a patient to make a list of questions to ask about a surgical procedure
    3. Identifies a problem with a broken side rail and contacts the maintenance department
    4. Keeps up to date with the latest information on medications and side effects
    5. Ensures that every patient gets a private room with a window and private bathroom
    6. Contacts the hospital's financial counselor if a patient has questions about the bill

29. An intoxicated patient comes to the walk-in clinic and verbally threatens a nurse with bodily harm. The nurse refuses to care for the patient and informs the supervisor about the threats. Which document/concept supports the nurse's right to refuse to care for this patient?
    1. Patient Care Partnership
    2. Position Paper of the American Nurses Association
    3. Health Care Providers' Rights
    4. Resident's Bill of Rights

30. Which action is outside the scope of practice for the LPN/LVN?
    1. Offers suggestions to improve the patient's fluid intake
    2. Collects data on the patient while giving medication
    3. Makes independent decision about altering the care plan
    4. Uses therapeutic communication with a patient's family

31. Which action would the LPN/LVN perform for primary prevention?
    1. Instructs the UAP to reposition a patient who has a pressure injury
    2. Administers prescribed medications to control hypertension and high cholesterol
    3. Gathers data about dietary habits from a patient with consistently high glucose levels
    4. Offers the patient brochures on colonoscopy and mammogram for cancer screening

CRITICAL THINKING ACTIVITIES

32. The nurse is interviewing a 65-year-old woman who has hypertension, which is well-controlled by blood pressure medication. She is retired, but recently started volunteering at her church. She describes herself as having some problems, but is happily coping and looking forward to spending time with her grandchildren. Describe this woman's state of health by placing an X on the Wellness-Illness continuum and give a rationale for the placement of the X.

Wellness ◄─────────────────────────► Illness

Highest level of optimal health

Diminished or impaired state of health

_____

_____

_____

_____

33. a. Compare and contrast the historical significance of the white pleated cap and the apron that were originally part of the nurse's uniform with contemporary mandatory dress codes for nursing students and nurses.

_____

_____

_____

_____

b. Compare and contrast your personal point of view about uniforms with patients' and families' points of view.

_____

_____

_____

_____

_____

NEXT-GENERATION NCLEX™ (NGN)

34. Drag and Drop

Cognitive Skill: Recognize Cues

Scenario: The 68-year-old patient is admitted for an exacerbation of a chronic respiratory disease and requires medication, oxygen therapy, and diagnostic testing. He ambulates but is unsteady and requires assistance for activities that require bending and lifting. He is overweight, smokes, and usually eats packaged frozen meals or fast foods. The patient lives alone in a second-story apartment and his primary source of income is from a small pension. A home health team will follow him upon discharge.

Which team member is **best** for each task?

Instructions: The left-hand column includes all of the members of the home health team. In the right-hand column in the space provided, write the letter that indicates which member is **best** to assign or delegate to each task. Note that letters will be used only once.

a. RN
b. LPN/LVN
c. UAP
d. Physical therapist
e. Respiratory therapist
f. Dietitian
g. Financial counselor
h. Social worker
i. HCP

_____ 1. Teaches techniques for safe ambulation, bending, and lifting

_____ 2. Determines medical diagnosis and prescribes treatments and medications

_____ 3. Oversees equipment for oxygenation and ventilation

_____ 4. Assists the patient with hygiene and other activities of daily living

_____ 5. Evaluates preferred foods and fluids

_____ 6. Provides direct patient care in the hospital and supervises care of any home health patient

_____ 7. Works under the supervision of the RN in providing patient care in the hospital or home health setting

_____ 8. Assists the patient to understand billing and paying out-of-pocket costs

_____ 9. Refers the patient to community resources

Legal and Ethical Aspects of Nursing

chapter

2

Answer Key: A complete Answer Key is provided in your Additional Learning Resources on Evolve.

MATCHING

Directions: Match the terms on the left to the correct definition on the right.

Terms	Definitions
_____ 1. malpractice	a. Defines acts whose performance is required, permitted, or prohibited
_____ 2. accountability	b. Legal responsibility
_____ 3. standards of care	c. Professional negligence
_____ 4. liability	d. Process of self-evaluation that helps gain insight into personal values
_____ 5. value clarification	e. Being responsible for one's own actions

MULTIPLE CHOICE

Directions: Select the best answer(s) for each of the following questions.

6. The nursing student needs to obtain patient information to prepare for the clinical experience and decides to stop and say hello to the patient. While they are talking, the patient suddenly stops breathing and becomes unresponsive. What should the student do **first**?
   1. Call the nursing instructor and write an incident report.
   2. Call the primary nurse and apply oxygen.
   3. Call the Rapid Response Team and get the crash cart.
   4. Call for help and initiate cardiopulmonary resuscitation.

7. In which case is the nurse **most** likely to be charged with malpractice?
   1. The nurse explains the restraint policy to the family, and later, the older adult patient climbs over the side rail and sustains a hip fracture.
   2. The patient becomes very angry when the nurse refuses to give an additional dose of pain medication before the prescribed time.
   3. The family wants the health care provider (HCP) called at 3:00 AM because "something is wrong;" the nurse waits until 7:00 AM, but the patient is unharmed.
   4. The patient is very demanding and unpleasant so the nurse ignores the call bell; the patient sustains tissue injury at the IV site.

8. The patient asked the unlicensed assistive personnel (UAP) to apply a heating pad to her back, despite the fact that the home health nurse had instructed both the patient and UAP to avoid using the device. The patient sustained a burn and decided to sue the UAP and the nurse. Which documents are likely to be used in this case? **Select all that apply.**
   1. Policies and procedures
   2. Standards of care
   3. Equipment maintenance records
   4. Patient's medical records
   5. UAP's personal health records
   6. Personnel files for UAP and nurse

9. The nurse recognizes that in today's health care climate, there is an increased likelihood of being involved in litigation. What action could the nurse take to improve the overall situation in the work setting?
   1. Agree to care for a limited number of high-acuity patients.
   2. Work on a committee to improve discharge teaching.
   3. Work at a facility that covers nurses with malpractice insurance.
   4. Ensure that others are accountable for their own actions.

10. A new UAP is assigned to do a task that was reviewed and demonstrated in orientation and practiced on a mannikin. The UAP tells the nurse that she does not know how to do the task. What should the nurse do **first**?
    1. Ask the UAP to recite the steps of the task and assess readiness to perform.
    2. Go with the UAP and perform the task while the UAP observes.
    3. Instruct the UAP to try to perform the task to the best of her ability.
    4. Pull the UAP's orientation file and see if competency was established.

11. The LPN/LVN is instructed by an HCP to start a unit of blood on a patient, but the institution's policy indicates that LPN/LVNs can monitor blood transfusions, but RNs must initiate blood transfusions. What should the LPN/LVN do?
    1. Start the blood transfusion as ordered because the HCP is supervising.
    2. Locate the RN in charge so that he/she can start the blood transfusion.
    3. Tell the HCP that hospital policy prohibits blood transfusion by LPN/LVNs.
    4. Obtain the unit of blood and assist the HCP as he/she initiates the transfusion.

12. A nursing student must write a clinical report about the care that was given to a patient in the hospital. What should the student do to prevent a Health Insurance Portability and Accountability Act (HIPAA) violation? **Select all that apply.**
    1. Do not use the patient's name in any section of the paper.
    2. If laboratory data are used, make sure no identification numbers are included.
    3. Avoid including the HCP's name in the report.
    4. Do not refer to the room number or the specific unit.
    5. Do not include the patient's vital signs.
    6. Avoid using details about the patient's medical condition.

13. Which unaccompanied minor requires parental consent prior to treatment?
    1. A 17-year-old who wants a prescription for insulin
    2. An 18-year-old who needs sutures for a laceration of the hand
    3. A 14-year-old who was sexually assaulted by a family member
    4. A 16-year-old who is independent and self-supporting and wants birth control

14. The nurse is working on the medical-surgical unit and answers the telephone. The caller wants to know, "How is Mr. Smith doing?" What is the **most** important factor that affects the nurse's response?
    1. The identity of the caller
    2. The stability of Mr. Smith's condition
    3. The hospital's policy for releasing information
    4. HIPAA

15. A mother brings her 8-year-old son to the clinic for a broken arm. There are no other apparent injuries and the child and mother appear to have a supportive relationship; however, review of the chart indicates that this child has frequently been treated for other fractures and injuries. What should the nurse do **first**?
    1. Ask the social worker to consult for possible child abuse.
    2. Call child protective services and make a report.
    3. Point out the history of injuries to the HCP.
    4. Take the child aside and assess his true feelings.

16. The nurse stops at a traffic accident and offers aid to victims. In which circumstance are Good Samaritan laws **less** likely to provide the nurse immunity from liability?
    1. The nurse initiates cardiopulmonary resuscitation after cardiac arrest occurs.
    2. The nurse directs bystanders to move a victim and a spinal cord injury occurs.
    3. The nurse uses the victim's coat and applies pressure to a bleeding wound.
    4. The nurse pauses to call 911 before assessing or assisting victims in distress.

17. Which action by the nurse is the **best** to avoid a lawsuit?
    1. Remain current on practice developments.
    2. Know the legal definition of terms such as *negligence.*
    3. Obtain professional malpractice insurance.
    4. Validate nursing actions with a supervisor.

18. The nurse performs a dressing change on a surgical wound. The procedure is routine and there are no signs of infection or excessive drainage. What should the nurse do about documentation?
    1. If using charting by exception, "dressing changed" is adequate.
    2. Document appearance of wound site and type of dressing used.
    3. There is no need to document because there are no problems with the wound.
    4. Read the previous entry about the wound and document "unchanged as above."

19. The nurse has to go before the state board of nursing because there is a question about her nursing license. Which type of insurance will provide a qualified attorney to represent the nurse?
    1. Claims-made policy
    2. Occurrence basis policy
    3. "Tail" agreement for extended coverage
    4. Disciplinary defense insurance

20. A newly graduated nurse has completed orientation and is assigned to take care of a patient who has a tracheostomy. The nurse has never done tracheostomy care. What should the nurse do **first**?
    1. Ask to be reassigned to a different patient.
    2. Review the procedure using a textbook or the Internet.
    3. Report that orientation did not include tracheostomy care.
    4. Seek instruction and supervision for any unfamiliar procedures.

21. An older adult patient begins to cry during review of the advance directive information and refuses to sign. What should the nurse do **first**?
    1. Encourage the patient to express his feelings about the advance directive.
    2. Reassure the patient that his wishes will be respected above all else.
    3. Alert the family to support the patient in the decision.
    4. Document in the patient's record that the information was given and declined.

22. A patient is in very critical condition and unable to make decisions about ongoing treatment. There is conflict among family members on what should be done. Which source, if followed, is the **most** likely to protect the health care team from liability?
    1. Agency's policy and procedure manual
    2. Patient's living will
    3. Patient Self-Determination Act
    4. Accreditation criteria of the Joint Commission

23. A mother and her pregnant 13-year-old daughter are arguing; the mother wants her to keep the baby and the girl wants to have an abortion. The nurse feels very angry toward the mother and very protective toward the girl. What should the nurse do **first**?
    1. Take the girl aside and assess her feelings and wishes regarding the pregnancy.
    2. Ask another nurse to assess the mother's rationale for opposing her daughter.
    3. Seek advice from a supervisor about who can legally make decisions about the pregnancy.
    4. Reflect on his or her own feelings and ability to be supportive and caring toward this family.

24. Which actions indicate that the nurse is practicing within the code of ethics developed by the National Federation of Licensed Practical Nurses (NFLPN)? **Select all that apply.**
    1. Collects data about the patient's skin and reports it to the RN
    2. Gives change-of-shift report to the oncoming nurse and the nursing student
    3. Wears professional attire and adheres to the facility's dress code
    4. Observes another nurse being rude and demeaning toward a patient
    5. Cares for a patient with an infectious disease and follows isolation precautions
    6. Uses a cell phone to text messages about another nurse's behavior toward coworkers

25. Nurse A knows that Nurse B is stealing small items from older residents in the long-term care facility, but Nurse A hesitates to report Nurse B because they are friends and Nurse B gives good care to the residents. Whom should Nurse A talk to **first**?
    1. Ask the residents if they have any complaints about Nurse B.
    2. Speak to the families of residents to see if the thefts can be substantiated.
    3. Speak to the supervisor and give facts; do not offer suspicions.
    4. Talk to an objective third party about personal values clarification.

26. Nursing Student Apple posts a detailed description of caring for an older patient on social media. Nursing Student Orange sees the Facebook post. What should Nursing Student Orange do **first**?
    1. Review the post to see if any patient identifiers are included.
    2. Give positive feedback to Student Apple for sharing the experience.
    3. Tell Student Apple that the nursing instructor should be informed.
    4. Do nothing; no harm is done if just a few people see the post.

27. Which nurse is appropriately incorporating cultural considerations while providing nursing care?
    1. Nurse A expects the patient to make better food choices to lose weight and thereby control his diabetes.
    2. Nurse B assumes that the patient understands English because the family is speaking English.
    3. Nurse C treats all patients the same, regardless of ethnicity or cultural background.
    4. Nurse D listens while a patient expresses feelings and thoughts related to a situation.

28. Which nursing action incorporates the ethical principle of nonmaleficence?
    1. Provides high-quality care to a homeless man who has no health insurance
    2. Advocates for better pain control for a patient who has cancer
    3. Encourages the patient to ask questions and make an informed choice
    4. Calls the HCP about a medication prescription because the dose seems too high

29. Which factors increase the risk for physical, emotional, or financial abuse among older adults? **Select all that apply.**
    1. Decreased strength and mobility
    2. Loss of independence
    3. Young or novice caregivers
    4. Declining physical health
    5. Isolation
    6. Loss of loved ones, friends, and relatives

30. Which member of the health care team has violated the patient's right to privacy?
    1. HCP closes the door before explaining the medical diagnosis to the patient.
    2. RN logs off the computer in the nurses' station after documentation is completed.
    3. UAP refers the family who has questions about the patient's health to the charge nurse.
    4. LPN/LVN leaves change-of-shift report sheets in the nurses' breakroom.

31. The surgeon verbally tells the new nurse to "get the surgical consent form signed." The surgeon is abrupt, and the nurse is unsure how to interpret the request but knows that nurses can witness consent but cannot explain the risks or benefits of the procedure. What would the new nurse do **first**?
    1. Ask the charge nurse for clarification of the nurses' role related to informed consent.
    2. Report the surgeon's request to the nursing supervision and risk-management department.
    3. Offer to go with the surgeon and act as a witness as the patient signs the consent form.
    4. Refuse to comply because the surgeon is responsible for the procedure and obtaining consent.

32. Which nurse has performed an action that would be considered "battery"?
    1. Nurse A leaves before giving a patient report to the oncoming nurses.
    2. Nurse B touches a patient to apply restraints without obtaining consent.
    3. Nurse C falsely documents physical assessment data to save time.
    4. Nurse D gossips about the charge nurse to undermine her reputation.

CRITICAL THINKING ACTIVITIES

33. Nurse A is assigned to care for a patient with AIDS, but asks Nurse B to switch patients. Nurse B readily agrees because Nurse A always helps other nurses and members of the health care team. Together, they inform the charge nurse, who gives the okay for the switch of assignments. At the end of the day, Nurse A thanks Nurse B for taking the patient with AIDS because "those kinds of people really bother me." Nurse B feels a little confused by the comment but shrugs it off.

    a. Discuss the behavior of Nurse A and Nurse B, as related to the NFLPN code of ethics.

    _____

    _____

    b. Nurse B goes home and thinks about the day and about Nurse A's comment. Nurse B realizes that the situation has created some uncomfortable feelings and a potential problem if Nurse A makes a future request to change patient assignments or makes additional comments. What should Nurse B do?

    _____

    _____

    _____

34. The nurse is caring for a patient who has been quadriplegic for 3 years following a diving accident. One morning, the nurse notes that the patient has redness on the sacral area and informs the patient that there is risk for a pressure injury and that careful turning and scheduled assessment will need to be started. The patient politely thanks the nurse but informs her that he intends to refuse any treatment for pressure injuries and is likely to start refusing other nursing measures as well. The nurse is stunned and upset because the patient has always been cooperative and generally very satisfied with the care.

   a. What should the nurse do? _____

   _____

   _____

   _____

   b. How can the nurse continue to interact with this patient if he continues to refuse therapies?

   _____

   _____

   _____

   c. How would you feel if a patient refused to allow you to meet basic needs such as food, hygiene, or preventive care like turning or receiving immunizations?

   _____

   _____

   _____

   _____

35. The nurse has been working for several years in the hospital. The patient assignments are always very heavy and there has been a continuous nursing shortage. Two patients have died within the past year, and although there have been no legal actions taken against the hospital or the staff, the general feeling among the nursing staff is that working conditions are going to result in more harm to the patients. The nurse has talked to her supervisor about her concerns for the patients' safety and the morale of the staff. The supervisor has assured her that everything that can be done has been done. Discuss the legal and ethical implications of these working conditions and the actions that the nurse could take.

   _____

   _____

   _____

NEXT-GENERATION NCLEX™ (NGN)

36. Matrix

Cognitive Skill: Recognize Cues

Scenario: The nurse manager informs the nurse that there is an investigation that may result in a malpractice lawsuit. Events and actions are displayed below. For liability to be established, four key elements (duty, breach of duty, harm, and proximate cause) must be present.

Instructions: Use an X to indicate which element is represented by the actions and events. All should be used and may be used more than once.

Actions and Events	Duty	Breach of Duty	Harm	Proximate Cause
7:00 RN assigns LPN/LVN to monitor an IV potassium infusion prescribed to infuse over 4 hours.				
7:45 Patient reports pain (1/10) at the site. LPN/LVN assesses the site and says, "Potassium is irritating to the veins, some discomfort is expected."				
8:30 Patient reports that pain (5/10) is increasing. LPN/LVN observes redness around insertion site, flushes IV with normal saline and notices that slight swelling occurs during flushing. Warm pack applied and nurse says, "Everything is fine. The warmth will relieve the pain."				
10:00 Patient reports severe pain (9/10). Redness and swelling are markedly increased. LPN/LVN stops infusion and notifies the RN.				
Several days later, extensive necrotic tissue damage is noted. The HCP informs the nurse manager that there may be permanent scarring or nerve damage.				

Documentation

Answer Key: A complete Answer Key is provided in your Additional Learning Resources on Evolve.

MATCHING

Directions: Match the abbreviations on the left to the correct terminology on the right.

Abbreviation		Terminology	
_____	1. CBE	a.	Plan, intervention, evaluation
_____	2. DRG	b.	Data, action, response, education
_____	3. EHR	c.	Identification, situation, background, assessment, recommendation
_____	4. HIPAA	d.	Charting by exception
_____	5. MDS	e.	Subjective, objective, assessment, plan, evaluation
_____	6. POC	f.	Electronic health record
_____	7. DARE	g.	Minimum data sets
_____	8. ISBAR	h.	Point of care
_____	9. PIE	i.	Diagnosis-related group
_____	10. SOAPE	j.	Health Insurance Portability and Accountability Act

SHORT ANSWER

Directions: Using your own words, answer the question in the space provided.

11. Briefly identify how long-term care and home health care documentation are different from acute care (hospital) documentation.

_____

_____

_____

TABLE ACTIVITY

12. In the right-hand column of the table, indicate all of the potential places where the examples of documentation could be recorded.

Nursing Process	Where to Document
Assessment	
Alert and oriented to person, place, and time.	
Ambulates independently to bathroom.	
Family assessed for knowledge of wound care.	
Diagnosis or Problem	
Risk for infection of surgical wound.	
Must independently perform wound care at home.	
Outcomes Identification/Planning	
Patient will participate in wound care prior to discharge.	
Family will demonstrate ability to perform wound irrigation.	
Implementation	
Wound care procedure demonstrated to patient and family.	
List of supplies and how to obtain reviewed with family.	
Referral made to home health agency.	
Evaluation	
Patient and family participated in wound care. They had questions about asepsis in the home setting; principles of hand hygiene and asepsis were reviewed. They acknowledged understanding of written and verbal information and agreed to follow up with the home health nurse.	

MULTIPLE CHOICE

Directions: Select the best answer(s) for each of the following questions.

13. The nurse does not have time to document a procedure after it was completed. Which action would the nurse take?
    1. Use an incident report to explain the circumstances related to documentation.
    2. Document the procedure anytime during the shift; this is acceptable practice.
    3. Computer documentation does not allow late entry; use a hand-written page.
    4. Note it as a "late entry" and then proceed with the documentation.

14. The nurse works at a facility that uses charting by exception. Which plan will the nurse use to accomplish the care and documentation?
    1. Instruct unlicensed assistive personnel (UAP) to take vital signs at least every 4 hours and record on the flow sheet; frequency of vital signs is increased as needed.
    2. Document a complete physical assessment at the beginning of the shift; during the shift, only changes in the patient's condition are documented.
    3. For each shift, all care must be documented; this includes a minimum of three detailed entries and a flow sheet that includes vital signs.
    4. Focus on an identified patient problem and document using the data (D), action (A), response (R), and evaluation (E) education and patient teaching.

15. Which actions by members of the health care team reflect the basic purposes of accurate and complete patient records? **Select all that apply.**
    1. Risk manager uses patient's records to investigate accusations of staff abuse of patient.
    2. Nursing instructor directs the students to look at nurses' notes written by expert nurses.
    3. Medicare auditor reviews patient records to observe for evidence of minimum data sets.
    4. Nursing student reads the patient's flow sheets to observe for trends in the vital signs.
    5. Nurse discusses the health care provider's (HCP) documentation with the patient to clarify medical diagnosis.

16. Which nurse is **most** likely to expect a peer review?
    1. Nurse A submits a research article to a nursing journal.
    2. Nurse B queries an HCP's medication prescription.
    3. Nurse C fills out an incident report for a patient fall.
    4. Nurse D completes an admission assessment and history.

17. In using the hospital's computer information system, where is the nurse **most** likely to find documentation about the patient's response to the last dose of pain medication?
    1. Individualized care plan
    2. Medication administration record (MAR)
    3. Automated Kardex form
    4. Narrative notes

18. An auditor is randomly reviewing the nurses' charts and the nurse manager has agreed that the auditor can ask questions and give feedback as necessary. Which example of documentation is the auditor **most** likely to query?
    1. Ambulated independently with steady gait to bathroom
    2. Instructed on method of clean midstream urine collection
    3. Discharged to home accompanied by spouse
    4. Placed side rails up x3 with call bell in place

19. The nurse is working on a medical-surgical unit in a large hospital and observes an unfamiliar person looking at a patient's chart. What would the nurse do **first**?
    1. Call hospital security and report the person's behavior and description.
    2. Ask for identification and determine if the person can look at the chart.
    3. Allow the person to continue unless there is suspicious behavior.
    4. Request that the chart be returned and contact the charge nurse.

20. The nursing student attempts to document am hygiene care, but several computers are broken and the remaining functional computers are being used. What would the student do?
    1. Make a note to self of time and relevant details and document at the end of the shift.
    2. Report to the instructor and ask for advice about what to do.
    3. Document the care on a hardcopy form and add it to the patient's chart.
    4. Jot down the time that care was given and document when a computer is available.

21. It is 10:00 AM, and the nurse needs to give a patient a blood pressure medication but would like to know what the morning vital signs were before administering the medication. The nurse looks at the flow sheet, but the vital signs are not there. Which action would the nurse take **first**?
    1. Give the blood pressure medication now and then check the blood pressure in 30 minutes.
    2. Find the UAP and ask why the morning vital signs have not been documented.
    3. Check the blood pressure, give the medication as appropriate, and then document both.
    4. Check in the nurses' notes to see if the vital signs were documented there.

22. The LPN/LVN phones the HCP to report a change in the patient's condition using the ISBARR (introduction, situation, background, assessment, recommendation, read back) method of communication; however, the HCP declines to listen to the "read back" and then hangs up. What would the nurse do **first**?
    1. Call the HCP back and insist on "read back."
    2. Carry out the orders if they are clear.
    3. Consult a supervisor about the incident.
    4. Document the HCP's exact words in the patient's chart.

23. The LPN/LVN is reading the documentation that was written by a newly graduated RN. There are numerous spelling mistakes and the grammar is terrible. What would the nurse do?
    1. Do nothing; an RN is not accountable to an LPN/LVN.
    2. Offer to teach the new nurse how to document.
    3. Ask the charge nurse to review the documentation.
    4. Correct the spelling errors and initial the changes.

24. The student nurse sees that it is time to give medication to a patient, but the patient is currently in radiology. The student is aware that there is a 30-minute time window to administer the medication, otherwise it will be considered late. What would the student do?
    1. Document that the medication was given at the correct time and then give it as soon as the patient returns from radiology.
    2. Call the pharmacy and inquire if a delay in administering the medication or holding it until the next dose is harmful to the patient.
    3. Document that the patient is in radiology, advise the charge nurse, and administer the medication when the patient returns to the unit.
    4. Hold the medication and fill out an incident report that explains the circumstances and details of why the medication was not administered.

25. A patient is admitted to the hospital for a total hip replacement. Care and documentation are performed according to the facility's clinical (critical) pathway for this condition. Which information is likely to appear in this documentation tool?
    1. Level of activity on a day-to-day basis following surgery
    2. Unusual events that have a potential for injury
    3. Nursing care plan with problem statement and interventions
    4. The LPN/LVN's role in monitoring the patient's progress

26. A patient comes to the nurses' station and demands to have his chart because he has decided to leave the hospital and seek care from a different facility. What is the **best** response?
    1. "Sir, all of the patient records are the property of the hospital."
    2. "Sir, let me contact your HCP so you can talk to him before leaving."
    3. "Sir, please wait and I will call the nurse manager right now."
    4. "Sir, please return to your room and I will make a copy of the chart."

27. The nursing student leaves a copy of a patient's Kardex on a bedside table. A visitor finds the copy and reads it. What should the student do?
    1. Take the Kardex out of the patient's room and immediately shred it.
    2. Apologize to the visitor and patient and explain the information on the Kardex.
    3. Obtain the copy of the Kardex and check for patient identifiers.
    4. Retrieve the Kardex, contact instructor, and complete an incident report.

28. The nurse is documenting with a black pen on the hardcopy nurses' notes about a patient's response to pain medication. The nurse suddenly realizes that she is writing the note in the wrong chart. What is the **best** action to take?
    1. Draw a line through the error and initial it.
    2. Report the error to the charge nurse.
    3. Use white correction fluid to cover the error.
    4. Discard the page that contains the error.

29. What types of inadequate or inappropriate documentation are likely to cause problems in malpractice cases? **Select all that apply.**
    1. Failed to document latex allergy
    2. Documented patient's complaint about care by using patient's remarks in quotes
    3. Charted medication that the patient claims he did not receive
    4. Documented amount of IV fluid, but no assessment of IV site
    5. Clustered information obtained from physical assessment
    6. Recorded verbal prescription using brand-name medication

30. Which nursing action/behavior would be considered a potential Health Insurance Portability and Accountability Act (HIPAA) violation?
    1. Faxes a patient's medical records to a consulting specialist
    2. Leaves the computer monitor display open for easy access
    3. Discusses a patient's problem during handover with oncoming staff
    4. Shares a copy of an incident report with the risk manager

31. The nurse sees a medication prescription for a patient who has acute postsurgical pain. The prescription reads "3 mg oral MS as needed for pain." What would the nurse do **first**?
    1. Report the prescribing HCP for using an inappropriate abbreviation.
    2. Correct the prescription to read "3 mg oral morphine sulfate as needed for pain."
    3. Call the prescribing HCP and ask for clarification of the abbreviation "MS."
    4. Ask the pharmacist to deliver the medication to the unit as soon as possible.

32. The nurse inadvertently gives the patient's 7:00 PM medication at 7:00 AM. What would the nurse do **first**?
    1. Call the pharmacist and ask if there are specific side effects related to the time of day the medication was administered.
    2. Observe for adverse effects, notify the prescribing HCP, and fill out an incident report.
    3. Notify the charge nurse and inform the patient about the medication error.
    4. Document the time and dose given and tell the evening shift not to give the pm dose.

33. The LPN/LVN arrives for her shift and is assigned to care for a patient who will soon return from surgery: acuity level 1. What would the nurse do **first**?
    1. Ask the offgoing nurse to give a comprehensive hand-off report about the patient.
    2. Prioritize the care of other assigned patients to accommodate the arrival of the postoperative patient.
    3. Check the patient's medical records to find out about the patient's condition and type of surgery.
    4. Consult with the charge nurse about the appropriateness of the patient assignment.

34. Which nursing students have violated the guidelines for safe computer documentation during their clinical rotation? **Select all that apply.**
    1. Shares password so that a classmate can collect preclinical information
    2. Logs on and leaves computer terminal to respond to a call light
    3. Records information on the wrong chart; reports to the charge nurse
    4. Positions the monitor display so that it is visible to patient and visitors
    5. Prints and takes a hardcopy of patient data to complete case study assignment

CRITICAL THINKING ACTIVITIES

35. Review the documentation samples below and then refer to Box 3.2, Basic Rules for Documentation, and Table 3.2, Legal Guidelines for Documentation to identify errors and examples of poor documentation.

    Sample #1

    Sept, 2014   Patient had a good night. Status was escendially unchanged. Family in to visit and asked about storage of patient's belongings. Reassured that diamond ring and gold watch were in the bedside table. Patient went with family to cafeteria. S. Smith, LPN.

    _____

    _____

    _____

    _____

    Sample #2

    Sept. 24, 2014 2100   J. Jones RN gave a 500-mL SSE; patient assisted to CC for a return of 600 mL with brown formed stool noted. Procedure well tolerated. J. Jones said that patient had relief of adominal distencion and discomfort. S. Smith, LPN

    _____

    _____

    _____

    _____

Sample #3

Sept 24, 2014   Patient reported pain. Noted in chart that HCP made an error and ordered MS. Consulted charge nurse who advised to give the dose morphine sulfate according to the written prescription. Patient was angry because he didn't get the pain medication as soon as he asked for it; called me a "stupid lazy fool." Pain medication given later in the shift.

_____

_____

_____

_____

36. Interview nurses during your clinical assignment and then compare and contrast electronic health record (EHR) systems to hardcopy (hand-written) record systems.

_____

_____

_____

_____

NEXT-GENERATION NCLEX™ (NGN)

37. Extended Multiple Response

Cognitive Skill: Recognize Cues

Scenario: The nurse is caring for a home health patient who is recovering from a mild stroke. Which documentation is required for reimbursement from Medicare, Medicaid, and other types of insurance?

Instructions: Place a check mark next to the documentation that the nurse would include. **Check all that apply.**

_____ a. Daughter reports that patient has some short-term memory loss that is worse when the patient is tired.

_____ b. Daughter requests that the home health service be extended while the family is away on vacation.

_____ c. Demonstrates difficulty with strength and balance when moving from a sitting to a standing position; physical therapist Ms. T notified

_____ d. Refuses to drink thickened liquids as prescribed; purpose of thickened liquids reviewed with patient; supervising RN, Nurse K, and speech therapist Mr. J notified.

_____ e. 2 cm skin flap noted on left forearm, "I bumped my arm." Gently cleaned with mild soap and water; covered with petroleum jelly and film dressing.

_____ f. Eager to independently ambulate; encouraged to use walker and handrails.

_____ g. Patient and daughter "dislike the HCP and want to change."

_____ h. Able to don pants and shirt, but unable to fasten buttons.

Communication

Answer Key: A complete Answer Key is provided in your Additional Learning Resources on Evolve.

MULTIPLE CHOICE

Directions: Select the best answer(s) for each of the following questions.

1. In which circumstance would it be **most** appropriate to incorporate the phrase 'patient problem statement' into the verbal communication?
    1. The nurse tells the health care provider (HCP) about a change in the patient's respiratory status.
    2. The nursing student and the nursing instructor discuss the patient's care plan.
    3. The home health nurse reviews the goals of rehabilitation with the patient and family.
    4. The off-going nurse gives hand-off report about several patients to the oncoming nurse.

2. What type of eye contact would be **best** to use if the nurse is trying to involve the patient in a discussion about sexuality without being threatening or intimidating?
    1. Lean slightly forward and maintain extended eye contact.
    2. Look downward if the patient uses slang terms related to sex.
    3. Maintain eye contact for 2 to 6 seconds during the discussion.
    4. Observe the patient and mimic the patient's eye contact.

3. A nursing student goes to an instructor's office to discuss an uncomfortable interaction that occurred with a patient during the last clinical experience. Which behaviors suggest that the instructor is failing to give the student full attention? **Select all that apply.**
    1. Instructor welcomes the student and offers 40 minutes for discussion.
    2. Instructor smiles and waves at others who walk past the office.
    3. Instructor offers advice before the student explains the details of the incident.
    4. Instructor appears relaxed and asks open-ended questions.
    5. Instructor frequently handles her cell phone.
    6. Instructor shuffles and rearranges papers on the desk.

4. The nurse is trying to interview a patient who is very hard of hearing. What strategy would the nurse try **first**?
    1. Talk to the patient's spouse.
    2. Shout loudly into the patient's good ear.
    3. Use simple language and avoid medical terminology.
    4. Use normal volume and lower tone of voice.

5. The patient says, "I trust you, so I am going to tell you a secret. I am going to end it all by going for a long swim in the ocean." What would the nurse do **first**?
   1. Tell the patient that intent to harm self must be reported to the health care team.
   2. Ask the patient to elaborate on the meaning of "end it all" and "long swim."
   3. Thank the patient for the trust and promise to keep the information confidential.
   4. Stay with patient and wait for him to express his thoughts and feelings.

6. The night nurse is giving report during shift change. A visitor passing by is an unintended receiver of the nurse's communication. What is the **best** method to prevent this type of occurrence?
   1. Ask visitors to leave the unit during shift change.
   2. Give report in a private room with the door closed.
   3. Eliminate negative connotations during report.
   4. Make written notes that are passed only to staff members.

7. The nurse is attempting to elicit the patient's state of mind about an upcoming surgery. Which approach is likely to be **most** effective?
   1. "Are you afraid of having the procedure?"
   2. "Let me give you information about the procedure."
   3. "Look at this series of pictures about the procedure."
   4. "What do you understand about the procedure?"

8. A patient is grimacing while trying to change his position in bed. He tells the nurse that he is feeling great and is ready to get up and go home. Which response **best** indicates that the nurse recognizes that the patient's communication is incongruent?
   1. "Going home is the goal, but let me help you get up and you can walk around for a while."
   2. "Let me help you sit up and then you can get dressed and pack up your belongings."
   3. "Would you like a dose of pain medication before you go home?"
   4. "That sounds great! I'll call your HCP and inform her that you are ready to go home."

9. The nurse is about to begin teaching a small group of adolescents about healthy eating habits. Which nonverbal behavior **best** indicates potential interest in listening to the nurse?
   1. Talking on a cell phone and smiling at the nurse
   2. Staring at the blackboard with a bored expression
   3. Using the Internet to search for topics of interest
   4. Removing a notebook and pen from a backpack

10. The patient tells the nurse, "I'm supposed to check my blood sugar at least three times each day, but I can't always find the test sticks and they're very expensive." Which response by the nurse is the **best** example of effective clarification?
    1. "When did you last check your blood sugar?"
    2. "I'll speak with the nurse practitioner about your situation."
    3. "I see that you know how important it is to check your blood sugar."
    4. "Let me make sure I understand what your concern is with the blood sugar testing."

11. The patient states, "I'm worried and don't know what to expect after my biopsy." Which question **best** encourages the patient to explain the problem to the nurse?
    1. "Would you like to talk to your surgeon before the procedure?"
    2. "Are you feeling anxious about the results of your biopsy?"
    3. "What are you worried about?"
    4. "How can I make you feel better?"

12. The nurse is trying to take a patient's history, but the patient makes frequent references to her aunt's health, a neighbor's illness, and events that happened many years ago to him or others. Which therapeutic communication technique is the nurse **most** likely to use with this patient?
    1. Clarifying
    2. Paraphrasing
    3. Restating
    4. Closed questioning

13. When communicating with a patient who has expressive aphasia, which communication strategy is the nurse **most** likely to use?
    1. Encourage the patient to speak as much as possible.
    2. Use eye blinks, one for "yes" and two for "no."
    3. Ask family members for information.
    4. Speak loudly and slowly with good enunciation.

14. The patient has a cultural background that is unfamiliar to the nurse. What would the nurse do when communicating with the patient? **Select all that apply.**
    1. Use formal names until preference is assessed.
    2. Realize that interpretation of social time versus clock time can differ.
    3. Be aware that touch varies according to gender and relationship.
    4. Assume that smiling and handshake are universal greetings.
    5. Use tone of voice that is soft and deferential.
    6. Understand that eye contact has different meaning among cultures.

15. When communicating with an older adult, what would the nurse do?
    1. Speak loudly and at a very slow pace.
    2. Allow time for processing information.
    3. Provide a dark, quiet environment.
    4. Discourage anecdotal or tangential replies.

16. Which nurse behavior/response **best** indicates to the patient that the nurse is actively listening to what he or she is trying to say?
    1. Says "Uh-huh"
    2. Smiles and nods at patient
    3. Says "So in other words, you are…"
    4. Looks at patient and leans forward

17. During the discharge teaching, the patient states, "I don't know how I will be able to care for myself after I leave the hospital." What is the **most** therapeutic response?
    1. "You don't know how you will take care of yourself when you leave the hospital?"
    2. "It sounds like you have some concerns. What do you think is going to happen?"
    3. "Would you like me to review the instructions so the information is clear?"
    4. "Could you get someone to stay with you until you are feeling better?"

18. The nurse is working with a patient from a different culture. Which action by the nurse is **most** likely to cause offense if patient's sense of intimate space differs from the nurse's?
    1. Assists the patient to transfer from bed to chair
    2. Sits in a chair and speaks with the patient
    3. Speaks to the family in the presence of the patient
    4. Hangs the patient's clothes in the closet

19. The nurse is completing the patient's history. Which question encourages the patient to provide a specific answer with relevant detail?
    1. "What type of surgeries have you had in the past?"
    2. "What kinds of problems do you have?"
    3. "Are you having any pain?"
    4. "How do you feel about your current health status?"

20. The patient tells the nurse that the unlicensed assistive personnel (UAP) is always making jokes. What is the **best** response?
    1. "Laughter is the best medicine."
    2. "What do you think about the UAP's jokes?"
    3. "Yes, the UAP really is a funny person."
    4. "Would you tell me a joke?"

21. The nurse is explaining a change in a patient's condition to an HCP. The HCP rudely and sarcastically replies, "Well, what do you want me to do about that?" What is the **best** response?
    1. "Well, mostly I just wanted you to know about the situation."
    2. "That's really your decision. I'm merely reporting the patient's condition."
    3. "Please come and examine the patient, because the condition has changed."
    4. "Sorry to bother you. I'll just keep monitoring the patient's condition."

22. The patient has just died. The wife and daughter are holding each other and crying at the bedside, while the little boy is standing apart staring out the window. Which communication approach would be the **best** to support everyone in the family?
    1. Talk to the little boy about what he is feeling and what he sees out the window.
    2. Stand beside the wife and daughter and direct the little boy to join the group.
    3. Use therapeutic touch with the wife and daughter and allow the little boy to have his space.
    4. Stand beside the little boy and keep an open body position toward the mother and daughter.

23. The nurse is present when the obstetrician informs a 17-year-old that she is pregnant. The adolescent shrugs, appears bored, and says, "That's no big deal to me." The nurse, who has been trying to get pregnant for several years, feels angry and hostile toward the patient. What would the nurse do **first**?
    1. Care for the patient and talk about the situation later with a friend.
    2. Perform a self-assessment of ability to convey acceptance.
    3. Be honest with the patient and express concern about her attitude.
    4. Ask another nurse to take over care of the patient.

24. An experienced UAP gives excellent care and is well-liked by all of the residents in the long-term care facility. She calls the female residents "Sweetie" and the male residents "Honeybunch." The nurse is newly graduated but recognizes that the UAP is using "elderspeak." What would the nurse do?
    1. Let a good thing continue because everyone seems happy and the care is good.
    2. Gain more experience and mimic the UAP's behavior and communication style.
    3. Report to the RN in charge about concerns for the UAP's disrespect of residents.
    4. Praise the UAP for giving excellent care and role-model use of "Mr.," "Mrs.," or "Ms."

25. Social isolation is one of the identified problems on the care plan for a resident with a hearing impairment in a long-term care facility. The nurse goes to the patient's room and finds that he is cheerful, conversant, and happy to engage. What would the nurse do **first**?
    1. Suggest to the RN that social isolation does not seem to belong on the problem list.
    2. Assess the patient to determine his social skills and the extent of his social network.
    3. Spend more time with the patient because trust and rapport are established.
    4. Suggest that the patient go into the common room and talk with other residents.

26. Which UAP is using the **best** communication in the care of an unresponsive patient?
    1. UAP positions patient toward the window and mentions the sunny summer day.
    2. Two UAPs who are turning the patient discuss the work duties for the shift.
    3. Two UAPs who are bathing the patient cheerfully discuss their boyfriends.
    4. UAP who is performing dental hygiene is silently attentive to detail.

27. For a patient who is receiving mechanical ventilation, which action would the nurse perform **first** to facilitate communication with the patient?
    1. Obtain a communication board that has an alphabet, phrases, and pictures.
    2. Tell the patient to blink once for yes and twice for no, then ask a series of yes/no questions.
    3. Obtain a computer and a keyboard and instruct the patient to types messages.
    4. Assess cognitive level, visual acuity, consciousness level, primary language, and motor skills.

CRITICAL THINKING ACTIVITIES

28. The nurse is having a very rough day. Another nurse called in sick; a physician's assistant was very rude; several patients have extremely complex care needs; and Mrs. M, who is an older adult widow, has repeatedly used the call bell all morning. The nurse goes to Mrs. M's room and stands in the doorway with her arms across her chest, saying nothing, but looking directly at the patient. Mrs. M says, "I'm sorry to bother you, dear, but I thought I heard my husband in the hallway. Could you check and see if he is here?" The nurse shakes her head and walks out. Analyze this situation and the factors that are influencing the communication between the nurse and the patient.

_____

_____

_____

_____

_____

29. Recall a conversation you recently had with a family member, friend, coworker, instructor, or patient in which you used responses that blocked communication. Such responses include false reassurance, giving advice, making false assumptions, giving approval or disapproval, automatic responses, defensive responses, arguing, asking for explanation, or changing the subject (see Table 4.4 for examples). Record two or three responses that you used and describe how the other person responded to you.

_____

_____

_____

_____

_____

_____

Rephrase your responses listed above so communication remains open. _____

_____

_____

_____

_____

_____

_____

NEXT-GENERATION NCLEX™ (NGN)

30. Matrix

Cognitive Skill: Take Action

Scenario: A 58-year-old man is admitted to the medical-surgical unit with a diagnosis of left-sided stroke. During the admission process, the nurse observes that the patient's speech is unclear, and his words are slurred. The nurse also observes that when the patient is asked a question that can be answered with a "yes" or "no" response, he answers the question by moving his head to indicate "yes" or "no." Which actions would the nurse use to facilitate communication with the patient?

Instructions: Use an X to indicate which actions are essential, nonessential, or contraindicated. All should be used and can be used more than once.

Action	Essential	Nonessential	Contraindicated
Collaborate with an occupational therapist.			
Avoid patronizing phrases.			
Shout or speak loudly.			
Give the patient time to understand.			
Offer pictures or a communication board.			
Direct comments toward family.			
Speak about topics of interest to the patient.			
Suggest speaking, rather than relying on yes/no responses.			

Nursing Process and Critical Thinking

Answer Key: A complete Answer Key is provided in your Additional Learning Resources on Evolve.

FIGURE LABELING

1. *Directions:* On the figure below, use a-f to indicate where the following patient problems would be according to Maslow's Hierarchy.

a. Acute pain
b. Insufficient cardiac output
c. Situational low self-esteem

d. Potential for injury
e. Ineffective relationship
f. Hopelessness

TABLE ACTIVITY

2. *Directions:* On the table below, list the conclusions that you would make based on the analysis of significant cues. The first block has been completed for you.

Determination of Significant Cues

Patient Values	Normal Range	Conclusion
10-month-old child not babbling	Babbling usually starts at 9 months	Babbling delayed
38-year-old patient with potassium 6 mEq/L	3.5 to 5.0 mEq/L	
45-year-old patient with Glasgow Coma score of 15	15 is normal; score of less than 8 is severe brain injury	
22-year-old patient with blood pressure 120/76 mm Hg	<120/80 mm Hg	
Adult male patient with sodium of 130 mEq/L	135 to 145 mEq/L	
Adult female patient with hemoglobin of 12 g/dL	12 to 16 g/dL	
65-year-old patient with 4+ pitting edema of lower legs	1+ is barely perceptible; 4+ is severe	
28-year-old female patient with pulse of 55 beats/min	60 to 100 beats/min	

SHORT ANSWER

Directions: Using your own words, answer each question in the space provided.

3. Identify six elements that are included in well-written patient-centered goals.

   a. _____

   b. _____

   c. _____

   d. _____

   e. _____

   f. _____

4. Identify four sources of evidence that are used to support evidence-based practice.

   a. _____

   b. _____

   c. _____

   d. _____

MULTIPLE CHOICE

Directions: Select the best answer(s) for each of the following questions.

5. Which patient goal statement contains a measurable verb?
   1. Patient will perform range-of-motion exercises twice a day.
   2. Patient will understand how to self-administer daily insulin.
   3. Patient will be advised about infection control in the home.
   4. Patient will know when to call the health care provider (HCP).

6. Which action would be considered a nurse-prescribed intervention?
   1. Adjusts the dosage of antihypertensive medication
   2. Explains the risks and benefits of a surgical procedure
   3. Administers scheduled antibiotic medication
   4. Gathers data and plans a bladder training schedule

7. What is a primary advantage of North American Nursing Diagnosis Association International (NANDA-I)?
   1. Lists thousands of predesigned interventions and activities that apply to common patient problems
   2. Includes measurement scales for baseline assessment and evaluation of patient outcomes
   3. Provides a standardized language that is recognized and applies to a variety of patient care settings
   4. Contributes to cost-effective outcomes for the patient and decreased out-of-pocket expenses

8. The nurse is caring for a patient who is 1 day postoperative for abdominal surgery. The patient reports, "Pain medicine didn't relieve my abdominal pain and it's getting worse." He also reports feeling dizzy, lightheaded, and slightly nauseated. Which objective data would the nurse collect **first**?
   1. Assess the dressing and observe for blood or drainage.
   2. Look at the most recent blood pressure and pulse.
   3. Check the last hematocrit and hemoglobin results.
   4. Assess the abdomen for distention and rigidity.

9. The nurse hears in report that the patient has a medical diagnosis of chronic obstructive pulmonary disease. Which data cluster does the nurse expect to find when assessing this patient?
   1. Low oxygen level, chronic cough, dyspnea with exertion
   2. Low blood pressure, ascites, shortness of breath
   3. Decreased range of motion in extremities, orthopnea, stridor
   4. Low carbon dioxide level; shallow, rapid respirations; pallor

10. Which patient problem would be considered a collaborative problem?
    1. The patient has sundown syndrome and the family is unsure what to do.
    2. The patient is reluctant to ambulate because of fear of falling.
    3. The patient has early Alzheimer's disease and shows early symptoms of dementia.
    4. The patient needs anticipatory guidance for transfer to long-term care.

11. Which intervention would be considered nurse-prescribed?
    1. Obtain and report peak and trough levels for vancomycin x3 days.
    2. Administer IV 5% dextrose and half normal saline at 125 mL/hour for 8 hours.
    3. Make a referral to physical therapy to teach the patient to transfer from bed to wheelchair.
    4. Encourage independence in hygiene by supervising while the patient washes face and hands.

12. The health care team is using a standardized clinical pathway in the care of patients who require cataract surgery and follow-up care. The nurse notes a "repetition of variances." What is the **best** rationale for the nurse to report this observation to the team leader?
    1. The clinical pathway is not consistent with patients' medical diagnosis.
    2. Team should review the clinical pathway and possibly make revisions.
    3. Some team members are not reliable about documentation and followup.
    4. The team is not consistently interpreting or applying the clinical pathway.

13. Place the nursing actions in correct order according to the six phases of the nursing process.
    _____ 1. Identifies outcome of "patient will demonstrate respiratory rate of 12-20 breaths/min after being positioned in high Fowler's."
    _____ 2. Assists RN to develop a plan of care that will improve the patient's ability to breathe and expand lungs.
    _____ 3. Collaborates with RN to make patient problem statement of ineffective breathing related to positioning that prevents lung expansion.
    _____ 4. Observes position and respiratory effort, counts rate, and auscultates lung fields.
    _____ 5. Assists to high Fowler's position or assists to sit in the bedside chair.
    _____ 6. Checks oxygen saturation and asks patient about subjective feelings of relief after being repositioned.

14. The nurse is performing the assessment phase of the nursing process. Which nursing action would be done during this phase?
    1. Observe a patient's ability to independently perform AM hygienic care.
    2. Adjust a standardized care plan to meet the needs of the individual patient.
    3. Take blood pressure 30 minutes after giving an antihypertensive medication.
    4. Assist the patient to make a list of questions to ask the HCP.

15. The nurse observes that the patient is pale; diaphoretic; slightly hunched over; and demonstrates deep, rapid breathing. Based on this objective data, which question will the nurse use to elicit the **most** relevant subjective data?
    1. "Do you feel chilled or feverish?"
    2. "Do you need some help to sit up?"
    3. "Are you having any pain?"
    4. "When did you start feeling like this?"

16. The nurse has identified six relevant patient problem statements that would apply to the patient's care. Which nursing action is the **most** important?
    1. Determine how the patient problem statements relate to the medical diagnoses.
    2. Plan interventions that will address the six problems that were identified.
    3. Prioritize the patient problem statements from most urgent to least urgent.
    4. Ask the patient if the identified problems are consistent with his/her view.

17. The nurse is caring for a patient who is newly diagnosed with asthma. On the care plan, there is the patient problem of ineffective breathing related to narrowing of airways, with a physician-prescribed intervention of "use inhaler as needed (PRN) for asthma attacks." How does the nurse implement this intervention?
    1. Consult the charge nurse to clarify the specific parameters for the intervention.
    2. Ask the patient how often he has asthma attacks and what triggers them.
    3. Keep the inhaler at the bedside and tell the patient to use it whenever he needs it.
    4. Observe baseline respiratory effort, frequently reassess, and instruct the patient to call for help.

18. Which data would be included in a cluster relevant to the patient problem of constipation? **Select all that apply.**
    1. Abdomen firm and nontender to touch
    2. Decreased bowel sounds
    3. Flat, brown, 1-cm lesion noted near umbilicus
    4. Takes opioid pain medications as needed
    5. Passed a small, hard stool yesterday
    6. Prefers to eat meat and potatoes, but lacks appetite

19. The nurse will perform a focused assessment on which patients? **Select all that apply.**
    1. Newly admitted to a long-term care facility
    2. Has a head injury that was sustained during a fall
    3. Reports sore throat and a low-grade fever
    4. Comes to the clinic for a physical examination for a job
    5. Reports pain in the left leg that worsens with walking
    6. Reports back pain, painful urination, and low-grade fever

20. What is the **best** rationale for collecting a patient's biographic data such as age, weight, and place of employment?
    1. Creates a complete and comprehensive legal document about the patient
    2. Is required by insurance companies and other third parties for reimbursement
    3. Helps the health care team identify potential risk factors for health problems
    4. Allows the patient to participate more fully and have a say in his/her own care

21. What is the advantage of using the nursing process to identify patient problem statements?
    1. Helps nurses identify a disease or illness that creates problems for the patient
    2. Allows nurses to use clinical judgment about actual or potential health problems
    3. Permits nurses to use standardized care plans for common patient problems
    4. Limits the type of problems that nurses are responsible for treating

22. The nurse has completed the assessment and reviewed the patient's record. The patient has potential for impaired skin integrity. Which datum supports this problem?
    1. A deep pressure injury is noted over the sacral area.
    2. Documentation includes descriptions of many skin lesions.
    3. The patient reports a painful, open sore on the left ankle.
    4. The patient is underweight and has trouble changing position.

23. What would be an example of a collaborative problem?
    1. Edema
    2. Coping
    3. Low self-esteem
    4. Social isolation

24. The home health nurse needs the patient's complete medication history, but the patient tells the nurse that many changes were made in the hospital and at discharge, so he is not sure what to tell her. What would be the **best** secondary source of this information?
    1. Patient's family
    2. Discharging HCP
    3. Medication reconciliation form
    4. Local pharmacist

25. The postsurgical patient reports that he is having lower abdominal pain. What would the nurse include in the focused physical assessment?
    1. Check peripheral pulses and sensation.
    2. Check for rigidity and rebound tenderness.
    3. Assess the patient's mental status.
    4. Auscultate the lung sounds.

26. The caregiver of a patient with Alzheimer's disease reports that the patient is unsteady and easily loses his balance, leaves the house, and needs coaching to accomplish tasks. Which patient problem statements will apply to this patient? **Select all that apply.**
    1. Acute confusion
    2. Self-care deficit for activities of daily living
    3. Wandering
    4. Potential for caregiver strain
    5. Potential for falls
    6. Potential for fluid overload

27. An older adult patient is wetting the bed because he is unable to independently get up to go to the bathroom. For this particular patient, which phase of the nursing process is **most** critical to address the patient's needs?
    1. Assessment
    2. Diagnosis
    3. Planning
    4. Evaluation

28. The home health nurse has been visiting a patient for several months. One of the patient's problems is that she is reluctant to leave the house. The goal of "patient will attend a social function two times per month" has not been met. What would the nurse do **first**?
    1. Document the interventions that were performed and the results
    2. Rewrite the goal and replace "two times per month" with "one time per month."
    3. Agree to visit the patient more frequently to decrease sense of isolation.
    4. Evaluate the factors that are affecting or interfering with the patient's response.

29. Which nursing action **best** demonstrates that the nurse believes that evidence-based practice is important for quality patient care?
    1. Routinely reads research articles and applies research to patient care
    2. Works on a committee to update policy and procedure manuals
    3. Looks on the Internet to find clinically relevant data
    4. Asks a clinical nurse specialist to validate nursing care decisions

30. A patient comes to the clinic for a broken toe. The nurse checks the patient's pulse and then attaches him to the cardiac monitor, which reveals an irregular heart rhythm. What is the **best** rationale for the nurse's action?
    1. The nurse saw that the patient had obvious risk factors for cardiac problems.
    2. Standard of care is a complete evaluation when patients first seek health care.
    3. A head-to-toe assessment is implemented when the patient is not distressed.
    4. Palpation of the pulse revealed irregularities, so the nurse considered pathophysiology.

31. The nursing student has diligently read all assignments, attended all lectures and skills practice sessions, but lacks clinical experience to improve critical thinking skills. What should the student do to improve critical thinking as it applies to patient care? **Select all that apply.**
    1. Mentally rehearse clinical scenarios: "What would I do if…"
    2. Develop the habit of formulating relevant questions when listening or reading.
    3. Ask the instructor or nurse preceptor to "think out loud."
    4. Discuss with classmates how they reached a certain decision.
    5. Advocate for more clinical time with patients.
    6. Scan for nursing information from a wide variety of sources.

CRITICAL THINKING ACTIVITIES

32. a. Discuss the LPN/LVN's role in the nursing process._____

    _____

    _____

    _____

    _____

    _____

    b. If the LPN/LVN disagrees with the RN about the choice or priority of a nursing diagnosis/patient problem statement, what should the LPN/LVN do?

    _____

    _____

    _____

    _____

    _____

33. The nurse is working on a busy medical-surgical unit, and today has been particularly hectic. Upon entering a patient's room, the nurse notes that the patient seems upset. The patient's body language suggests that she would like to talk to the nurse. Discuss how the nurse would use critical thinking in the decision to stay (or not) and sit with the patient to talk.

_____

_____

_____

_____

_____

NEXT-GENERATION NCLEX™ (NGN)

34. Cloze

Cognitive Skill: Recognize Cues

Scenario: Ms. M, age 48 years, was just transferred from the surgical recovery unit and is being admitted to the medical-surgical unit after an abdominal hysterectomy. She is alert and conversant but is anxious to see her family and reports severe pain (9/10). IV normal saline is positional but infuses at the prescribed rate of 125 mL/hr if the left arm is straight and extended. No reports of discomfort or tenderness at the IV site, no swelling or redness are noted. The abdominal dressing has a small amount of light-pink staining in the middle of the dressing. An indwelling urinary catheter is draining clear, yellow urine. Vital signs are: T 100.3° F (37.9° C), pulse 100, R 30, BP 140/90, O_2Sat 98% on room air.

Instructions: Choose the most likely options to complete the statement below.

During assessment, the nurse recognizes that assessment finding in need of immediate attention is the ___1___. First, the nurse will ___2___. Interventions are then used to address the immediate needs. To evaluate the efficacy of nursing actions, the ___3___ is the primary source of information.

Options for 1	Options for 2	Options for 3
patient's anxiety related to seeing her family	call the HCP	supervising RN
report of severe pain (9/10)	give pain medication	HCP
IV because it is positional	check the policy and procedure manual	patient
abdominal dressing because it shows pink staining	do a focused assessment on the problem area	electronic medical record
vital signs because they are all slightly elevated	reassure the patient that everything will be OK	family
	repeat the vital signs	

Cultural and Ethnic Considerations

chapter

6

Answer Key: A complete Answer Key is provided in your Additional Learning Resources on Evolve.

1. Crossword Puzzle

Directions: Use the clues to complete the crossword puzzle.

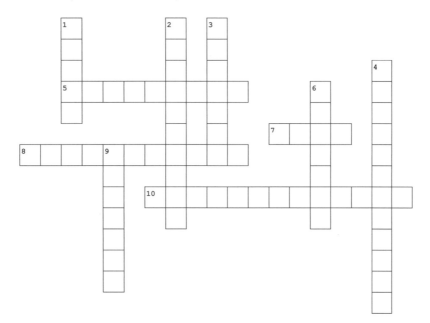

Across

5. Common social and cultural heritage based on shared traditions, national origin, and physical and biologic characteristics
7. Shares biologic physical characteristics
8. Preventable negative outcomes that disproportionately affect socially and economically disadvantaged populations
10. Understanding cultural variables and integrating that understanding during interaction

Down

1. Accepted traditional customs, moral attitudes, or manners of a particular social group
2. Shares characteristics with primary culture, but behaviors and ideals distinguish it from the rest of a cultural group
3. Learned beliefs, customs, and practices shared by a group and passed to another generation
4. Belief that one's own beliefs and cultural practices are the best
6. Nation, community, or broad group of people who establish particular aims, beliefs, or standards of living and conduct
9. Discrimination and prejudice toward people with disabilities

MULTIPLE CHOICE

Directions: Select the best answer(s) for each of the following questions.

2. The nurse observes a young, friendly unlicensed assistive personnel (UAP) giving the "thumbs up" hand gesture as he passes by the doorway of his assigned patients. What would the nurse do **first**?
   1. Ask the patients what they think about the "thumbs up" gesture.
   2. Suggest that the UAP talk to the charge nurse before someone complains.
   3. Observe the UAP for evidence of additional culturally biased behavior.
   4. Talk to the UAP about the hand gesture and the response from the patients.

3. A nursing student has to rely on public transportation and she is late several times for class and clinical. The instructor is very unhappy with the tardiness. What should the student do **first**?
   1. Promise never to be late for the remainder of the semester.
   2. Ask for a transfer to another instructor and a different clinical site.
   3. Explain transportation issues and ask for help to problem-solve.
   4. Ask for lenience and offer to do additional make-up assignments.

4. Which behavior **most** strongly suggests that the patient has a future time orientation?
   1. Patient declines a recommended cancer screening test because she has no family history of cancer.
   2. Patient goes to the emergency department for acute-onset abdominal pain.
   3. Patient asks the nurse if his daughter can stay overnight with him in the hospital.
   4. Patient initiates a program of regular exercise and healthy eating habits.

5. Which situation **most** strongly indicates a patriarchal family structure?
   1. Oldest son makes medical decisions for older adult father and provides emotional support for his mother.
   2. Family requests that diagnosis of cancer be withheld from the patient, who is an older adult female.
   3. Female family members sit at the patient's bedside; male members sit in the waiting room.
   4. At immunization clinic, mother gives her son emotional support and comfort.

6. Based on the nurse's knowledge of health disorders found among persons of American Indian ancestry, which question is the nurse **most** likely to ask?
   1. "Have you experienced any unintentional weight loss?"
   2. "Has anyone in your family ever been told they have diabetes?"
   3. "When was the last time you had a complete physical?"
   4. "Do you know if you have a family history of sickle cell disease?"

7. The nurse is assisting a patient to change position in bed. The patient has a limited understanding of English. What would the nurse do?
   1. Speak loudly to emphasize key information.
   2. Keep instructions brief and simple.
   3. Wait for an interpreter.
   4. Provide directions with detailed rationale.

8. Which cultural differences does the nurse need to be aware of when caring for older adults? **Select all that apply.**
   1. They may be less tolerant of other cultures.
   2. They may say hurtful things if cognitive impairment is present.
   3. They are less likely to be well-educated.
   4. They are more likely to use home remedies.
   5. They belong to a cultural group of shared historical experiences.

9. The surgeon informs the patient about a risk of blood loss during the planned surgical procedure and advises that a blood transfusion may be needed during the surgery. The patient refuses to sign the consent form because of religious beliefs. Which nursing action is in the **best** interest of the patient?
   1. Support the patient's decision to refuse the procedure.
   2. Discuss realistic alternatives to blood transfusion with the surgeon.
   3. Document the patient's decision in the medical record.
   4. Contact the risk manager for advice about convincing the patient.

10. To respect the Muslim woman's religious beliefs, what would the nurse do?
    1. Provide privacy and a place to pray before each procedure.
    2. Stay with the woman until a family member arrives.
    3. Keep her head, arms, and legs covered as much as possible.
    4. Have a female escort present if the health care provider (HCP) is male.

11. The nurse is from a small town in the United States and is starting a new job in a large urban area with a diverse population. What strategies can the nurse use to develop cultural competence? **Select all that apply.**
    1. Perform a self-assessment of beliefs and practices.
    2. Adapt personal beliefs to match those of individual patients.
    3. Keep an open mind about cultural differences.
    4. Treat everyone equally and act the same toward all patients.
    5. Ignore the differences and focus on exhibiting kindness and care.
    6. Understand own values, preferences, and cultural heritage.

12. The nurse is caring for a patient who is dying. What does evidence-based practice indicate about cultural beliefs and rituals that surround death?
    1. The family should be encouraged to pray at the bedside.
    2. Respect and protection of the dying person's soul are important.
    3. Lack of religious preference increases problems with coping.
    4. Rituals and ceremonies to delay or ward off death should be discouraged.

13. The patient, who is in no apparent distress, is accompanied to the clinic by several family members who cluster around. All are attempting to talk to each other and the nurse at the same time. The nurse can hear a mixture of English and another language being spoken. What would the nurse do **first**?
    1. Try to determine who speaks the best English.
    2. Escort the patient to an examination room and shut the door.
    3. Project a calm manner and try to identify the leader of the family.
    4. Physically assess the patient and take vital signs to ascertain condition.

14. A older male patient says to the nurse regarding the UAP, "That young Asian woman who helped me with my bath was really nice, but she seemed scared and never looked up; just kept her head down. Did I do something to scare or offend her?" What would the nurse do **first**?
    1. Find the UAP and ask her to explain her behavior to the patient.
    2. Reassure him that he did nothing wrong and that the UAP's behavior is cultural.
    3. Tell the patient that you will check with the UAP and then get back to him.
    4. Apologize to the patient and give then give feedback to the UAP.

15. The nurse is a happy and outgoing person, and comes from a family where hugging, touching, patting, or playfully punching are part of normal everyday interaction. What is the **best** strategy for the nurse to combine her personal strengths and giving culturally appropriate care?
    1. Assess her own behaviors and try to understand the origin of her personal style.
    2. Consider different patient care settings and observe interactions.
    3. Learn which cultures can accept touch by health care personnel.
    4. Request to care for patients who are from her own culture.

16. The nurse is working in an assisted-living facility and most residents take their meals in a common dining area. What is the **best** method for seating the residents?
    1. Assign seating so that each resident has a consistent place at mealtimes.
    2. Encourage the residents to continuously sit with someone new for stimulation.
    3. Observe how self-mobile and ambulatory residents seat and group themselves.
    4. Ask each resident where he/she would like to sit at the beginning of each meal.

17. The nurse is trying to give all of his patients the 9:00 AM medications. An older Hispanic woman needs 15 medications every morning but is consistently preoccupied whenever the nurse enters the room. What would the nurse do?
    1. Administer the medications to other patients first and then help this patient.
    2. Give the patient a 15-minute warning and then stick to the promised time.
    3. Try to find out why the woman is so consistently preoccupied.
    4. Start giving this patient the medications at 8:00 AM so there is extra time.

18. The nursing student is trying to explain the importance of taking blood pressure medication every day to an older patient who is on a fixed income. Which question from the patient is the **best** indication that his perception of time tends to be present-oriented?
    1. "Can I save the medication on the days when I feel okay?"
    2. "What should I do if I am running out of medication and have no money?"
    3. "My wife takes blood pressure medication too. Can I share her pills?"
    4. "Would you take this medication if you were in my position?"

19. The nurse is discussing the parents' beliefs and use of folk medicine, which they would like to use to treat their child's respiratory infection. Which health care practice is the cause for **greatest** concern?
    1. Placing a religious medal on the bedside table
    2. Having a folk healer come to heal with touch and faith
    3. Giving the child an herbal tea that gives strength and health
    4. Bathing at night instead of in the morning

20. On visiting the patient at home, the nurse finds that the patient is not following the dietary instructions. The nurse discovers that the wife, who shops and cooks, believes that her husband needs "nutritious home-cooked meals from his native country." What would the nurse do **first**?
    1. Change the dietary plan to meet the patient's and family's cultural preferences.
    2. Consult a nutritionist for ways to adapt the wife's cooking to the dietary plan.
    3. Revise the patient's nutritional goal to incorporate the cultural dietary patterns.
    4. Ask the wife to describe a typical 24-hour day of meal preparation and snacks.

21. The nurse is assessing a patient who reports, "It feels like there is something inside me that wants to come out." Which questions would the nurse ask to assess the patient's belief system? **Select all that apply.**
    1. "When did you first notice the feeling?"
    2. "Why do you think this is happening right now?"
    3. "What do you think is causing the problem?"
    4. "Why do you think this is happening to you?"
    5. "What do you think will help clear up the problem?"

CRITICAL THINKING ACTIVITIES

22. Every morning the same day-shift nurse is late for work, so giving handover report is always delayed. The night-shift nurses have mentioned this to the nurse manager, who has promised to take care of the problem, but the late behavior continues. One of the night nurses tries to talk to the day-shift nurse about her behavior, but the nurse says, "Oh, you Americans are always so worried about time. Just relax. You know I will always be here." Analyze this situation and make suggestions about how the problem can be addressed. Ask your clinical instructor if you can discuss this topic in a postconference.

_____

_____

_____

_____

_____

23. Nursing students who grow up and work in the United States sometimes have difficulty describing their own culture and identifying how "American" culture is viewed by people who did not grow up in the United States.

    a. If you are an American who grew up in the United States, describe the how "American" culture affects your values and belief system.

    _____

    _____

    _____

    _____

    _____

    _____

b. If you are not originally from the United States, discuss how your view of "American" culture and how living in the culture is currently affecting you.

_____

_____

_____

_____

_____

_____

NEXT-GENERATION NCLEX™ (NGN)

24. Extended Multiple Response

Cognitive Skill: Recognize Cues

Scenario: The nurse is caring for an older patient who has recently emigrated from another country. The patient's family is at the bedside and the nurse overhears them speaking in English and Spanish. The nurse's first language is English and she understands and speaks a little Spanish. What are the disadvantages of asking family members to translate?

Instructions: Place a check mark next to the disadvantages of asking family members to translate. **Check all that apply.**

_____ 1. The nurse loses the opportunity to practice using Spanish.

_____ 2. There is a potential for violation of privacy and confidentiality.

_____ 3. The presence of family members hinders the nurse-patient relationship.

_____ 4. Family may intentionally withhold information from the nurse and patient.

_____ 5. Family may or may not be able to accurately convey the nurse's meaning to the patient.

_____ 6. The hospital must provide room and board for family members who are translating.

_____ 7. The nurse must spend extra time responding to the family's questions and comments.

_____ 8. Miscommunication may lead to poor patient outcomes or cause legal problems.

_____ 9. Patient has less opportunity to decide whether the information should be shared with family.

Asepsis and Infection Control

Answer Key: A complete Answer Key is provided in your Additional Learning Resources on Evolve.

SHORT ANSWER

Directions: Using your own words, answer each question in the space provided.

1. Describe the procedure for gowning for contact isolation._____

_____

_____

_____

_____

_____

_____

LABELING

2. Review the following nursing tasks and identify whether medical asepsis (MA) or surgical asepsis (SA) is necessary to prevent the spread of infection. Label each task as MA or SA.

_____ a. Assisting a patient with a meal tray

_____ b. Helping a patient brush the teeth

_____ c. Obtaining a urine specimen from an existing catheter

_____ d. Obtaining a throat swab for a culture

_____ e. Inserting a urinary catheter

_____ f. Changing the bed linens

_____ g. Replacing a colostomy bag

_____ h. Drawing up medication in a syringe

_____ i. Removing medication from a bubble pack

_____ j. Dressing change of a new surgical incision

_____ k. Suctioning the lower airway

_____ l. Suctioning the oral cavity

ORDERING

3. Place steps 1-7 of opening a wrapped sterile package in the correct order.

   _____ Grasp the outer surface of the last and innermost flap; pull the flap back, allowing it to fall flat.

   _____ Place the wrapped sterile package flat in the center of the work surface.

   _____ Grasp the outside surface of the first side flap; open the side flap; allow it to lie flat on the table surface.

   _____ Grasp the outer surface of the tip of the outermost flap; open the outer flap away from your body.

   _____ Grasp the outside surface of the second side flap; allow it to lie flat on the table surface.

   _____ Remove the tape or seal indicating the sterilization date.

   _____ Perform hand hygiene.

MULTIPLE CHOICE

Directions: Select the best answer(s) for each of the following questions.

4. What is included in the proper method for disposal of sharps? **Select all that apply.**
   1. Everyone is responsible for disposing of sharps immediately after using them.
   2. Dispose of sharps in a puncture-proof container in the patient area.
   3. Drop sharps into container, avoid touching the rim.
   4. Carefully recap used needles in the home setting before disposing.
   5. Avoid pushing items into the container or overfilling it.
   6. Avoid leaving sharps on procedure trays or among bed linens.

5. The unlicensed assistive personnel (UAP) is assigned to disinfect equipment. Which instructions will the nurse give to the UAP about maintaining personal safety? **Select all that apply.**
   1. Wear gloves to protect skin and prevent breakdown.
   2. Follow manufacturer's instructions for dilution and use.
   3. Avoid using disinfectant if equipment is contaminated with spores.
   4. Assume equipment is contaminated and use Standard Precautions.
   5. Use an antiseptic solution if the disinfectant is not removing the debris.
   6. Discard any equipment that cannot be readily and safely cleaned and disinfected.

6. A visitor enters the nursing home without a mask. The nursing student politely hands her a disposable mask and suggests that social distancing decreases spread of the COVID-19 virus. The visitor refuses to comply. Which action is **best** for the nursing student to take?
   1. Give the visitor a brochure that explains the COVID-19 virus.
   2. Contact the charge nurse about the situation.
   3. Escort the visitor and the resident to a private room.
   4. Allow the visitor to have free choice and document the incident.

7. Which patient is **most** likely to need neutropenic precautions?
   1. Has hepatitis A and is incontinent of bowels and bladder
   2. Has chronic wound with methicillin-resistant *Staphylococcus aureus* (MRSA) infection
   3. Has leukopenia with fewer than 3,500 white blood cells per microliter.
   4. Has a flat red rash and cold symptoms and sibling has measles.

8. The patient has a large midline abdominal incision. With the specific purpose of reducing a possible reservoir of infection, what would the nurse do?
   1. Wear gloves and mask at all times.
   2. Isolate the patient's personal articles.
   3. Direct the patient to cover mouth when coughing.
   4. Change the dressing when it becomes soiled.

9. What would be included in the care of a patient with incontinence and rotavirus?
   1. A private room with negative airflow
   2. Hand hygiene after filtration masks are removed
   3. Use of gloves and gown upon entering the room
   4. Use of a surgical mask on the patient during transfers

10. A patient with rubella needs to be transported to the radiology department. What would the nurse do to prepare the patient for transport?
    1. Advise the patient to immediately wash hands after returning from procedure.
    2. Call the radiology department and inform them to wear gloves at all times.
    3. Dress the patient in an isolation gown and then apply a mask.
    4. Instruct the patient to wear a mask and follow cough etiquette.

11. Which action by the nursing student requires correction because it contributes to the potential transmission of pathogens?
    1. Uses a dampened cloth to wipe off the overbed table
    2. Shakes linens to remove debris and then places them in laundry bag
    3. Holds soiled linens at a distance to prevent touching uniform
    4. Washes hands with soap and water after emptying and cleaning a bedpan

12. When caring for a patient with tuberculosis who is on airborne precautions, what would the nurse routinely use?
    1. Regular mask and eyewear
    2. Gown and gloves
    3. Surgical handwashing and gloves
    4. Particulate respirator mask

13. The nurse is observing a nursing student who is preparing to do a sterile dressing change. Which action requires correction and additional instruction?
    1. Opening the outer flap of the sterile package by moving it toward the body
    2. Placing the cap of the sterile solution inside up on a clean surface
    3. Opening sterile items and dropping them directly onto the sterile field
    4. Maintaining a 1-inch border around the sterile drape

14. The nurse is aware that the body has normal defenses against infection. Which medication can affect the acidic environment, which is one defense mechanism?
    1. Ciprofloxacin
    2. Aluminum/magnesium antacid
    3. Doxycycline
    4. Chlorhexidine gluconate

15. The patient has been receiving antibiotic therapy. Which laboratory result indicates the need to contact the health care provider (HCP) for a reevaluation of prescribed therapy?
    1. Sensitivity results are positive.
    2. Blood titer is positive for antibodies.
    3. White blood cell count is elevated.
    4. Blood cultures are negative for growth.

16. For which circumstance would it be appropriate to contact the infection-control nurse for assistance?
    1. Results of a blood culture are needed to validate antibiotic therapy.
    2. Contaminated waste material needs to be properly disposed.
    3. An unusual cluster of infection is seen in the emergency department.
    4. A newly admitted patient requires droplet and isolation precautions.

17. What is the **best** rationale for the consistent use of Standard Precautions?
    1. Centers for Disease Control and Prevention (CDC) recommend "universal blood and body fluid precautions."
    2. It is difficult to accurately identify all patients infected with blood-borne pathogens.
    3. Studies show that infection rates are unaffected by use of protective measures.
    4. Hand hygiene, gloves, masks, eye protection, and gowns are appropriate for patient contact.

18. The patient has tuberculosis and has been placed in a negative-pressure isolation room with airborne precautions. Despite patient education, he slips out of his room and goes outside to smoke cigarettes. What would the nurse do **first**?
    1. Obtain an order for an around-the-clock sitter.
    2. Report the patient's behavior to the infection-control nurse.
    3. Ask the HCP to prescribe a nicotine patch.
    4. Discuss the behavior with the patient.

19. Which patient needs to be placed into contact precautions?
    1. Has a draining wound colonized with multidrug-resistant bacteria
    2. Has cancer and currently has leukopenia
    3. Has meningitis caused by invasive *Neisseria meningitidis*
    4. Has tuberculosis caused by *Mycobacterium tuberculosis*

20. A patient comes into the clinic and tells the nurse that he has a sore throat and would like to see an HCP. For which tasks does the nurse need to wear gloves? **Select all that apply.**
    1. Interview and taking a history
    2. Taking the patient's radial pulse
    3. Measuring an oral temperature
    4. Taking a throat swab for culture
    5. Reviewing the patient's home medications
    6. Using a tongue blade to look at the throat

21. Immediately after donning a pair of gloves, a family member develops red, watery eyes and contact dermatitis with itching of the hands. What would the nurse do **first**?
    1. Inform the person that these are the signs/symptoms of latex allergy.
    2. Instruct the person to remove the gloves and wash thoroughly with soap and water.
    3. Contact the HCP and observe for any signs of anaphylaxis.
    4. Assess for a personal or family history of latex allergy or other allergies.

22. The nurse sees the UAP trying to take an overly full laundry bag from the patient's room to the dirty utility room. The UAP is struggling to manage the bag and is partially dragging it on the floor. What would the nurse do?
    1. Allow the UAP to continue because she is completing her duties.
    2. Report the UAP for creating a situation where proper handling is impossible.
    3. Assist the UAP to carry the bag and then find out how it got so overfilled.
    4. Remind the UAP that overfilling the bag creates a problem for proper disposal.

23. The nurse is assigned to care for some patients who are in isolation and some who are not. What would the nurse do to meet the needs of all the patients?
    1. Provide care for patients who are not in isolation first.
    2. Ask the charge nurse to reassign at least one of the isolation cases to another nurse.
    3. See if patients with same type of isolation can be rearranged to be roommates.
    4. Organize and cluster care of isolation patients to minimize donning and doffing gowns.

24. Which patient is the **most** challenging regarding maintaining sterile technique throughout the procedure?
    1. 4-month-old infant is crying and upset, and needs routine immunization
    2. 75-year-old woman is obese and confused and needs an indwelling urinary catheter inserted
    3. 50-year-old man is continuously coughing and needs a dressing change on upper chest
    4. 15-year-old cheerful patient with Down syndrome "wants to help" insert the IV

25. The nurse is assisting an HCP by setting up a sterile tray for a procedure at the bedside. When the nurse opens the tray, there is moisture on a piece of equipment. What would the nurse do?
    1. Continue to set up the tray, because everything inside the kit is considered sterile.
    2. Return the entire tray to the supply area for resterilization and obtain a new tray.
    3. Put on a sterile glove and remove the moist piece of equipment and set it aside.
    4. Inform the HCP and obtain a new order for additional equipment.

26. The nurse is supervising a nursing student who is setting up a sterile tray to suction a patient. When would the nurse intervene?
    1. Student sets up the field on a clean overbed table that is at waist-level.
    2. Student touches the outside of the sterile wrapper when handling the package.
    3. Student picks up a sterile drape by the corner and lets it unfold by itself without touching any object.
    4. Student puts on sterile gloves, opens the bottle, and sets the cap on the sterile field.

27. A patient is positive for human immunodeficiency virus (HIV) and ready for discharge. He expresses fears about exposure of other family members, particularly young children, to the disease. What is the **best** response to help decrease the patient's fears and concerns?
    1. Review general principles of infection control in the home setting.
    2. Review principles of mode of transmission for HIV.
    3. Encourage expression of fears and concerns and validate feelings.
    4. Suggest that the patient maintain contact with family using phone calls, email, or video conferencing.

28. The new nurse observes an HCP who routinely comes out of a patient's room, goes to the sink, quickly soaps her hands, rinses, and then shakes water from her hands so that it splashes on the floor, sink, and her clothing. What would the new nurse do?
    1. Contact the infection-control nurse for advice.
    2. Do nothing because the HCP is not accountable to the nurse.
    3. Check on the patient's status and then write up an incident report.
    4. Offer the HCP a paper towel and assess understanding of hand hygiene.

29. Which patient is **most** likely to be susceptible to infection because of factors affecting immunologic defense mechanisms?
    1. A 5-year-old child who is not up to date on school immunizations
    2. A 35-year-old woman who has recently returned from Japan
    3. A 73-year-old man who recently had chemotherapy and radiation treatments
    4. A 55-year-old man who has a high-stress job and is overweight

30. The nursing student has been diagnosed with "strep throat." Under what circumstances can the student go to the clinical unit and care for patients and complete the clinical objectives?
    1. Has been taking prescribed antibiotics for at least 24 hours
    2. Agrees to wear a mask whenever caring for patients
    3. Cares only for patients who are not susceptible to infection
    4. Can return to clinical if the instructor is aware of the condition

31. Which patient has a condition that will be **most** challenging for the health care team to manage?
    1. The patient is immunocompromised and has a wound infected with MRSA.
    2. The patient has a throat infection and throat culture shows β-hemolytic group A streptococci.
    3. The patient has pelvic inflammatory disease caused by *Neisseria gonorrhoeae*.
    4. The patient handles an exotic animal hide and develops a skin lesion; culture shows *Bacillus anthracis*.

32. Which health care worker is **most** likely to be a vector of infection?
    1. A UAP removes a bag full of dirty laundry from a patient's room.
    2. A clinic nurse places a child exposed to measles at school in an isolated area.
    3. A nursing student has mild influenza symptoms but feels okay to go to the clinical experience.
    4. An HCP sees the last patient at the clinic and forgets hand hygiene before going home.

33. Nurses are assigned a mixture of patients a who need isolation or just routine Standard Precautions. Which nurse has exposed his/her patients to infection via the indirect method of transmission?
    1. Nurse A first provides care for all of her patients who are not in isolation.
    2. Nurse B uses her personal stethoscope to assess all of her patients.
    3. Nurse C dons and doffs a new mask, gown, and gloves in caring for all of his patients.
    4. Nurse D washes his hands upon entering and exiting each patient's room.

34. The first-year nursing students are going to the hospital for their first clinical experience. What is the **most** important thing that the students would do to prevent exposing patients to health care–associated infections (HAIs)?
    1. Understand how to care for patients who are in different kinds of isolation.
    2. Ensure that personal immunizations are up to date and health status is good.
    3. Know the steps for sterile technique and practice before going to clinical.
    4. Perform hand hygiene using recommendations from the CDC.

35. Which patient is showing signs of an inflammatory response in the absence of infection?
    1. The patient has sore throat and hoarse voice that are resolving with antibiotic therapy.
    2. The patient has burning with urination and urine appears cloudy with a strong odor.
    3. The patient's ankle is swollen, red, and tender; symptoms started after falling.
    4. The patient's eye is red and irritated; he wakes with a crusty, yellow drainage.

36. The nurse performs hand hygiene before donning gloves, completes the procedure, and then doffs the gloves. What is the **best** rationale for performing hand hygiene after doffing the gloves and before leaving the patient's room?
    1. The patient sees that the nurse is cautious and consistent about hand hygiene.
    2. The nurse may suddenly have to attend to another patient immediately upon exiting the room.
    3. The CDC recommends this final step to complete the procedure.
    4. There is a risk of perforating the gloves during use and the perforation may not be obvious.

37. The nurse is supervising a new UAP in performing care for isolation patients. When is the nurse **most** likely to intervene? **Select all that apply.**
    1. The UAP wears a mask dangling around the neck and repositions it before entering patient's room.
    2. The UAP changes the mask every 20 to 30 minutes because it takes a long time to assist a patient.
    3. The UAP removes the mask by grasping the front portion that covers the mouth and pulling if off.
    4. The UAP wears an isolation gown over the uniform to provide an extra layer of warmth.
    5. The UAP pushes the sleeves of the isolation gown up while bathing a patient.
    6. The UAP reuses a mask when reentering the patient's room.

38. The nurse is interviewing a patient at a walk-in clinic. The patient reports fatigue, weight loss, dyspnea, fever, night sweats, and coughing up small flecks of blood. What would the nurse do **first**?
    1. Put a mask on the patient and escort him to an isolation room.
    2. Don a mask, gown, and gloves and put a mask on the patient.
    3. Assess for history of respiratory disease or family history of cancer.
    4. Alert the HCP about the patient's symptoms.

39. Which actions require intervention? **Select all that apply.**
    1. A nursing student uses hot water to clean fecal material from a bedpan.
    2. A new nurse uses a mask, protective eyewear, fluid-resistant gown, and gloves when handling a bedpan.
    3. A UAP dons gloves before performing perineal care.
    4. An HCP puts a blood-encrusted instrument into the patient's sink.
    5. A nurse uses a small brush and applies friction to remove dried blood in the grooves of an instrument.

40. The patient has a urinary tract infection. Which nursing intervention would enhance the normal defense mechanism of the urinary system?
    1. Instruct the patient to complete the prescription of antibiotics.
    2. Direct the patient to drink extra fluids to flush the urinary system.
    3. Monitor for and report fever and pain in the back or lower abdomen.
    4. Tell the patient that she will be notified about the urine culture.

CRITICAL THINKING ACTIVITIES

41. The nurse is caring for several patients. The patients include a frail 87-year-old woman with a hip fracture; a 78-year-old woman with advanced Alzheimer's disease who is being treated for dehydration secondary to incontinence of watery diarrhea; and a 60-year-old man who sustained a small perforation during a routine colonoscopy, which was recommended as part of his annual physical examination.

    a. Explain conditions that promote the onset of HAIs for these patients._____

    _____

    _____

    _____

    _____

    b. What measures can be used to prevent HAIs? _____

    _____

    _____

    _____

    _____

    c. Although the HCP has not currently ordered isolation precautions for any of these patients, the nurse should consider initiating isolation precautions for which patient? Identify the type of isolation that the nurse would choose and give the rationale that supports the decision.

    _____

    _____

    _____

    _____

42. The nurse is caring for a 35-year-old patient who sustained a penetrating abdominal wound and multiple bruises and contusions in a farming accident. The abdominal wound was very contaminated, but cleaned before and during surgery. The wound-care specialist has been consulted and has taught the nursing staff how to do the dressing changes. The patient has a peripheral IV and is receiving IV antibiotics and pain medication. The nurse identifies that the patient is at risk for infection.

    a. Give examples of questions that the nurse could use to collect data about factors that would affect the patient's immunologic defense mechanisms.

    _____

    _____

    _____

    _____

    b. Explain why this patient is likely to have an inflammatory response and describe the physiologic process that will occur.

    _____

    _____

    _____

    _____

    c. Describe the signs and symptoms that would occur if the patient developed a localized infection at the abdominal wound site or at the IV site.

    _____

    _____

    _____

    _____

    d. Describe the signs and symptoms that would signal a systemic infection. _____

    _____

    _____

    _____

    _____

NEXT-GENERATION NCLEX™ (NGN)

43. Matrix

Cognitive Skill: Recognize Cues

Standard Precautions are guidelines designed to reduce the risk of transmission of microorganisms from known and unknown sources of infection and prevent the spread of organisms present in blood, all other body fluids, nonintact skin, and mucous membranes. Based on clinical judgment in applying the Standard Precautions guidelines, which actions would be considered essential, nonessential, or contraindicated?

Instructions: Use an X to indicate which actions are essential, nonessential, or contraindicated. All should be used and can be used only once.

Action	Essential	Nonessential	Contraindicated
Performs hand hygiene after completing wound care and dressing change			
Washes hands and changes gloves between cleaning for perineal area and rectum			
Wears a mask and eye protection or a face shield while performing venipuncture			
Dons a clean, unsterile gown before caring for a patient with copious vomiting			
Handles laboratory specimens from all patients as if they are infectious			
Uses an alcohol-based hand cleanser after caring for a patient who has diarrhea related to *Clostridium difficile*			
Isolates patient with suspected airborne communicable disease and notifies the HCP			

Body Mechanics and Patient Mobility

chapter

8

Answer Key: A complete Answer Key is provided in your Additional Learning Resources on Evolve.

MULTIPLE CHOICE

Directions: Select the best answer(s) for each of the following questions.

1. A nurse walks into the patient's room and notices that the patient is having trouble breathing. Which position will the nurse use to help relieve the patient's respiratory distress?
   1. Lower the head of the bed and place the patient in a supine anatomical position.
   2. Position the patient on the side with knee and thigh drawn up toward the chest.
   3. Lower the patient's head and place the body and legs on a slightly inclined plane.
   4. Raise the head of the bed to 90 degrees and have the patient lean forward on the overbed table.

2. Which position would be **most** comfortable for the patient and provide the **best** access for the nurse to insert a rectal suppository?
   1. Modified left lateral recumbent position
   2. Lithotomy
   3. Trendelenburg
   4. Orthopneic

3. Which medications are **most** likely to contribute to orthostatic hypotension?
   1. Medications used to treat osteoporosis
   2. Medications used to prevent thrombophlebitis
   3. Medications used to reduce high blood pressure
   4. Medications used to treat arthritis pain

4. The nurse is assisting a patient who has poor balance to move from the bed to the chair. What is included in the correct technique for assisting the patient to stand and pivot to the chair?
   1. Keep the knees slightly bent.
   2. Maintain a narrow base with the feet.
   3. Keep the stomach muscles loose.
   4. Stand at arm's length from the patient.

5. The patient had a surgical procedure and is getting up to ambulate for the first time. While ambulating down the hallway, the patient says, "I'm going to faint." What would the nurse do **first**?
   1. Call out for someone to obtain a wheelchair.
   2. Pull the patient close and lower him gently to the floor.
   3. Lean the patient against the wall until the episode passes.
   4. Support the patient and move quickly back to the room.

6. The patient will be immobilized for an extended period due to extensive injuries. Which intervention will the nurse use to prevent respiratory complications?
    1. Suction the airway every hour.
    2. Change the patient's position every 4-8 hours.
    3. Use oxygen and nebulizer treatments regularly.
    4. Encourage deep-breathing and coughing every hour.

7. Patients who are immobilized in health care facilities have psychosocial needs that must be met along with their physiologic needs. Which statement by the nurse acknowledges these needs?
    1. "Visiting hours will be limited so you can rest."
    2. "We will help you do everything so you don't have to worry."
    3. "Let's talk about what you used to do at home during the day."
    4. "A private room can be arranged for you."

8. The patient experienced a stroke that left her with severe left-sided paralysis and very limited mobility. Which device would prevent plantar flexion?
    1. Footboard
    2. Bed board
    3. Trapeze bar
    4. Trochanter roll

9. When assessing the neurovascular status of a patient, what is an expected finding?
    1. Capillary refill after 8 seconds
    2. Pulses strong and easily palpated
    3. Loss of sensation to an affected area
    4. Mild localized discomfort

10. Which range-of-motion (ROM) exercises can be safely performed on the neck? **Select all that apply.**
    1. Flexion
    2. Supination
    3. Lateral flexion
    4. Rotation
    5. Hyperextension

11. Which patient has a contracture?
    1. Patient has abnormal extension of a finger joint.
    2. Patient's wrist is abnormally flexed and joint is fixed.
    3. Patient's knee is hyperextended.
    4. Patient has abnormal lateral movements of ankle joint.

12. What is the **most** likely complication when an older adult patient gets pulled across the bed when changing wet linens?
    1. Dislocation of a joint
    2. Increased stress to the joints
    3. Abnormal hyperextension of a joint
    4. Shearing or tearing of the skin

13. For an older female patient who is at risk for osteoporosis, which associated complication can be minimized by participating in a regular exercise program as prescribed by the health care provider (HCP)?
    1. Bone loss that results in fractures
    2. Immobility secondary to joint degeneration
    3. Tissue ischemia and pressure injuries
    4. Thrombophlebitis secondary to blood clots

14. The nurse is preparing to assist the patient to transfer from the bed to the chair. Which action demonstrates the nurse's proper use of body mechanics?
    1. Stands by the chair and reaches out to guide the patient toward the chair
    2. Stands by the side of the patient and pulls up on the stronger arm
    3. Stands directly in front of the patient and places hands at the patient's waist level
    4. Stands to the side of patient and assists as the patient pivots

15. Which situation is the **best** example of proper ergonomic principles?
    1. Nurse A raises the head of the bed, supports the patient's shoulders, and helps to swing the legs around and off the bed using a pivoting motion.
    2. Nurse B rolls the patient onto his/her side. The nurse then stoops, and when standing, brings the patient along with the nurse.
    3. Nurse C gradually lowers the patient into the chair; the nurse bends his hips and knees as the patient leans slightly forward and sits down.
    4. Nurse D assesses for equipment such as IV lines, urinary catheters, or tubes and positions them to avoid tension during the transfer.

16. Which patient behavior should be corrected to reduce the risk of thrombophlebitis?
    1. The patient gets out of bed and forgets to put on slippers.
    2. The patient sits in chair and crosses legs while reading a book.
    3. The patient forgets to rise slowly when getting out of bed.
    4. The patient sits in a slouched position on a soft couch.

17. The patient has a cast on the left lower leg. Which assessment is performed to prevent compartment syndrome?
    1. Assess the patient's ability and willingness to assist with mobility.
    2. Assess muscle strength, activity tolerance, body position, and ROM.
    3. Assess skin color, temperature, movement, sensation, pulses, capillary refill, and pain.
    4. Assess patient's understanding of cast care and complications of immobility.

18. Which health care facility is using evidence-based practice to protect patients and health care workers from musculoskeletal injuries?
    1. Hires unlicensed assistive personnel (UAP) who have at least 3 years experience and demonstrate proficiency in transferring and moving patients
    2. Has mechanical lifts available for use; there is at least an 80% compliance rate and nurses and UAP are trained in the use of devices
    3. Uses National Institute for Occupational Safety and Health (NIOSH) Division of Safety Research guidelines for designing exercise programs for older adults
    4. Places any patient who takes blood pressure medication on fall precautions and UAPs help those patients ambulate

19. Which nurse is using the **key** factor in body mechanics?
    1. Nurse A keeps head aligned and bends straight over at the waist to assist the patient to tie his shoelaces.
    2. Nurse B puts one leg slightly behind other, bends knees, and uses large leg muscles to boost a box to a high shelf.
    3. Nurse C reaches across the bed to support patient's back and shoulders as he dangles his feet for several minutes.
    4. Nurse D keeps head erect and aligns and balances weight on both feet when assisting a patient to stand up.

20. The nurse had a previous back injury and knows that she should avoid twisting her spine as she cares for patients. What is the **best** strategy for the nurse to use?
    1. Ask to be assigned to patients who are self-mobile.
    2. Direct the UAP to do any heavy lifting.
    3. Stand directly in front of the person or object being worked with.
    4. Take antiinflammatory pain medication before assisting patients.

21. What is an **early** sign of acute compartment syndrome?
    1. Pain upon stretching
    2. Numbness
    3. Paralysis
    4. Cold, pale skin

22. Which patient is the **most** likely candidate for active assisted ROM exercises?
    1. Patient A is difficult to arouse but is responsive to painful stimuli.
    2. Patient B is able to move but is very depressed and reluctant to participate.
    3. Patient C has right-sided weakness in the upper body due to a stroke.
    4. Patient D is alert and oriented but is very frail and debilitated.

23. The nurse is helping plan an activity schedule for an older adult resident at a long-term care facility who is at risk for disuse syndrome. Which plan is the nurse **most** likely to suggest?
    1. Ten minutes of warmup and stretching, followed by 45 minutes of mild aerobic exercise, followed by 10 minutes of cool-down exercises performed 3 days a week
    2. Twenty minutes of walking on Mondays, Wednesdays, and Fridays and 10-15 minutes of moderate weight training on Tuesdays and Thursdays
    3. Patient participation in active assisted ROM for uninvolved joints for 10 minutes; alternate every 2 hours with passive assisted ROM on involved joints for 10 minutes
    4. Patient participation in activities of daily living (ADLs) (e.g., combing hair, walking to bathroom) for 10-15 minutes every 2-3 hours while awake for a total of 2 hours of activity per 24 hours

24. Which instructions would the nurse give to a new home health aide about helping the patient who has problems of immobility? **Select all that apply.**
    1. Ensure that the patient wears shoes with a nonslip sole during ambulation and transfer.
    2. Assist the patient to make gradual position changes.
    3. If the patient has orthostatic hypotension, advise him to stay in bed.
    4. If the patient becomes faint or dizzy when walking, ease him to the floor or a chair.
    5. Be sure the home is free of clutter, wet areas, or rugs that may slide.

CRITICAL THINKING ACTIVITIES

25. The nurse is caring for a patient who is comatose after sustaining a severe head injury several months ago. He is breathing on his own and his vital signs are stable but he shows no purposeful movements.

    a. What are the complications of immobility for this patient? _____

    _____

    b. What nursing interventions may be implemented to prevent the occurrence of complications of immobility?

    _____

    _____

    _____

c. During morning hygiene, the nurse notes a reddened area on the patient's sacrum. What nursing interventions can be used to address this finding?

_____

_____

NEXT-GENERATION NCLEX™ (NGN)

26. Extended Drag and Drop

Cognitive Skill: Take Action

Scenario: The nurse is caring for a patient who has had a stroke with right-sided impairment. The patient has a problem with physical mobility related to right-sided paresis. He has difficulty moving his right arm and leg and this interferes with ADLs. Before moving the patient, the nurse assesses for the patient's ability to assist in the move and the necessary safety measures that should be taken. The nurse is aware that immobility creates risk for complications. Which action would the nurse take to address each potential complication?

Instructions: Indicate which nursing intervention listed in the right column would be used to address the potential complication of immobility listed in the left column. Each intervention will be used only once.

Potential Complication	**Nursing Interventions**
_____ 1. Contractures	a. Range-of-motion exercises
_____ 2. Disuse osteoporosis	b. Deep-breathing and coughing exercises
_____ 3. Disorientation	c. Frequent ambulation
_____ 4. Hypostatic pneumonia	d. Suitable diversion, stimulation, socialization
_____ 5. Muscle atrophy	e. Meticulous skin care
_____ 6. Orthostatic hypotension	f. Footboard, trochanter roll, hand rolls, splinting devices
_____ 7. Pressure injury	g. Up to bathroom at regular intervals
_____ 8. Thrombophlebitis or deep vein thrombosis (DVT)	h. Dangle over side of bed
_____ 9. Urinary tract infection	i. Antiembolism measures (thromboembolic deterrent [TED] hose or decompression boots)

Hygiene and Care of the Patient's Environment

Answer Key: A complete Answer Key is provided in your Additional Learning Resources on Evolve.

MULTIPLE CHOICE

Directions: Select the best answer(s) for each of the following questions.

1. The nurse is teaching a patient who has diabetes about foot care. What would be included in the self-care instructions?
   1. Carefully cut corns and apply moleskin.
   2. Inspect feet daily for breaks in the skin.
   3. Wear loose shoes or sandals to air the feet.
   4. Use alcohol on a gauze pad to clean between toes.

2. The nurse will delegate denture care to the unlicensed assistive personnel (UAP). What instructions would the nurse give to the UAP about the patient's dentures?
   1. Use hot water and a mild soap.
   2. Let the patient wear them at night.
   3. Brush dentures with a soft toothbrush.
   4. Wrap them in a soft towel when not worn.

3. In delegating the early morning care that should occur before breakfast, what does the nurse remind the UAP to do for the patient?
   1. Shampoo the patient's hair and comb it.
   2. Assist the patient with a bath and clean gown.
   3. Offer the patient a backrub with warmed lotion.
   4. Help the patient wash hands and face.

4. A patient who is paralyzed from the waist down is at risk for developing a pressure injury on the sacral area. Which intervention would the nurse use for this patient?
   1. Frequently check and change the bed linens.
   2. Teach to shift weight every 15 minutes.
   3. Obtain an order for a donut cushion for sitting.
   4. Keep skin moist and frequently reapply lotion.

5. The nurse notices a reddened area on the patient's sacrum. What would the nurse do **first**?
   1. Cleanse the skin with alcohol.
   2. Wash the area with warm water and soap.
   3. Massage the area to stimulate blood flow.
   4. Assess for other areas of erythema.

6. The nurse is assessing the oral cavity of an unconscious patient and sees tenacious, dried exudate on the tongue, teeth, and gums. Which instructions would be given to the UAP?
   1. Use a moistened sponge applicator and gently clean crusts several times per shift.
   2. Spray the mouth with a bulb syringe and use oral suction to remove the fluid.
   3. Use a toothbrush with paste and scrub the area until the crusts are removed.
   4. Wrap a gauze sponge around a tongue blade and apply hydrogen peroxide.

7. The nurse is evaluating the eye care that has been delegated to and is being provided by a new staff member. Which action is appropriate?
   1. Removing dried secretions with moist gauze
   2. Using soap and water on a washcloth
   3. Cleansing the eyes from the outer to the inner canthus
   4. Wiping plastic eyeglasses with a clean paper towel

8. The nurse observes the patient performing ear care. Which behavior indicates a need for additional teaching?
   1. Cleans the pinna with a cotton-tipped swab
   2. Turns the hearing aid off when not in use
   3. Leaves the hearing aid by a sunny window
   4. Rotates a clean washcloth to clean ear canal

9. The nurse is caring for a postpartum patient. Which assessment would the nurse perform **first** before starting perineal care?
   1. Note presence of accumulated secretions.
   2. Evaluate the appearance of the perineum.
   3. Assess ability to perform own care.
   4. Ask about burning with urination.

10. The nurse is caring for an older adult patient who requires assistance with elimination. He can walk very slowly, but is frequently incontinent of urine before he can get to the toilet. What would the nurse do to help the patient with elimination? **Select all that apply.**
    1. Instruct the UAP to be alert for the call signal and answer promptly.
    2. Obtain an order for an indwelling catheter until bladder training is achieved.
    3. Show the patient how to use a urinal and place it within his reach.
    4. Obtain an order for a commode chair and place it close to the bed.
    5. Restrict fluids to exact intervals to establish a voiding pattern.
    6. Make a plan with the patient to call sooner, rather than delaying.

11. The nursing student is told to observe the bowel movements of an adult patient and report any abnormalities to the nurse. What would the student report as an **unexpected** finding?
    1. Stool was a dull clay color.
    2. Stool had soft, formed consistency.
    3. Patient reported three bowel movements this week.
    4. Stool had the shape of the rectum.

12. The nurse is caring for an obese patient who needs assessment of skin and self-care abilities. The patient also needs perineal care, partial bath, and the bed linen changed. What is the **best** strategy to meet the needs of the patient?
    1. Instruct the UAP to perform all tasks except the skin assessment.
    2. Ask the UAP to call when the patient's back is positioned for assessment.
    3. Assess skin and self-care abilities while working with the UAP to complete care.
    4. Assess skin and self-care abilities, then tell the patient to perform her own care.

13. Which patient is **most** likely to request that the room temperature be turned down?
    1. Has chronic obstructive pulmonary disease
    2. Has alternating chills and fever
    3. Has peripheral vascular disease
    4. Has end-stage pancreatic cancer

14. The nurse is caring for older adult residents in an assisted living facility. What is the **best** strategy to prevent skin breakdown among this vulnerable group?
    1. Make daily rounds and assess skin condition.
    2. Instruct UAP to help residents out of bed as much as possible.
    3. Plan a toileting schedule for the residents at greatest risk.
    4. Ask the dietary department to serve high-quality protein foods.

15. A family member tells the nurse that the staff is spending too much time laughing and chatting at the nurses' station and it is disturbing the patient's rest and comfort. What would the nurse do **first**?
    1. Instruct the staff to be more discreet and move conversation to the breakroom.
    2. Assess other environmental factors that are interfering with patient's comfort.
    3. Apologize to the family member and assure that the situation will be corrected.
    4. Assess the patient's discomfort and ask what other things are interfering with rest.

16. The nurse is supervising a nursing student who is giving a patient a bed bath. The nurse would intervene if the student performed which action?
    1. Lowers the side rail to perform care
    2. Raises the head of the bed to a semi-Fowler's position
    3. Bathes arms using long, firm strokes
    4. Puts up all four side rails after completing the bath

17. The care plan indicates that all caregivers should encourage the patient's independence in accomplishing activities of daily living (ADLs). What is the **best** indication that the nurses and UAP are successful with this part of the care plan?
    1. The UAP waits until the patient uses the call light for assistance.
    2. The nurse sees that the commode chair is close to the bed.
    3. The nurse observes that the patient is brushing his own teeth.
    4. The UAP tells the patient to independently complete ADLs.

18. An unconscious patient needs oral care. What instructions would the nurse give to the UAP to ensure the safety of the patient? **Select all that apply.**
    1. Put the patient in a side-lying position; use pillows for support as needed.
    2. Report bleeding, sores in the mouth, or obvious problems with teeth or gums.
    3. Check for gag reflex by gently inserting a tongue blade into the throat.
    4. Use a soft toothbrush to clean inner and outer surfaces of teeth; swab mouth and tongue
    5. Have an oral suction device ready and check function prior to starting.
    6. Perform hand hygiene before donning clean gloves.

19. A neighbor tells the nurse that he has muscle soreness and stiffness after performing a new exercise program. What would the nurse recommend?
    1. A tub bath with the proper temperature of 113° to 115° F (45° to 46° C).
    2. A bath with the water temperature at a tepid 98.6° F (37° C).
    3. A sitz bath that lasts 20-30 minutes for soaking and relaxing.
    4. A shower with a recommended water temperature of approximately 110° F (43° C).

20. A patient with dementia needs assistance with bathing. What strategies are **best** to help the patient accomplish this task? **Select all that apply.**
    1. Maintain a relaxed demeanor, smile frequently, and use a calm tone of voice.
    2. Demonstrate and explain the desired behavior, such as how to turn on the water.
    3. Reassure frequently and say things such as, "You are doing well. We are almost done."
    4. Try to repeat the same hygiene pattern every day and wash the same body parts.
    5. Use distraction rather than trying to negotiate or making demands.
    6. Attempt to have the same caregivers as often as possible for hygienic care.

21. What is a general principle to consider when using heat and cold therapy for patients?
    1. The patient should be assessed for ability to perceive temperature in the area of the application.
    2. The patient should adjust the temperature settings for comfort.
    3. The patient should move the application around for relief.
    4. Application is positioned for convenient observation.

22. A cold application is ordered for the patient. What is a positive effect of this treatment?
    1. Vasodilation
    2. Local anesthesia
    3. Reduced blood viscosity
    4. Increased metabolism

23. The nurse applies heat to a large area on the patient's trunk. The patient reports feeling slightly dizzy and his pulse is rapid. What is the **best** physiologic explanation for this systemic reaction?
    1. The heat application has triggered a fever.
    2. The trunk contains some large blood vessels.
    3. The application is causing vasodilation.
    4. Antibodies and leukocytes are activated.

24. What instructions would the nurse give to the UAP about applying a warm, moist compress to a small abscess in the patient's axilla? **Select all that apply.**
    1. Compress should be 105° to 110° F.
    2. Apply for 30-40 minutes.
    3. Report pain, exudate, or redness.
    4. Notify about completion of therapy.
    5. Evaluate the response to therapy.

25. The home health nurse is observing a family member assist the patient with a heating pad. The nurse would intervene if the family member performs which action?
    1. Assists the patient to lie on the heating pad
    2. Adjusts the pad to the lowest temperature setting
    3. Places a cloth between the skin and the heating device
    4. Checks electrical cord for fraying or kinks

26. The patient was diagnosed with a sprained ankle and the provider recommended a cold application for 20 minutes. Which condition would cause the nurse to question the order?
    1. The patient's ankle is already slightly swollen.
    2. The pain medication has not had time to work.
    3. The patient has a history of peripheral vascular disease.
    4. The patient tells the nurse that 20 minutes is too long.

27. With appropriate instructions and supervision, which tasks related to hygienic care could be delegated to experienced UAP? **Select all that apply.**
    1. A patient with diabetes wants to soak his feet in warm water.
    2. A patient with an indwelling urinary catheter needs assistance with pericare.
    3. A patient who is bed-bound would like to have his legs massaged after a bed bath.
    4. A patient on anticoagulant therapy is too unsteady to hold his disposable razor for shaving.
    5. A patient who is unconscious has secretions along the margins of the eyelids.
    6. A patient with peripheral vascular disease would like to have her toenails trimmed.

28. What is an expected change related to aging that necessitates more frequent oral hygiene for older adults?
    1. Older adults don't recognize that good dental health helps preserve their ability to eat.
    2. There is a decreased production of saliva and commonly an alteration in the sense of taste.
    3. Older adults tend to have more dental caries because teeth are less resistant to bacteria.
    4. There is a decreased ability to chew and digest raw fruits and vegetables that contribute to dental health.

29. A new resident has been admitted to a long-term care facility. What is the **most** important thing for the nurse to assess before delegating oral hygiene to the UAP?
    1. Does the resident have adequate supplies, such a soft-bristled toothbrush and nonalcohol-based mouthwash?
    2. Does the UAP understand how to assist the resident and maximize the resident's independent efforts?
    3. Does the resident actually want and need assistance or is self-care more appropriate?
    4. Does the resident have a gag reflex and is he able to spit out residue from toothpaste and mouthwash?

30. The nurse is assessing a patient who is immobile because of injuries sustained in a car accident. What areas does the nurse pay special attention to for the prevention and early detection of pressure injuries? **Select all that apply.**
    1. Sacrum
    2. Scapulae
    3. Trochanteric areas of the hips
    4. Heels
    5. Back of the head
    6. Sternum

31. A sitz bath has been ordered for a patient with a history of recent vaginal delivery with extensive perineal lacerations. How would the nurse explain this treatment to the patient?
    1. The water should be as warm as possible.
    2. The purpose of the sitz bath is to cleanse and reduce inflammation.
    3. If sitz bath equipment is not available, a shower can be substituted.
    4. The patient should remain in the sitz bath for 5-10 minutes.

32. Which of the following patients have an increased risk of a skin pressure injury? **Select all that apply.**
    1. A patient with obesity
    2. A patient who is underweight
    3. An incontinent patient
    4. A patient with a nasogastric tube in place
    5. A patient with a diagnosis of renal calculi
    6. A patient with a spinal cord injury

33. Which would be the **most** important factor to consider when planning personal hygiene for a patient from a cultural background that the nurse has not previously worked with?
    1. The country of origin of the patient
    2. The language the patient prefers to speak
    3. The patient's individual preferences
    4. The reports that came with the patient from a previous institution

34. Which instructions would the nurse provide to the UAP who will be bathing a patient with a hearing aid ? **Select all that apply.**
    1. Leave the hearing aid in place throughout the bathing process so the patient can hear instructions.
    2. Remove the hearing aid when washing the patient's hair.
    3. Clean the hearing aid with a soft dry cloth.
    4. Place the hearing aid on a sunny windowsill to air dry.
    5. Allow the patient to attempt to put the hearing aids back in after the bath.
    6. Notify the nurse if any drainage is noted in the ear.

35. The nurse is assessing a patient being admitted from another institution for the presence of pressure injuries. Which of the following statements is correct?
    1. A reddened area of the skin is considered a pressure injury.
    2. Pressure injuries are apparent upon inspection of the skin.
    3. Documentation should include measurements and description of any injuries.
    4. The patient should be assessed in prone position as most pressure injuries are on the back.

CRITICAL THINKING ACTIVITIES

36. For the following patients, identify how bathing may be affected or altered.

    a.   The patient is extremely fatigued. _____

    _____

    b.   The patient is on complete bedrest. _____

    _____

    c.   The patient has right-sided paralysis following a stroke. _____

    _____

    d.   The patient has inflammation of the perianal tissue. _____

    _____

    e.   The patient is an East Indian Hindu. _____

    _____

    f.   The patient is an older adult who is incontinent. _____

    _____

37. A 30-year-old female patient has quadriplegia secondary to a diving accident that occurred 5 years ago. She was very healthy and athletic prior to the accident, but within the last several months, she has been hospitalized several times for recurrent urinary tract infections and significant weight loss. She currently has a poor appetite.

    a.   Identify possible risk factors that will contribute to development of pressure injuries for this patient.

    _____

    _____

    b.   The nurse observes a stage I pressure injury on the patient's sacral area. Describe the criteria for a stage I pressure injury.

    _____

    _____

    _____

    c.   The nurse observes suspected deep tissue injury on the patient's right heel. Describe the criteria for suspected deep tissue injury.

    _____

    _____

    d.   How can the nurse prevent the development of pressure injuries? _____

    _____

    _____

e. Identify general guidelines for care of pressure injuries. _____

_____

_____

_____

_____

NEXT-GENERATION NCLEX™ (NGN)

38. Cloze

Cognitive Skill: Analyze Cues

Scenario: The nurse has received report on a patient admission for possible sepsis resulting from a urinary tract infection. The patient is a 75-year-old male with very limited mobility. His medical history is significant for diabetes, hypertension, stroke, and asthma. His BMI is 20. He has an indwelling bladder catheter in place due to recent urinary retention. He also has a stage 2 pressure injury on his sacral area.

Instructions: Choose the most likely option to complete the statements below.

The factors in the patient's history that put him most at risk for pressure injury are ___1___. The characteristics of the stage 2 pressure injury that the nurse would note on assessment would include ___2___. In addition to the ointment ordered by the health care provider, the nurse would provide the following interventions for the care of the pressure injury: ___3___.

Options for 1	Options for 2	Options for 3
immobility, age 75, and asthma	undermining or tunneling	turn and reposition patient every 3 hours
age 75, BMI 20, and diabetes	shallow, shiny pink wound bed	instruct patient to reposition himself every 15 minutes
immobility, possible sepsis, and age 75	skin intact with nonblanchable redness	place patient in full lateral position
urinary retention, immobility, hypertension	subcutaneous fat is visible	assure adequate nutrition and fluid intake

Safety

Answer Key: A complete Answer Key is provided in your Additional Learning Resources on Evolve.

ABBREVIATIONS

Directions: For each abbreviation, write out the full term or phrase.

1. RACE: _____

2. CDC: _____

3. OSHA:_____

4. PASS: _____

5. SRD: _____

MULTIPLE CHOICE

Directions: Select the best answer(s) for each of the following questions.

6. The older adult tells the nurse that he is having trouble reading the labels on his medication bottles. What is the **best** strategy that the nurse could suggest to reduce the risk of an accidental medication error?
   1. Recommend that a younger family member assist in handling the pills.
   2. Teach the patient to use a medication organizer to manage the medication.
   3. Tell the patient to have the pharmacist read the label information to him.
   4. Assist the patient to memorize the shape and color of each pill.

7. In which clinic setting is the nurse **most** likely to need knowledge of how to apply safety reminder devices (SRDs) and manage the care of these patients?
   1. Pediatric walk-in clinic
   2. Outpatient surgery clinic
   3. Mental health walk-in clinic
   4. Adult ambulatory care clinic

8. A confused patient is yelling at the unlicensed assistive personnel (UAP). As the nurse enters the room, the patient throws the food tray at the UAP. What would the nurse do **first?**
   1. Ask the UAP to explain what is happening with the patient.
   2. Instruct the UAP to move toward the door and then slowly shut it.
   3. Slowly walk toward the patient and use a gentle touch to soothe him.
   4. Calmly talk to the patient and respectfully address him by name.

9. The nurse is teaching a new group of UAP how to evacuate residents from a long-term care facility in case of a fire or other emergency. Which item would be needed for the universal carry method?
   1. A blanket
   2. A wheelchair
   3. A stretcher
   4. A mechanical lift

10. The older adult residents in a nursing home must be evacuated because the facility is at risk for flooding and damage due to a hurricane that will pass through the area in several days. The nurse is assigned to keep a log to document the events. Which information is **most** important to record? **Select all that apply.**
    1. How each resident was transported
    2. Names of residents
    3. Where the residents were sent
    4. What personal belongings were sent
    5. Who transported each resident
    6. Notification of family members and health care providers (HCPs)

11. In the event of a mercury spill, what is the **priority** nursing action?
    1. Evacuate everyone from the room.
    2. Close the interior doors and open windows.
    3. Vacuum the mercury and the glass shards.
    4. Mop the floor with hot water and soap.

12. The nurse is caring for a patient who relies on mechanical ventilation. The nurse hears a fire alarm and flames are visible in a back corridor. What would the nurse do **first**?
    1. Seek assistance to move the patient and the ventilator to safety.
    2. Turn off the oxygen supply and provide manual respiratory support.
    3. Close the patient's door, call 911, and fight the fire in the corridor.
    4. Delegate the UAP to move ambulatory patients toward the exit.

13. The nurse is planning to teach a community group about fire safety in the home. Which information would be included in the presentation? **Select all that apply.**
    1. No smoking by the patient, family, or visitors in areas where oxygen is used.
    2. Use safety matches to light candles or fireplaces.
    3. Install fire alarms, smoke detectors, and carbon monoxide detectors.
    4. Practice fire escape routes from each room and practice exit drills.
    5. Use one electrical circuit to facilitate monitoring of cords and appliances.
    6. Cover electrical cords with a secure carpet to prevent falls.

14. An older adult patient in a long-term care facility has been wandering around outside of the room during the late evening hours. The patient has a history of falls. How would the nurse intervene?
    1. Obtain an order for a bed and chair alarm.
    2. Keep the light on and play the television all night.
    3. Put up the side rails and frequently check on the patient.
    4. Have the family come to check on the patient at night.

15. The nurse applies a gait belt to a male patient of average build who has some weakness on the left side. How does the nurse position herself before assisting the patient to ambulate?
    1. On the patient's left side and holding the weak left arm.
    2. On the patient's right side and holding the front of the gait belt.
    3. On the patient's left side and holding the back of the gait belt.
    4. On the patient's right side and holding one arm around his waist.

16. The nurse is considering the use of an SRD to prevent a patient from self-injury. When using an SRD, what would the nurse do? **Select all that apply.**
    1. Obtain an order from the HCP for the SRD.
    2. Explain the purpose of the SRD to the patient.
    3. Explain the purpose of the SRD to the family.
    4. Obtain consensus of nursing staff for type of SRD.
    5. Exhaust all alternatives before using an SRD.

17. The nurse notices smoke coming from the wastebasket in a patient's room. Upon entering the room, the nurse sees a fire that is starting to flare up. What would the nurse do **first**?
    1. Extinguish the fire.
    2. Remove the patient from the room.
    3. Close the door to the room.
    4. Turn off all electrical equipment.

18. Which occurrence is **most** likely to be investigated as a "sentinel event"?
    1. Patient leaves the hospital against medical advice because she gets angry with the nurse.
    2. An older patient sustains a broken arm related to the use of an SRD.
    3. A nurse is 2 hours late administering routine scheduled medications.
    4. During a follow-up phone call, a patient reports that care in the hospital was poor.

19. The nurse is conducting a fall risk assessment on an older adult patient who is moving into an assisted living center. Which questions would the nurse ask? **Select all that apply.**
    1. "Have you had any falls in the past year?"
    2. "Are you able to independently get up after a fall?"
    3. "Do you feel unsteady when you stand up?"
    4. "Are you able to independently walk from room to room?"
    5. "What medications are you taking?"
    6. "Do you use a cane or other assistive device?"

20. The nurse is giving instructions to the UAP about patient safety and fall prevention. What would the nurse tell the UAP about helping the older adult patient to go to the bathroom?
    1. "Help the patient whenever she needs help."
    2. "Ask her if she wants to walk or use the bedpan."
    3. "Have her put on her glasses before getting up."
    4. "Help her to the commode chair if she seems weak."

21. For the care of a patient who has an SRD in place, which task can be delegated to a UAP?
    1. Observe for circulation distal to the SRD.
    2. Check for respiratory effort and breathing.
    3. Change position every 2 hours.
    4. Determine when the SRD can be removed.

22. Which instructions would be given to the UAP who is assigned to assist in the care of a patient who is being treated with internal radiation?
    1. "Do not go into the room unless the patient uses the call bell."
    2. "Help children to don a lead shield apron before entering the room."
    3. "Wear a mask, eye shield, and isolation gown when entering the room."
    4. "Wear your personal dosimeter during care or when handling patient items."

23. A patient begins to have a grand mal seizure. What is the **priority** action?
    1. Monitor the patency of the airway.
    2. Protect against falls and other injuries.
    3. Suction the mouth to prevent aspiration.
    4. Gently insert an oral airway between the teeth.

24. The nurse is talking to a young mother who has an infant who has just started to crawl. Based on knowledge of growth and development, which safety issue is currently the **most** important to discuss with the mother?
    1. What to do when using pots and pans on the stove
    2. How to ensure backyard pool safety measures
    3. How to manage electrical sockets and cords
    4. Where to obtain safety labels for cleaning products

25. Which newly obtained piece of equipment creates the **greatest** risk for falls for an older adult?
    1. Gait belt
    2. Prescription lenses
    3. Safety bar in shower
    4. Walker

26. The postoperative patient demonstrates some mild dizziness and mild shortness of breath when moving from sitting to standing position. Which action would the nurse perform **first**?
    1. Assist the patient to get into bed.
    2. Assist the patient to sit back down.
    3. Check vital signs and assess symptoms.
    4. Call the provider for an order for oxygen.

27. The patient reports dizziness when standing up too fast. Which over-the-counter medication is **most** likely to be contributing to the patient's orthostatic hypotension?
    1. Nonaspirin pain reliever
    2. Antihistamine
    3. Vitamin supplement
    4. Medicated cough drop

28. An infant has a wound with a dressing on the left upper arm. He repeatedly attempts to remove the dressing. Which SRD would the nurse select?
    1. Mummy wrap
    2. Wrap jacket
    3. Bilateral wrist SRDs
    4. Right elbow SRD

29. A mother brings her alert and playful child to the clinic because she "found him playing with this empty bottle of baby aspirin." Which question is the **most** important to ask the mother?
    1. "Has he ever done anything like this before?"
    2. "How many times has he vomited since the ingestion?"
    3. "How many pills do you think were in the container?"
    4. "Did you contact poison control before you drove to the clinic?"

30. A patient with a latex allergy is exposed to latex. Which sign or symptom is cause for the **greatest** concern?
    1. Hives
    2. Laryngeal edema
    3. Runny eyes and nose
    4. Localized swelling

31. Before the nurse can intervene, the UAP pushes contaminated material into an over-filled sharps container and sustains a puncture wound. What would the nurse do **first**?
    1. Tell the UAP to immediately report to the infection-control nurse.
    2. Assist the UAP to scrub the wound with copious amounts of soap and water.
    3. Report the UAP for improper handling of hazardous material.
    4. Dispose of the sharps container to prevent any additional injuries to others.

32. The nurse started a new job in a small long-term care facility in a rural area. The back exit hallway is being used as a storage area while a new storage area is being planned. What would the nurse do **first**?
    1. Report the facility for unsafe conditions.
    2. Express unwillingness to work in unsafe conditions.
    3. Review the facility's policies/procedures for emergencies.
    4. Check the building for other safety issues.

33. The nurse is sitting at the front desk at a walk-in clinic. A patient comes in and reports fever, malaise, and muscle aches with a rash on the tongue, mouth, and throat. The nurse notes pustules on the patient's palms. What would the nurse do **first**?
    1. Notify the public health department.
    2. Isolate the patient.
    3. Put on personal protective equipment (PPE).
    4. Call the HCP to triage the patient.

34. It is suspected that a patient has been exposed to cyanide gas. The nurse is alert for which symptom?
    1. Erratic behavior
    2. Nausea and vomiting
    3. Respiratory distress
    4. Vesicle formation

35. The nurse is reviewing the disaster preparedness plan for a small nursing home. What would be included in the plan? **Select all that apply.**
    1. Emergency treatment for the most critically injured
    2. Possible admission to a hospital or transfer to a temporary shelter
    3. Log to document residents' names and locations
    4. System to notify families and providers
    5. Designation of an area for decontamination
    6. Method of patient identification, such as a bracelet or picture ID

36. The nurse is working in a local health department and has noted an unusually large number of phone calls about food-borne illness. Which question is the nurse **most** likely to ask callers to differentiate the possible involvement of the bioterrorist agent that causes botulism from other more common causes of food-borne illness?
    1. In addition to gastrointestinal symptoms, have you had drooping eyelids or difficulty swallowing or speaking?
    2. Have you experienced a low-grade fever, sweating, fatigue, and a nonproductive cough?
    3. How soon after eating did the abdominal cramping, vomiting, and diarrhea start?
    4. Have you had fever, malaise, and muscle aches with a rash on the tongue, mouth, throat, and palms?

37. The nurse is preparing to give an intramuscular injection to a patient. What factors would increase the risk of needlestick injury to the nurse? **Select all that apply.**
    1. Using a needleless device
    2. Disposing the needle device in the needle disposal container
    3. Applying a Band-Aid to the injection site immediately after administering injection
    4. Using a new type of safety device injection system
    5. Recapping the needle after the injection
    6. Cleansing the skin with an alcohol swab after uncapping the needle

38. The patient with mild cognitive impairment is being discharged from the hospital with several new medications. Which action by the nurse would be **most** effective in reducing the risk of accidental poisoning by medication misuse?
    1. Teach the patient the names, doses, potential side effects, and indication for use for each medication.
    2. Request that the patient have their adult son come to safely set up the medications each day.
    3. Teach the patient how to use a medication box and reminders.
    4. Teach the patient how to organize the medications on the day of discharge.

39. The hospitalized patient is confused and has a history of falls. Which actions would the nurse take to help avoid the use of SRDs? **Select all that apply.**
    1. Review the patient's medication list.
    2. Assign the patient to a quiet room far from the nurses' station.
    3. Use a sitter if needed if family members are not available.
    4. Use a bed alarm.
    5. Restrict visitors because the patient becomes upset when they leave.
    6. Use relaxation techniques such as massage or music to create a calm atmosphere for the patient.

CRITICAL THINKING ACTIVITIES

40. The nurse is caring for a patient in a long-term care facility. The patient has a history of falls in the home.

   a. To prevent falls, identify a patient outcome and three nursing interventions. _____

   _____

   _____

   _____

   _____

   b. Describe how the nurse can promote safe ambulation for the patient in a health care facility.

   _____

   _____

   _____

   _____

   c. Identify three additional factors that influence the safety of the older adult in the home or health care environment.

   _____

   _____

   _____

41. The nurse is working in a small urban outpatient clinic. The nurse manager has just informed the staff that the disaster plan may have to be activated because the emergency department of a nearby hospital has identified a possible bioterrorism-related event.

   a. What is the role of the nurse in a disaster event? _____

   _____

   _____

   b. What indications would alert the nurse to a possible bioterrorism-related event? _____

   _____

   _____

42. List your personal fears or concerns about safety for family, friends, and self that might occur during a bioterrorism event. Discuss these fears and concerns with a classmate or your instructor.

   _____

   _____

   _____

   _____

   _____

NEXT-GENERATION NCLEX™ (NGN)

43. Extended Drag and Drop

Cognitive Skill: Generate Solutions

Scenario: The student nurse is preparing for his first clinical educational experiences on a medical-surgical floor. He is 25 years old and healthy. He lives with his wife who is diabetic, his child who has survived leukemia, and his mother-in-law who has an autoimmune disease. He is very concerned about keeping his family safe from infectious diseases while he does his clinical education.

Instructions: Use an X to indicate which items would be recommended for the student nurse.

Items	Recommended for Student Nurse
Hepatitis B vaccine	
Standard Precautions with all patients	
Flu vaccine	
Sterile glove use for any potential contact with body fluids	
Human papillomavirus (HPV) vaccine	
Recap needles immediately after administration of injection	
COVID-19 vaccine	
Pneumococcal vaccine	
Rotavirus vaccine	
Tetanus, diphtheria, pertussis (TDAP) vaccine	

Admission, Transfer, and Discharge

Answer Key: A complete Answer Key is provided in your Additional Learning Resources on Evolve.

IDENTIFYING PATIENTS' REACTIONS TO ADMISSION TO A HEALTH CARE FACILITY

1. *Directions:* In the blanks provided, identify and record the patient's reaction to admission to a health care facility; then on the figure below (use a, b, c, or d), indicate where each patient would be on Maslow's Hierarchy. The first item is completed for you as an example.

   a. Patient appears anxious as he enters the exam room for the first time. He nervously begins to ask the nurse a series of questions about what will happen to him. Reaction: Fear of the unknown

   b. A preschooler who is admitted to the hospital is happily engaged in playing with the toys that the nurse has provided, but when her parents prepare to leave, she begins to cry and clings to them. Reaction: _____

   c. An older adult woman who has just moved into an assisted living facility seems to need a lot of social interaction. She becomes very talkative when the nurse tries to leave the room. Reaction: _____

   d. An adolescent is admitted to the hospital, but refuses to take off his clothes and put on a hospital gown. Reaction: _____

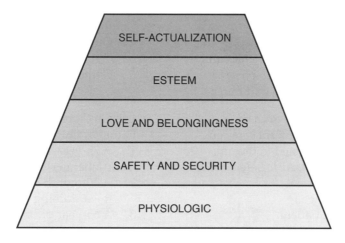

MULTIPLE CHOICE

Directions: Select the best answer(s) for each of the following questions.

2. The nurse is admitting a new patient to the diagnostic and surgical center. What would the nurse do **first**?
   1. Assess immediate needs.
   2. Take vital signs.
   3. Check identification band.
   4. Orient patient to the facility routines.

3. An experienced LPN/LVN is working on a medical-surgical unit. The LPN/LVN sees that a new RN has not completed the admission assessment on a patient who arrived 20 hours ago. What would the LPN/LVN do **first**?
   1. Wait to see if the new RN completes the admission assessment.
   2. Mention the incomplete admission assessment to the nurse manager.
   3. Remind the RN that the Joint Commission requires admission assessment within 24 hours.
   4. Offer to collect data so that the new nurse can complete the admission assessment.

4. An older adult patient is postoperative for hip surgery. He is transferred by ambulance from the hospital to a rehabilitation (rehab) unit. One hour after he is assisted into bed at the rehab unit, he dies in his sleep. Which documentation provides the **best** legal protection for the transferring nursing staff?
   1. The provider's discharge summary and order to transfer the patient to the rehab unit
   2. The discharge assessment that was performed just before the patient left the hospital
   3. The assessment that was performed by the ambulance team in route to the rehab unit
   4. The partially completed admission assessment performed by the rehab unit nurse

5. The patient is being transferred from the medical-surgical unit to a long-term care center. Which tasks can be delegated to the unlicensed assistive personnel (UAP)? **Select all that apply.**
   1. Change soiled dressings.
   2. Bathe an incontinent patient.
   3. Assist to collect personal items.
   4. Take a final set of vital signs.
   5. Review transfer details with family.

6. A rational patient wishes to leave the hospital against medical advice (AMA), despite the nurse's best attempt at therapeutic communication. What is the nurse's **first** responsibility?
   1. Notify the health care provider (HCP).
   2. Document the incident.
   3. Detain the patient.
   4. Obtain an AMA form.

7. The patient has an old head injury and demonstrates occasional intermittent episodes of belligerence and confusion interspersed with appropriate behavior. He is currently angry and wants to leave AMA. The nurse is unable to reach the HCP. What would the nurse do **first**?
   1. Explain the AMA form and consequences to the patient.
   2. Call the supervising RN, because the patient now has acute needs.
   3. Notify the family and ask them to take responsibility.
   4. Contact the risk manager and ask for permission to detain.

8. During the admission of a patient to a health care facility, what are the responsibilities of the admission department representative? **Select all that apply.**
   1. Obtaining identifying information
   2. Giving information on the Health Insurance Portability and Accountability Act
   3. Placing the correct identification band on the patient's wrist
   4. Obtaining a list of current medications
   5. Obtaining emergency contact information
   6. Gathering insurance information

9. Which newly admitted patient is **most** likely to need and benefit from an individualized explanation of the bathroom facilities?
   1. A 75-year-old woman with advanced Alzheimer's disease
   2. A 20-month-old child who has just started toilet training
   3. A 65-year-old man who recently emigrated from a remote rural area in a poor country
   4. A 50-year-old woman who has stress incontinence

10. The nurse is placing an identification band on a patient who was admitted through the emergency department. What is **best** to say as the band is applied?
    1. "This is your assigned hospital identification number."
    2. "The primary purpose of the band is to maintain safety."
    3. "All patients have to wear these; it's standard procedure."
    4. "We don't want to lose you while you are in the hospital."

11. The patient is newly admitted and seems anxious, but also appears very hesitant to ask questions. Which statement by the nurse **best** demonstrates empathy?
    1. "Call me if you need anything; I'll be happy to help you."
    2. "There's nothing to worry about; we'll take good care of you."
    3. "I know you must have a lot of questions; I know I would."
    4. "You seem a little uncertain; do you have some questions?"

12. The nurse is trying to explain the bed controls and the call button and other items related to hospitalization, but the older adult patient keeps telling the nurse to "wait for my son to get here." What would the nurse do **first**?
    1. Go find the son or other available family members.
    2. Leave written information at the bedside.
    3. Give brief information using very simple language.
    4. Offer comfort measures and ensure patient safety.

13. Which tasks related to admitting a new patient can be delegated to the UAP? **Select all that apply.**
    1. Obtain personal care items, such as water pitcher or packaged cleansing cloths.
    2. Position the bed for transfer from stretcher or wheelchair.
    3. Hang signs above the bed related to care, such as "nothing by mouth."
    4. Ask the patient if he/she needs special equipment, such as a walker.
    5. Store belongings, such as jewelry, watch, or wallet, in bedside table.
    6. Assist the patient to arrange desired items, such as eyeglasses, within reach.

14. The patient tells the nurse that he would like to be transferred to hospital X, because his cardiologist doesn't come to hospital Y. What would the nurse do?
    1. Obtain an AMA form and have the patient sign it.
    2. Call hospital X and advise that the patient desires transfer.
    3. Advise the patient that the cardiologists in hospital Y are good.
    4. Advise the patient that a transfer requires an order from the HCP.

15. A patient with Alzheimer's disease is being transferred from a long-term care facility to an acute care hospital for possible sepsis and change in mental status. Which question is the **most** important to ask the nurse who is giving the report?
    1. "Has the family been advised about the reason for the transfer?"
    2. "What is the patient's baseline mental status and behavior?"
    3. "When is the patient scheduled to be transferred?"
    4. "Will the patient be accompanied by a nurse or family member?"

16. Which patient is likely to have the **most** complex discharge plan?
    1. A 73-year-old man with chronic disease who has no family in the area
    2. A 23-year-old mother who just delivered her first healthy baby
    3. A 17-year-old adolescent who broke his leg during a ski trip
    4. A 35-year-old woman who had an emergency appendectomy

17. The nurse is giving instructions to a family caregiver of an older patient who will need help after discharge from the hospital. The nurse senses tension, resentment, and unwillingness from the caregiver. What would the nurse do **first**?
    1. Continue to give the instructions and ask for feedback from the caregiver.
    2. Notify the provider for an order for home health nursing.
    3. Get a social service consult to resolve family tensions and problems.
    4. Assess the caregiver's attitude toward the patient and the circumstances.

18. The nurse is admitting a patient with limited English language ability who smiles and nods in response to the nurse's questions. What would be the **best** action by the nurse?
    1. Ask the patient's teen daughter who is present to translate.
    2. Call the patient's English-speaking husband and ask him to check that his wife has understood everything.
    3. Ask the UAP on the floor who speaks the patient's language to translate.
    4. Utilize the video translation service provided by the hospital.

19. A frail older woman has been admitted to the hospital during a time of pandemic with a no visitor policy in place. The patient's daughter asks to accompany her mother just to " help her get settled and decrease her fear." How would the nurse respond to this request?
    1. "You can come in just for a few moments, to help her; but then, I am sorry, you must leave."
    2. "I'm sorry, but due to the pandemic, you cannot come in, but I will set up a video visit with your mother in just a few minutes so you can help her with the admission process."
    3. "There is a pandemic going on, and I am sorry, but you cannot enter the hospital. I will call you later with information about how your mother is doing."
    4. "I will ask your mother if she feels the need to have you with her during her admission."

20. There are orders to transfer a patient from the hospital to a long-term care facility. The nurse comes into the room to prepare the patient for transfer and finds the patient crying and stating she wants to go home. What would the nurse do **first**?
    1. Talk to the patient and listen to her concerns about the transfer.
    2. Inform the HCP that the patient does not want to be transferred.
    3. Ask the hospital social worker to speak again with the patient about the transfer.
    4. Call the family of the patient and inform them of the patient's wishes.

CRITICAL THINKING ACTIVITIES

21. The patient is admitted through the emergency department for an exacerbation of a chronic respiratory disorder. When the patient arrives at his room on the medical-surgical unit, he appears very tired. He has oxygen per nasal cannula and demonstrates labored breathing. He is able to speak, but his sentences are short and he takes a breath after every few words. How would the nurse modify the nursing actions related to the admission to meet the needs of this particular patient?

    a. Checking and verifying the identification band: _____

    _____

    b. Assessing immediate needs: _____

    _____

    c. Explaining hospital routines, such as visiting hours, mealtime, and morning wake-up: _____

    _____

    d. Orienting the patient to the room:_____

_____

_____

22. A 45-year-old woman was admitted to the hospital for chronic infection of a stasis ulcer on her leg. She will be discharged after completing antibiotic therapy and consultation with the wound care specialist.

    a. Identify examples of health care disciplines other than nursing that are involved in referrals and explain their role in the discharge process.

_____

_____

_____

_____

    b. Discuss the importance of discharge instructions for patients who have chronic conditions.

_____

_____

_____

NEXT-GENERATION NCLEX™ (NGN)

23. Drag and Drop

Cognitive Skill: Recognize Cues

Scenario: The hospital nurse is calling report to the receiving nurse at the rehabilitation facility where the patient will be transferred. The nurse is using the ISBARR format to give report.

Instructions: Place the information for the ISBARR report in the correct order. In the right-hand column, write the number (1-7) to indicate the correct order.

Information to Include in ISBARR Report	Order of Information
Please repeat back the vitals that I read to you.	
His temperature is 99.2° F.	
I am the nurse from X hospital calling to give report on patient Y.	
He will be transferring to the rehabilitation facility today.	
The patient fell at home 4 days ago, sustained a right hip fracture, and underwent hip replacement surgery 3 days ago.	
His goal is to continue physical therapy as soon as possible as he is highly motivated to recover and return to independent living.	

Vital Signs

Answer Key: A complete Answer Key is provided in your Additional Learning Resources on Evolve.

MATCHING

Directions: Match the term to the correct definition or characteristic listed below.

Term	Definition or Characteristic
_____ 1. bradycardia	a. Irregularity in the normal rhythm of the heart
_____ 2. dyspnea	b. Normal finding for well-conditioned athlete
_____ 3. hyperthermia	c. Represents the ventricles contracting, forcing blood into the aorta and the pulmonary arteries
_____ 4. bradypnea	d. Expected respiratory pattern while exercising
_____ 5. systolic	e. Laboring with difficulty to get enough oxygen
_____ 6. tachypnea	f. Slow respiratory rate, fewer than 10 per minute
_____ 7. dysrythmia	g. Above-normal body temperature
_____ 8. hypothermia	h. Expected heart rate if very frightened or angry
_____ 9. tachycardia	i. The silent killer
_____ 10. hypertension	j. Oral temperature of 93.2° F (34° C)

FIGURE LABELING

11. *Directions:* Label the figure below with the names and sites for assessment of peripheral pulses.

Posterior view

FIGURE LABELING

12. *Directions:* Identify on the aneroid gauge where the Korotkoff's sounds are heard for a blood pressure of 136/78 mm Hg.

TABLE ACTIVITY

13. *Directions:* Complete the table below with the expected vital signs for different age groups.

Age Group	Heart Rate (per Minute)	Respiratory Rate (per Minute)	Blood Pressure (mm Hg)
Neonate			Systolic:
Infant			Systolic:
Toddler			Systolic:
School-age (6-10 years)			Systolic: Diastolic:
Adolescent (10-18 years)			Systolic: Diastolic:
Adult			Systolic: Diastolic:
Older adult			Systolic: Diastolic:

MULTIPLE CHOICE

Directions: Select the best answer(s) for each of the following questions.

14. The nurse is taking blood pressures (BPs) at a community health fair and screening people for risk factors for hypertension. Which person has the **most** risk factors for developing hypertension?
    1. 23-year-old athletic Asian American woman with a BP of 120/80 mm Hg and a family history of hypertension
    2. 32-year-old African American mother of two children with a BP of 134/70 mm Hg who exercises regularly
    3. 66-year-old thin Jewish American male with a BP of 124/80 mm Hg; he regularly drinks alcohol and has a sedentary lifestyle
    4. 45-year-old African American man with a BP of 130/80 mm Hg who smokes, is overweight, and eats a vegetarian diet

15. The unlicensed assistive personnel (UAP) just reported patients' vital signs to the nurse. For which patient is an increased pulse an expected finding?
    1. Patient received antihypertensive medications 4 hours ago.
    2. Patient needs scheduled routine medication for hypothyroidism.
    3. Patient who has a fever had a dose of antipyretic medication 6 hours ago.
    4. Patient's medications are being managed by the cardiac rehabilitation team.

16. The nurse needs to get an apical pulse on an older woman who has large, pendulous breasts. What would the nurse do **first**?
    1. Lift the left breast and place the bell or diaphragm at the fifth intercostal space.
    2. Lift the breast and place palm of hand over the point of maximal impulse.
    3. Use the bell of the stethoscope to make a tight seal against the lateral chest wall.
    4. Obtain the ultrasonic Doppler and position it where breast tissue is most flattened.

17. The nurse observes that the patient has an elevated temperature. What questions would the nurse ask to collect data about a systemic infection? **Select all that apply.**
    1. "Do you feel thirsty?"
    2. "Do you have a headache?"
    3. "Are you having trouble resting or getting comfortable?"
    4. "Would you like some medication to reduce your fever?"
    5. "Have you experienced any chills?"

18. The UAP reports to the nurse that the "pulse oximeter might be broken" because some of the patients had low readings. What would the nurse do **first**?
    1. Instruct the UAP to go back and retake the readings on any patient who had a low value.
    2. Ask the UAP if the patients who had a low reading were having any problems breathing.
    3. Examine and troubleshoot the pulse oximeter and test it on several healthy staff members.
    4. Assess the patients who had low readings and determine if extraneous factors are present.

19. The nurse hears in report that the patient has peripheral arterial disease that affects his lower extremities. What would the nurse expect to find during assessment?
    1. Popliteal pulses are full and bounding and there is some mild edema in the posterior calf.
    2. Dorsalis pedis and posterior tibial pulses are weak, and toes are cooler than upper leg.
    3. Patient reports severe pain with loss of sensation and decreased strength and movement in legs.
    4. Brachial and radial pulses are weak compared to dorsalis pedis and posterior tibial pulses.

20. The nurse notes that a patient occasionally sighs during the morning assessment. What is the clinical significance of occasional sighing?
    1. The patient had trouble breathing during the night and sighing is related to lower blood oxygen levels.
    2. This is a behavior that many people demonstrate when they are bored or frustrated.
    3. The patient has a chronic lung disease and deep breathing is characteristic of the disorder.
    4. Occasional sighing is considered normal and allows all alveoli to be aerated.

21. An experienced UAP reports that the patient is alert and asking for breakfast. Vital signs have been completed and recorded as follows: axillary temperature of 100.6° F, pulse of 80 beats/min, respirations 16/min, and BP 120/70 mm Hg. What is the nurse's **first** action?
    1. Instruct the UAP to obtain a breakfast tray for the patient.
    2. Ask the UAP to repeat the temperature using the oral or tympanic method.
    3. Direct the UAP to repeat all of the vital signs and observe technique.
    4. Ask the UAP to explain the choice of axillary method to measure the temperature.

22. A new nurse has taken a job on a medical-surgical unit. According to the shift report, the four assigned patients are stable and should have a predictable clinical stay. Based on the report, how often does the nurse plan to take the vital signs?
    1. Every hour until the nurse verifies for self that the patients are stable.
    2. Before and after administering any oral or intravenous medications.
    3. According to facility policy for frequency unless status changes.
    4. At the beginning and end of the shift, unless the health care provider (HCP) orders otherwise.

23. The nursing student takes a BP on a patient who has been in a coma for several months. The student reports to the nurse that the BP seems too low. What would the nurse do **first**?
    1. Direct the student to retake the BP on the opposite extremity.
    2. Go with the student and assess the patient for other signs/symptoms.
    3. Instruct the student to check the chart to see what is baseline for the patient.
    4. Remind the student that a prolonged coma will cause changes in vital signs.

24. A patient who is brought to the emergency department was discovered lying in an alley. He is cold and wet and demonstrates slurred speech. His temperature is 94° F. How does his condition affect his pulse rate?
    1. Tachycardia is likely due to the stress of cold exposure.
    2. Since he is conscious, there should be no effects on pulse.
    3. A decreased heart rate reflects lowered metabolism.
    4. Palpating pulses will be impossible because of vasoconstriction.

25. The UAP takes vital signs at 3:00 AM and reports to the nurse that the patient's temperature is 97.6° F (36.4° C). The nurse sees that the patient's temperature at 6:00 PM was 99.6° F (37.5° C) and at 11:00 PM was 98.2° F (36.8° C). What would the nurse do?
    1. Thank the UAP and explain that lower temperatures occur between 1 AM and 4 AM.
    2. Repeat the temperature, but use a different method than what the UAP used.
    3. Tell the UAP to document the temperature and not to worry about it.
    4. Ask the UAP to get the patient a warm blanket and increase the room temperature.

26. Two nurses simultaneously assess to determine if a patient has a pulse deficit. One nurse counts the apical pulse at 105 beats/min. The other nurse takes the radial pulse and counts 96 beats/min. What is the pulse deficit?

27. When assessing the apical pulse, how does the nurse count the pulse rate?
    1. Counts for 20 seconds and multiplies by 3
    2. Counts for 60 seconds and does not multiply
    3. Counts for 30 seconds and multiplies by 2
    4. Counts for 15 seconds and multiplies by 4

28. The nurse is supervising a first-year nursing student who is checking the patient's peripheral pulses. The nurse would intervene if the student performed which action?
    1. Palpated all of the pulses, including carotids and femorals bilaterally
    2. Positioned the patient in the prone position to assess the popliteal artery
    3. Palpated the point of maximal impulse and assessed the apical pulse for 60 seconds
    4. Palpated the radial pulse with the pads of the index and third fingers

29. Which factor/condition is **most** likely to increase the patient's respiratory rate?
    1. Opioid medication
    2. Acute pain
    3. Hypothermia
    4. Brainstem injury

30. The nurse counts respirations immediately following measurement of the radial pulse while the fingers are still in place over the artery. What is the **best** rationale for this technique?
    1. Rapport has been established so the patient is likely to be less anxious.
    2. Therapeutic touch of the nurse's fingers on the patient's wrist is soothing.
    3. Patients may voluntarily alter respiratory rate if they know they are being monitored.
    4. Counting respirations immediately after pulse check is an efficient timesaver.

31. A nursing student is preparing to take the BP on a patient who has excessive adipose tissue on the upper arm. If the student uses a normal-sized cuff, what is likely to occur?
    1. The BP will be falsely elevated.
    2. The patient will be uncomfortable during the procedure.
    3. The systolic pressure will be artificially lower.
    4. The BP is likely to be very close to baseline.

32. The nurse receives the end-of-shift report from the off-going nurse. Based on the vital sign information for the assigned adult patients, which patient would the nurse check on **first**?
    1. BP 120/80, P 68, R 16
    2. BP 110/74, P 72, R 14
    3. BP 130/90, P 80, R 18
    4. BP 120/90, P 62, R 9

33. The nurse sees in the patient's documentation that the patient has a radial pulse of 4+. What assessment would the nurse plan to make for this patient?
    1. Doppler assessment of pulses for hands and feet
    2. Observe for pallor or cyanosis in the hands
    3. Assess BP for hypertension
    4. Assess apical and radial pulse for a pulse deficit

34. The patient's pulse oximetry reading appears to be lower than expected. The patient is breathing easily, the lungs are clear, the oxygen is delivered as ordered, and the patient reports, "feeling fine." What would the nurse do **first**?
    1. Check the position of the pulse oximeter.
    2. Feel the patient's fingers for coolness or warmth.
    3. Apply the pulse oximeter to own finger to test function.
    4. Ask the patient if he has any circulation problems.

35. The nurse needs to take the temperature of a baby who was brought to the clinic for his 6-month well-baby visit. Which method of measuring the temperature is the **best** choice for this patient?
    1. Oral
    2. Axillary
    3. Rectal
    4. Temporal arterial

36. The nurse received a new stethoscope as a graduation present. What will he/she do to care for and appropriately use the stethoscope?
    1. Drape the stethoscope around the neck to have it readily available.
    2. Clean the tubing with alcohol swabs after every patient contact.
    3. Remove the earpieces regularly and clean off cerumen, dust, and oils.
    4. Frequently rub the tubing between the palms to keep it soft.

37. The nurse is caring for a patient who is several days postoperative for major abdominal surgery. The UAP reports that the pulse is 120 beats/min. The nurse rechecks the pulse and gets 122 beats/min. What will the nurse assess for? **Select all that apply.**
    1. Pain
    2. Infection
    3. Anxiety
    4. Hemorrhage
    5. Substance abuse
    6. Hypothermia

38. The patient has a sudden deterioration in condition with confusion; diaphoresis; pallor; and cold, clammy skin. Which peripheral pulse site is the **best** to quickly determine the pulse rate?
    1. Radial
    2. Femoral
    3. Carotid
    4. Brachial

39. The nurse hears in report that the patient has bilateral dorsalis pedis pulses 3+. How does the nurse use this information in planning care?
    1. Allots time to check circulation and sensation on both feet every 2 hours
    2. Plans to follow up and ensure that the HCP is aware of the finding
    3. Instructs UAP to do range-of-motion exercises to hands every 3 hours
    4. Plans to do routine change-of-shift assessment and observe as needed

40. The UAP tells the nurse that the patient has a respiratory rate of 40/min and "is having trouble breathing." What additional signs or symptoms is the nurse **most** likely to observe? **Select all that apply.**
    1. Pursed-lip breathing
    2. Flared nostrils
    3. Epistaxis
    4. Costal retractions
    5. Fatigue
    6. Shortness of breath

41. The nurse checks the patient's BP and obtains a reading of 160/90 mm Hg. What is the pulse pressure? _____

42. The nurse hears in report that the patient has an auscultatory gap. The nurse plans to adapt the technique for measuring which vital sign?
    1. Temperature
    2. Pulse
    3. Respiratory rate
    4. BP

43. The patient states she has a history of an eating disorder and does not want her weight taken while being admitted to the hospital for treatment of pyelonephritis. How would the nurse **best** handle this request?
    1. Review the chart for the most recent weight from a past admission and enter it with a notation of the reason.
    2. Discuss the history of the eating disorder with the patient to understand why she would avoid a weight now.
    3. Offer to have the patient stand backwards on the scale so as not to see the weight when taken.
    4. Explain that weight is an important part of the data collected upon admission.

44. The student nurse is checking BPs at the community health fair. Which situations would require the nurse to review BP measurement techniques with the student? **Select all that apply.**
    1. The patient is seated in a comfortable chair.
    2. The patient's arm is extended on his lap.
    3. The student is quietly conversing with the patient during the process.
    4. The cuff size is 80% of the circumference of the upper arm.
    5. The patient's feet are flat on the ground.
    6. The patient's hand is palm down.

45. The nurse is checking orthostatic BP on a patient. Which of these steps would be done **first**?
    1. Obtain a standing BP.
    2. Obtain a supine BP.
    3. Obtain a left lateral BP.
    4. Obtain a sitting BP.

MATH AND CONVERSION

46. Convert the following temperature readings.

   a.   37° C   =   _____ ° F

   b.   101.2° F   =   _____ ° C

   c.   39.2° C   =   _____ ° F

   d.   97.8° F   =   _____ ° C

47. Convert weight in pounds to the equivalent in kilograms.

   a.   A patient who weighs 44 lbs weighs _____ kg.

   b.   A patient who weighs 210 lbs weighs _____ kg.

48. Convert weight in kilograms to the equivalent in pounds.

   a.   A patient who weighs 6 kilograms weighs _____ lbs.

   b.   A patient who weighs 16 kilograms weighs _____ lbs.

49. Convert height in feet and inches to the equivalent in centimeters.

   a.   A patient who is 5 feet 9 inches tall is _____ centimeters.

   b.   A patient who is 2 feet 3 inches tall is _____ centimeters.

50. Fluid balance may be assessed by weighing the patient. If the patient weighs 2 kg less today than yesterday, how much fluid was lost? _____ mL

CRITICAL THINKING ACTIVITIES

51. A 58-year-old female patient was admitted with pneumonia 2 days ago. The nurse recognizes that the patient must be monitored for signs of worsening infection. The patient's temperature, taken at 7:00 AM, is 101.2° F.

   a.   Discuss factors that may be affecting the body temperature of this patient. _____

   _____

   _____

   b.   What systemic signs and symptoms are associated with an elevated temperature? _____

   _____

   _____

   c.   What would the nurse do if the patient's temperature is above normal? _____

   _____

   _____

52. The nurse is caring for a patient who was admitted for a chronic respiratory problem. Upon entering the room, the nurse observes that the patient is struggling to move from a supine position to a sitting position and breathing is rapid and labored. The nurse notes tension in neck and shoulder muscles with each inspiration. The patient is anxious and repeatedly apologizes for "being a bother" while trying to explain why he came to the hospital and how his disease is affecting his life and his family.

   a. For this patient, what factors may be contributing to the increased respiratory rate? _____

   _____

   _____

   _____

   b. What would the nurse do if the patient's respirations are rapid and labored? _____

   _____

   _____

   _____

   c. Write a response that the nurse could use to help this patient deal with the immediate respiratory problem.

   _____

   _____

   _____

53. Discuss how the nurse uses clinical judgment to determine the frequency, method, and interpretation of vital signs.

   _____

   _____

   _____

   _____

   _____

   _____

   _____

   _____

NEXT-GENERATION NCLEX™ (NGN)

54. Matrix

Cognitive Skill: Analyze Cues

Scenario: The nurse works on a floor with a patient population of various ages and diagnoses. The UAP is reporting the findings of morning vital signs and patient issues to the nurse.

Instructions: Use an X to indicate if the finding for the age group described falls into normal or abnormal categories.

Vital Sign or Assessment Finding	Normal	Abnormal
Infant pulse 130		
Older adult oral temperature 97° F (36.1° C)		
Child tympanic temperature 38.5° C (101.3° F)		
Older adult pulse 120		
Adult blood pressure 180/105		
School-age child blood pressure 100/64		
The older adult is refusing food today		
The pulse pressure of the older adult is 50		
The adult patient reports feeling really weird		

Physical Assessment

Answer Key: A complete Answer Key is provided in your Additional Learning Resources on Evolve.

TABLE ACTIVITY

1. *Directions:* Complete the table by supplying the correct terms that you would use to document the physical assessment findings described on the right. Aim for correct spelling!

Term	Description
	Lack of appetite resulting in the inability to eat
	Heart rate of less than 60 beats per minute
	Difficulty passing stools or infrequent passage of hard stools
	Bluish discoloration of the skin and mucous membranes
	Profuse sweating
	Shortness of breath or difficulty breathing
	Extravasation of blood into the subcutaneous tissues
	Abnormal accumulation of fluid in interstitial spaces
	Redness or inflammation of the skin or mucous membranes
	The protective response of the tissues of the body to irritation or injury
	Yellow tinge to the skin
	State or quality of being indifferent, apathetic, or sluggish
	Sensation often leading to the urge to vomit
	Must sit upright or stand to breathe comfortably
	Unnatural paleness or absence of color in the skin
	Itching and an uncomfortable sensation leading to an urge to scratch
	Creamy, viscous, pale yellow, or yellow-green exudate; liquefied necrosis of tissues
	Unhealthy yellow color; usually said of a complexion or skin
	Heart rate greater than 100 beats per minute
	Abnormally rapid rate of breathing
	Expulsion of the contents of the stomach out of the mouth

MULTIPLE CHOICE

Directions: Select the best answer(s) for each of the following questions.

2. The patient sprains his ankle. During the inflammatory response, damaged tissue releases chemicals that increase the permeability of the capillary walls, which allows white blood cells and plasma to move into the area. What does the nurse expect to be included in the subjective and objective data?
   1. Patient reports pain and obvious swelling around ankle.
   2. Patient reports numbness and skin is cool and pale.
   3. Patient reports pruritus and there is a fine red rash.
   4. Patient reports weakness and peripheral pulses are weak.

3. The nurse is almost finished doing a routine head-to-toe assessment on a newly admitted patient. Suddenly, the patient starts coughing and reports "trouble breathing." What would the nurse do **first**?
   1. Quickly complete the head-to-toe assessment and then call the health care provider (HCP).
   2. Switch to a focused respiratory assessment and listen to lung sounds.
   3. Assist the patient to sit upright and give oxygen per mask or nasal cannula.
   4. Stay with the patient and reassure him that the coughing episode will pass.

4. The nurse needs to assess a patient who had a head injury. Which neurologic assessment would the nurse perform **first**?
   1. Vital signs
   2. Motor function
   3. Pupillary response
   4. Level of consciousness

5. The nurse hears in shift report that an older patient has "tenting" over the sternum. Based on this information, what is **most** important for the nurse to monitor and assess?
   1. Auscultate lung sounds and respiratory status.
   2. Monitor intake and output and check electrolyte values.
   3. Observe the anterior trunk for redness or ecchymoses.
   4. Monitor for tenting on other areas of the body.

6. An older adult woman walks into the interview room. She smiles at the nurse and looks around the room. The nurse says, "Please take a seat," and the woman takes a brochure from the display case. The nurse says, "Why have you come to see us today?" The woman says, "Yes dear, tea is fine. Thank you." Based on this interaction, which assessments will the nurse perform **first**?
   1. Head-to-toe assessments to detect any problems
   2. Mental status and family structure/support
   3. Cultural, age, and gender influences on behavior
   4. Auditory sensory perception and cognitive function

7. The patient is diagnosed with sickle cell trait. Based on the nurse's knowledge of pathophysiology, which intervention is **most** likely to be recommended for the patient?
   1. Review of allergens in the home environment
   2. Referral for genetic counseling
   3. Dietary evaluation to identify deficiencies
   4. Prescription for broad-spectrum antibiotics

8. The nurse is examining the patient's eyes. Which finding is the **most** important to report to the HCP?
   1. Eyes appear asymmetric; left eyelid has a fold, right eyelid does not.
   2. Sclerae of both eyes are white and the conjunctivae are pink.
   3. Right pupil constricts when light is applied and left pupil also constricts.
   4. There is similar puffiness and periorbital edema around both eyes.

9. The nurse hears in report that the patient had a Glasgow Coma Scale score of 15 during the night shift. What is an **early** sign that indicates deterioration in neurologic status?
    1. Patient knows his own name, but does not recognize his spouse.
    2. Patient is unable to move hands or fingers on command.
    3. Patient's right pupil is slightly larger and more sluggish than the left.
    4. Patient has widening pulse pressure, bradycardia, and irregular breathing.

10. To decrease the risk for lung disease, which lifestyle modification is the **most** important to recommend to patients?
    1. Seek cancer screening.
    2. Exercise regularly.
    3. Stop smoking.
    4. Limit dietary fats.

11. While obtaining the vital signs of an adult, the nurse observes that the patient is diaphoretic and flushed. Which change in vital signs would the nurse expect to accompany this observation?
    1. Respiratory rate of 10/min
    2. Pulse of 65 beats/min
    3. Blood pressure of 100/60 mm Hg
    4. Temperature of 101° F (38.3° C)

12. The nurse hears in report that the patient has had occasional episodes of cyanosis and dyspnea. Which physical assessment does the nurse plan to frequently perform during the shift?
    1. Check for abdominal pain.
    2. Assess respiratory effort.
    3. Monitor urinary output.
    4. Assess for headache.

13. While assessing the patient, the nurse observes that the patient experiences orthopnea. What instruction will the nurse give the unlicensed assistive personnel (UAP) about assisting the patient?
    1. The patient is too weak to walk to the bathroom.
    2. Dizziness will occur if the patient stands up too quickly.
    3. Keep the head of the bed elevated at all times.
    4. The dominant hand is not functioning properly.

14. The patient's oral temperature is 101.2° F (38.4° C). The patient tells the nurse that he doesn't feel well, but has no known health conditions. Which question would the nurse ask **first** to try to localize the source of infection?
    1. "What other symptoms are you having?"
    2. "Do you have any known allergies?"
    3. "Have you ever felt like this before?"
    4. "When did you first notice the fever?"

15. The nurse hears in report that a patient who has cancer is experiencing anorexia. Which assessment does the nurse plan to conduct during the shift?
    1. Assess need for supplemental oxygen.
    2. Evaluate ability to independently ambulate.
    3. Review efficacy of PRN pain medication.
    4. Assess need for supplemental nutrition.

16. The nurse is interviewing an older patient and notices that the patient is slumping and irritable and frequently sighs. Which question would the nurse ask to validate the **most** likely interpretation of the patient's behavior?
    1. "Are you short of breath?"
    2. "Are you feeling tired?"
    3. "Would you like some water?"
    4. "Are you having pain?"

17. A patient tells the nurse that she is "afraid of the doctor." How could this affect the objective data?
    1. Description of pain will be exaggerated.
    2. Patient is likely to experience nausea.
    3. Blood pressure could be higher than expected.
    4. Pupils will be constricted and nonreactive.

18. The HCP tells the nurse that the patient has pruritus. Which objective finding is the nurse **most** likely to observe?
    1. Scratch marks on skin
    2. Abdominal distention
    3. Abnormal breath sounds
    4. Low-grade temperature

19. The nurse uses the OPQRSTUV method of obtaining the most information about the patient's pain. Which question addresses the P in the OPQRSTUV?
    1. On a scale of 1 to 10, what number is the pain?
    2. What causes the pain to increase or decrease?
    3. When did you first notice the pain?
    4. Is the pain spreading out to other areas?

20. The nurse reads in the patient's chart that the patient has crackles in the posterior lower lobes. What does the nurse expect to hear during auscultation if the patient's condition is unchanged?
    1. Short, discrete, bubbling sounds on inspiration
    2. High-pitched, musical sounds on inspiration
    3. Grating sounds on expiration
    4. Coarse gurgling on expiration

21. Which evaluation statement indicates that the antibiotic therapy has successfully resolved the patient's leg infection?
    1. The patient reports that pain is decreased compared to previously.
    2. The patient is observed independently ambulating in the hallway.
    3. The wound site shows no signs of erythema; white cell count is normal.
    4. The wound site shows edema, redness, and white cell count is elevated.

22. Which method would be **best** to assess an older patient's ability to accomplish activities of daily living?
    1. Accompany the patient during ambulation to the bathroom.
    2. Ask the patient what he normally eats during the day.
    3. Take a full set of vital signs and include pain assessment.
    4. Observe the patient's level of consciousness and orientation.

23. The nurse is assessing an older patient. Which explanation would the nurse use?
    1. "I am going to auscultate the posterior lung fields."
    2. "I will be checking your motor function."
    3. "I would like to check your perineal area."
    4. "I am going to listen to your heartbeat."

24. The nurse is **most** likely to use the Glasgow Coma Scale for which patient?
    1. Recently had a myocardial infarction
    2. Sustained a serious head injury
    3. Shows some signs of septic shock
    4. Has risk for respiratory failure

25. The nurse observes jugular venous distention on a patient who is sitting in the interview chair. What other signs or symptoms would the nurse check to validate suspicion of heart failure?
    1. Low heart rate
    2. Increased urinary output
    3. Dependent edema in legs
    4. Jaundice of sclera

26. A new nurse documents PERRLA in the patient's chart. When the preceptor nurse asks him to describe the findings, the new nurse is unable to explain. What would the preceptor nurse do **first**?
    1. Show the new nurse how to perform the assessment.
    2. Ask the new nurse how he knew to document PERRLA.
    3. Instruct the new nurse to seek out the nurse educator.
    4. Report the new nurse for falsifying the documentation.

27. The nurse is assessing the patency of the nostrils. What is the **best** method to use?
    1. Use a penlight and observe for blockage or excess mucus.
    2. Press against one nostril and ask the patient to breathe.
    3. Give the patient a tissue and instruct to blow the nose.
    4. Ask the patient to breathe quietly and listen for air movement.

28. What is the UAP's role in assessing the respiratory system?
    1. Observe and report changes in rate and depth.
    2. Determine a position that accommodates orthopnea.
    3. Auscultate the lung sounds every 4 hours or as needed.
    4. Monitor and interpret the pulse oximeter readings.

29. What would be considered a normal finding when assessing the patient's spine?
    1. A gentle inward curvature of the lumbosacral curve
    2. A large posterior curvature of the thoracic spine
    3. An increased curvature of the lumbar spine
    4. A right or left lateral spinal curvature

30. The nurse is unable to palpate the popliteal pulse. Which pulse would the nurse assess before informing the HCP?
    1. Femoral pulse
    2. Dorsalis pedis pulse
    3. Brachial pulse
    4. Apical pulse

31. Which adventitious breath sound would the nurse expect to auscultate in the patient with upper airway obstruction?
    1. Stridor
    2. Crackles
    3. Wheezing
    4. Pleural friction rub

32. Which environmental factor(s) may contribute to a patient's poor health? **Select all that apply.**
    1. Air quality
    2. Water quality
    3. Housing condition
    4. Crime rate
    5. School quality
    6. Age

33. The nurse is doing a health assessment on the patient. Which items are subjective data or symptoms? **Select all that apply.**
    1. Rash
    2. Elevated blood pressure
    3. Pain
    4. Vertigo
    5. Pus
    6. Bleeding

CRITICAL THINKING ACTIVITIES

34. A 40-year-old man comes to the clinic. He desires a general physical check-up and reports, "not feeling quite 100%." This is the patient's first visit to the clinic, so there are no medical records available for comparison. Provide examples of questions that the nurse could ask to obtain information during a review of systems.

    a. Respiratory: _____

    b. Endocrine: _____

    c. Gastrointestinal: _____

    d. Cardiac: _____

    e. Neurologic: _____

    f. Genitourinary: _____

35. A 30-year-old woman comes to the emergency department. She reports pain in the lower abdomen. She appears very uncomfortable and is walking in a slightly bent-over position. Her hands are supporting her lower abdomen as she moves toward the examination room.

   a. Use the OPQRSTUV method to elicit information about the abdominal pain. _____

   _____

   _____

   _____

   _____

   _____

   _____

   b. Describe how the nurse performs the physical assessment of the abdomen. _____

   _____

   _____

   _____

   _____

36. How does the nurse generate subjective and objective data when the patient says, "I have a really bad headache"?

   _____

   _____

   _____

   _____

   _____

37. The nurse is conducting an interview with a patient who was just admitted to the medical-surgical unit. The nurse stands at the bedside and initially smiles at the patient, but as she is asking the questions, the nurse frequently glances out the window and shifts restlessly back and forth. She diligently fills out the admission form while reading the questions from the form. When the patient tries to explain a point, she cuts him off and moves on to the next question. She checks the equipment necessary for the patient's care while the patient is trying to explain his symptoms. Discuss this nurse-patient interaction from the patient's point of view.

   _____

   _____

   _____

   _____

   _____

   _____

NEXT-GENERATION NCLEX™ (NGN)

38. Cloze

Cognitive Skill: Analyze Cues

Scenario: The nurse is performing a physical assessment on a 68-year-old woman being admitted to the hospital. Her admitting diagnosis is pyelonephritis. Her recent past medical history is significant for asthma, bladder infections, atherosclerosis, and dehydration.

Instructions: Choose the best option to complete the statements below.

Based on the recent past medical history, the nurse would be likely to note the following during physical assessment: ___1___. The finding of ___2___ would be common with the current admitting diagnosis. The nurse would anticipate the following laboratory orders relating to the current admitting diagnosis: ___3___.

Options for 1	Options for 2	Options for 3
wheeze, tenting, and bruit	tenderness with palpation of right upper quadrant of abdomen	complete blood count (CBC), urine culture
crackles, edema, and tachypnea	tenderness with percussion of flank areas	urinalysis, prothrombin time
stridor, jaundice, and hypotension	decreased breath sounds with auscultation of lungs	urinalysis, fasting blood sugar
tachypnea, pallor, and presence of S_4 heart sound	increased bowel sounds with auscultation of abdomen	ova and parasites test, blood chemistry profile

Oxygenation

Answer Key: A complete Answer Key is provided in your Additional Learning Resources on Evolve.

CROSSWORD PUZZLE

1. *Directions:* Use the clues to complete the crossword puzzle.

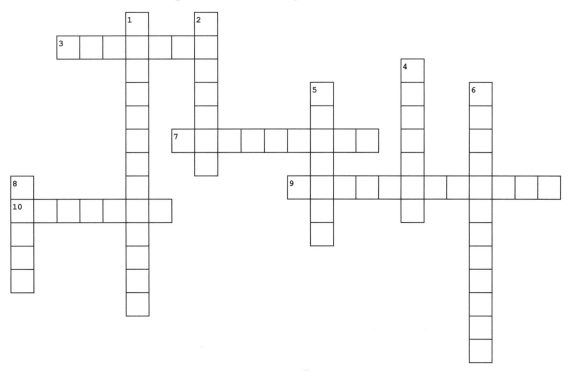

Across

3. Reduced oxygen content in tissue and cells
7. A device used to set the prescribed rate of oxygen
9. A(n) _____ tube is inserted through the patient's mouth and into the upper airway to provide a patent airway
10. When a(n) _____ rebreathing mask functions properly, the reservoir fills on exhalation and almost collapses on inhalation

Down

1. A(n) _____ can deliver 6 to 15 L/min = 70% to 100% O_2
2. A nasal _____ is a device consisting of small tubes inserted into the nares
4. A(n) _____ mask offers a precise, controlled concentration of oxygen
5. Openness
6. An artificial opening made by a surgical incision into the trachea
8. Cessation of breathing

MULTIPLE CHOICE

Directions: Select the best answer(s) for each of the following questions.

2. For a patient who is receiving oxygen through an oxymizer, which intervention is the **most** important?
    1. Clean and dry the skin every 2 hours.
    2. Observe for fine mist or bubbling in humidifier.
    3. Allow the patient to fit or adjust the device in the nares.
    4. Check the reservoirs to ensure that they do not deflate.

3. In performing nursing skills and procedures for patients, which action demonstrates the nurse's understanding and use of Standard Precautions?
    1. Always checks the patient's armband and asks the patient to state his or her name
    2. Assesses the patient's understanding and teaches accordingly
    3. Performs hand hygiene before and after every patient encounter
    4. Evaluates the patient's response to and tolerance of the procedure

4. The patient requires suctioning of pulmonary secretions. Which problem statement is the **most** accurate for this patient's condition?
    1. Potential for fluid volume excess
    2. Inability to maintain breathing pattern
    3. Potential for inadequate tissue perfusion
    4. Inability to clear airway

5. What is included in the preparation for tracheostomy care in the acute care environment?
    1. Using clean technique and supplies for cleaning
    2. Preparing cotton balls to clean inside the ostomy
    3. Removing and cleaning the outer cannula
    4. Placing the patient in a semi-Fowler's position

6. The nurse is caring for a patient who is on 3 L oxygen per nasal cannula. Which tasks can be delegated to the unlicensed assistive personnel (UAP)? **Select all that apply.**
    1. Ensuring that the oxygen flow is set at 3 L/min throughout the shift
    2. Helping the patient clean area around nares and ears
    3. Counting the respiratory rate and taking the pulse oximeter reading
    4. Listening to breath sounds before and after the patient coughs
    5. Assisting the patient to a semi-Fowler's position
    6. Observe the nares, external nasal area, and ears for breaks in skin integrity

7. The nurse is reviewing laboratory results and sees that the PaO_2 level for a 75-year-old patient is 80 mm Hg. What would the nurse do **first**?
    1. Notify the health care provider (HCP) about the unusually low level.
    2. Contact the clinical laboratory to verify the low result.
    3. Check the previous laboratory values for comparison.
    4. Assess patient for signs/symptoms of respiratory distress.

8. Which patient is the **most** likely candidate for an endotracheal tube?
    1. The patient is discovered in the bathroom, unresponsive and pulseless.
    2. The patient is choking on a foreign body that cannot be dislodged.
    3. The patient needs long-term mechanical ventilation for oxygenation.
    4. The patient needs precise, controlled concentration of oxygen.

9. The nurse walks into the room and notices that the patient is anxious, demonstrates labored breathing, and seems to be struggling to get out of bed. What would the nurse do **first**?
   1. Gently advise the patient to calm down, then and ask him what is wrong.
   2. Count the respiratory rate, note rhythm, and auscultate breath sounds.
   3. Assist him to sit upright and calmly instruct him to take slow, deep breaths.
   4. Stay with the patient, apply oxygen, and have another nurse call the HCP.

10. The nurse must be vigilant for signs of hypoxia in an older patient who has dementia and also has risk for decreased oxygenation because of chronic respiratory disease and immobility. What is an **early** sign that warrants additional assessment of respiratory status?
    1. Lips are cyanotic, fingers are cool, and capillary refill is sluggish.
    2. Respirations are slow and shallow.
    3. Patient seems restless and anxiously picks at linens.
    4. Pulse is slower than normal and is thready and weak.

11. The nurse is caring for a patient with a tracheostomy. What signs/symptoms indicate the need for suctioning? **Select all that apply.**
    1. Fine crackles in posterior lobes
    2. Gurgling sounds heard during respiration
    3. Restlessness or anxiety
    4. Emesis in the oral cavity
    5. Drooling excessive secretions
    6. Patient indicates need for suctioning

12. The patient had an uneventful hip surgery several days ago and will soon be transferred to a rehabilitation unit. The patient says to the nurse, "I feel silly complaining about this, but I feel a little short of breath and a little anxious and fuzzy-headed." The patient has no known history of respiratory or cardiac problems. What would the nurse do **first**?
    1. Reassure the patient that she is not being silly, and that anxiety is normal.
    2. Take the vital signs, apply a pulse oximeter, and listen to breath sounds.
    3. Ask the patient to describe what she is feeling and what she thinks is going on.
    4. Apply oxygen per nasal cannula, notify the charge nurse, and call the HCP.

13. In caring for a patient with a tracheostomy, which interventions will the nurse use to reduce the risk for infection? **Select all that apply.**
    1. Evaluate the patient for excess secretions and suction as often as necessary.
    2. Provide constant airway humidification.
    3. Provide frequent mouth care.
    4. Assist the patient to perform hand hygiene.
    5. Remove water that condenses in equipment tubing.
    6. Change or clean all respiratory therapy equipment every 8 hours.

14. Which fluid would be the **best** choice for a patient who needs to drink fluids to thin and liquefy secretions?
    1. 10 ounces of water
    2. 8 ounces of cold milk
    3. 1-2 cups of black coffee
    4. 6 ounces of unsweetened iced tea

15. Which family members need to be cautioned about fire safety around an older patient who recently started to use home oxygen therapy? **Select all that apply.**
    1. Brother-in-law arrives smoking a cigarette.
    2. Toddler is excited to show grandpa his new friction toy car.
    3. Son-in-law suggests that drinking a cold beer would be refreshing.
    4. Wife offers to help her husband learn how to use an electric razor.
    5. Daughter wants to help her father wash his face with a warm washcloth.
    6. Sister-in-law has brought several new wool blankets to place on the bed.

CRITICAL THINKING ACTIVITIES

16. The nurse is caring for an older patient who has chronic obstructive pulmonary disease (COPD). The family comes in and spends several hours with him. The patient is in good spirits and introduces the nurse to his family when he comes in to give the patient his medication. The family leaves and the nurse observes that the patient is resting and assumes that he is very tired after the long visit. Two hours later, the nurse goes into check on the patient; his breathing is very shallow, and he is very difficult to arouse. The nasal cannula is in place and the oxygen is flowing at 7 L/min.

a. What does the nurse suspect? _____

_____

_____

_____

_____

_____

b. What should the nurse do? _____

_____

_____

_____

_____

_____

c. What should the nurse have done to prevent this situation? _____

_____

_____

_____

_____

_____

d. Discuss how the "hypoxic drive" affects patients with COPD. _____

_____

_____

_____

_____

_____

NEXT-GENERATION NCLEX™ (NGN)

17. Cloze

Cognitive Skill: Analyze Cues

Scenario: The older patient is being treated for pneumonia and will be discharged back to the long-term care facility in the afternoon. During the morning assessment, the nurse observes that the patient has pulled out the IV and removed his clothes and the oxygen nasal cannula. He seems unusually anxious and appears to be trying to sit up and get out of bed.

Instructions: Choose the most likely options to complete the statement below.

The nurse knows that for older adults, ___1___ is a common early sign of hypoxia. The nurse assists the patient to a ___2___ position to facilitate breathing. The nurse replaces the nasal cannula and adjusts the flowmeter to ___3___, which is the maximum oxygen percentage for this device.

Options for 1	Options for 2	Options for 3
bradycardia	Sims	1 L/min = 24% O_2
cyanosis	Trendelenburg	5 L/min = 35% O_2
apnea	prone	6 L/min = 44% O_2
shallow, slow respirations	supine	8 L/min=55% O_2
digital clubbing	Semi-Fowler's	10 L/min = 55% O_2
restlessness	recumbent	12 L/min = 90% O_2

Elimination and Gastric Intubation

chapter
15

Answer Key: A complete Answer Key is provided in your Additional Learning Resources on Evolve.

CLINICAL APPLICATION OF MATH AND CONVERSION

Directions: Calculate or make the necessary conversions for math problems encountered in performing skills for patients.

1. At the beginning of the shift, the nurse inserts a urinary catheter and observes 300 mL of urine output into the drainage bag. One hour later, there is an order to send a urine sample, so the nurse uses the appropriate sterile technique and draws 20 mL from the port. At that time, the nurse notes 350 mL of urine in the bag, empties the bag, and records the urine output. At the end of the shift, the drainage bag contains 500 mL. How many mL of urine are recorded as the total output for the shift? _____ mL

2. The patient vomits 200 mL of green bile drainage. Twenty minutes later, he vomits 100 mL. The health care provider (HCP) orders the insertion of a nasogastric tube to decompress the stomach. During the procedure, the patient vomits 50 mL. At the end of the shift, there is 150 mL in the drainage container. What does the nurse record as the output of emesis for the shift? _____ mL

3. Using sterile technique, the nurse inserts a straight catheter into the patient, allows some urine to pass into the drainage container, then collects 15 mL in the specimen container (midstream sample), then allows the bladder to empty by placing the end of the catheter in the drainage container. The nurse removes the catheter and measures the urine in the drainage container at 750 mL. What does the nurse record as output? _____ mL

4. The patient is receiving continuous bladder irrigation through a three-way indwelling urinary catheter. Prescribed and administered: 350 mL of normal saline irrigating solution. There are 475 mL in the urinary drainage bag. What is the patient's urinary output? _____ mL

5. The HCP has ordered nasogastric tube irrigation with 100 mL of normal saline. After confirming tube placement and assessing bowel sounds, the nurse instills 30 mL of normal saline and then withdraws the fluid and measures 25 mL. The nurse instills another 30 mL and withdraws and measures 20 mL. The nurse instills another 30 mL and withdraws 30 mL. The nurse instills the last 10 mL and withdraws and measures 10 mL. How does the nurse record the intake and output? _____ mL

6. The nurse is irrigating a nasogastric tube to maintain the patency of the tube. The nurse instills 30 mL of normal saline and withdraws 35 mL. How does the nurse record intake and output? _____ mL

FIGURE LABELING

7. *Directions:* label the figure below with the names of the three landmarks that are used to measure the length of insertion of a nasogastric tube.

MULTIPLE CHOICE

Directions: Select the best answer(s) for each of the following questions.

8. The nursing student has the opportunity to perform urinary catheterization on a patient. What would the student do **first**?
    1. Perform hand hygiene and don gloves.
    2. Explain the procedure to the patient.
    3. Obtain the necessary equipment.
    4. Check the HCP's order.

9. The nurse must perform catheter care. Prior to starting the procedure, the nurse raises the bed and lowers one side rail. What is the **best** rationale for this action?
    1. Ensures patient safety and comfort
    2. Promotes good body mechanics
    3. Facilitates visualization of the patient's body
    4. Adheres to standard procedure

10. The nurse has inserted the urinary catheter into the patient and while the balloon is being inflated, the patient expresses discomfort. What would the nurse do?
    1. Remove the catheter and begin the procedure again.
    2. Pull back on the catheter to determine tension.
    3. Draw fluid out of the balloon and move the catheter forward.
    4. Continue to inflate the balloon since discomfort is expected.

11. Which instruction will the nurse give to the unlicensed assistive personnel (UAP) about catheter care for the patient?
    1. Maintain continuous tension on the external catheter tubing.
    2. Empty the drainage bag once a day or sooner if necessary.
    3. Attach the drainage bag to the side rails, below the level of the bladder.
    4. Clean the urinary meatus and 2 inches down the catheter.

12. The charge nurse delegates the removal of an indwelling urinary catheter to a new staff member. Which action requires correction?
    1. Explaining the burning sensation with the first voiding
    2. Obtaining a final urine specimen from the drainage bag
    3. Deflating the balloon and pinching the catheter
    4. Using clean gloves and performing perineal care

13. The home health nurse is assessing whether a patient with a spinal cord injury would be a candidate for intermittent self-catheterization. Which criteria would support this choice for this patient? **Select all that apply.**
    1. The patient and family understand the use and cost of sterile supplies.
    2. The patient understands how to recognize signs/symptoms of infection.
    3. The patient has the manual dexterity to perform the cleaning and insertion.
    4. The patient and family are seeking ways for the patient to maintain independence.
    5. The family wants noninvasive and natural methods to maintain bodily functions.

14. The nurse has just removed a urinary catheter from a postsurgical patient. What is the **most** important instruction to give the UAP?
    1. Be especially gentle when performing perineal care, because area is likely to be irritated.
    2. Report the amount of food and fluids that the patient consumes for the remainder of the shift.
    3. Measure the amount of the first voiding and report the time and amount to the nurse.
    4. Assist the patient to ambulate because the patient is likely to be sore and uncomfortable.

15. What is the **most** important thing for the nurse to assess in caring for an older patient who has a condom catheter?
    1. Inspect the skin underneath the catheter.
    2. Monitor for a urinary tract infection.
    3. Measure the daily urinary output.
    4. Assess for urinary retention.

16. The patient has an indwelling urinary catheter. The UAP reports that no new urine is collecting in the bag since it was measured and discarded at the beginning of the shift. What would the nurse do **first**?
    1. Irrigate the system using sterile closed technique.
    2. Call the HCP for an order to discontinue the catheter.
    3. Give the patient oral fluid to flush the bladder and catheter.
    4. Check for kinks in the tubing system and reposition the patient.

17. The nurse is assessing the insertion site of the patient's indwelling urinary catheter and notices exudate. What other assessment is the nurse **most** likely to perform before notifying the HCP?
    1. Look at the trends of intake and output for the past several days.
    2. Gently palpate the patient's suprapubic area to assess for bladder distention.
    3. Check the patient's temperature and draw fresh urine from the drainage port.
    4. Observe the clarity, odor, and color of urine in the collection bag.

18. The student nurse is obtaining a urine specimen from a patient who has had an indwelling catheter for several days. Which actions require correction? **Select all that apply.**
    1. Disconnects the catheter from tubing and collects urine in a sterile container
    2. Obtains the urine from the collection bag using the drainage tube on the bag
    3. Draws urine directly from the catheter by using a sterile small-gauge needle
    4. Applies clean gloves and scrubs the drainage port with an alcohol swab
    5. Uses a sterile needle and syringe and collects 10 mL from the drainage port

19. For a patient on a bladder retraining program, which dietary/fluid intervention is the **best**?
    1. Encourage black coffee for breakfast.
    2. Help the patient identify high-fiber foods.
    3. Restrict fluid intake to control bladder.
    4. Encourage at least 2000 mL of fluid each day.

20. An older adult resident in a long-term care facility is incontinent of urine. The nurse observes that the resident always asks for assistance to go to the toilet after eating breakfast. Based on this observation, what would the nurse do **first**?
    1. Instruct UAP to apply incontinence pants before breakfast.
    2. Note times that the resident asks for help to the bathroom or requires changing of underwear.
    3. Suggest that the health care team plan and initiate a bladder training program.
    4. Obtain an order for a condom catheter or an indwelling urinary catheter.

21. The nurse hears in report that a patient receiving tube feedings has been having trouble with dumping syndrome. Based on the report, which action is the nurse **most** likely to perform?
    1. Ensure that the feeding is administered very slowly.
    2. Auscultate bowel sounds before and after the feeding.
    3. Stay with the patient while the feeding is infusing.
    4. Offer the feeding through a straw instead of the tube.

22. The postsurgical patient has a Salem sump tube for decompression of the stomach. The nurse observes fluid leaking out of the pigtail. What would the nurse do?
    1. Remove the tube and reinsert it.
    2. Introduce 30 mL of air into the pigtail.
    3. Pull the tube back a few centimeters.
    4. Increase the pressure of the wall suction.

23. Which evaluation statement indicates that the polystyrene sulfonate enema was a successful therapy?
    1. The patient evacuated 300 mL of light-brown fluid after the third enema.
    2. Removal of hard fecal mass was followed by a small, soft, brown stool.
    3. The patient reports resumption of normal bowel pattern after enema.
    4. The patient's serum potassium level is within normal limits.

24. Which patient is **most** likely to need extra teaching about how to protect the skin around an ostomy?
    1. The patient has an ileostomy.
    2. The patient has a colostomy of the transverse colon.
    3. The patient has a colostomy of the descending colon.
    4. The patient has a percutaneous endoscopic gastrostomy.

25. The patient tells the home health nurse that he is doing fine and has been irrigating his colostomy 5-6 times a week with 2000 mL each time. What is the **immediate** concern that needs to be followed up?
    1. The patient needs to have blood drawn for possible low electrolyte levels.
    2. The patient needs review of teaching points about colostomy care.
    3. The patient needs to have laboratory studies to rule out peritonitis.
    4. The patient needs to have psychological evaluation for failure to cope.

26. The patient begins to cough and gag when the nurse inserts a nasogastric tube. The nurse instructs the patient to breathe easily and take a few sips of water, but the patient continues to cough. What would the nurse do **first**?
    1. Remove the tube and let the patient rest before reinsertion.
    2. Attach a syringe to the tube and aspirate for stomach contents.
    3. Use a flashlight and tongue blade to look at the throat.
    4. Pull the tube back just slightly and instruct the patient to breathe slowly.

27. Before the digital removal of a fecal impaction, the nurse checks the medical record. Which part of the patient's history alerts the nurse to be especially observant during the procedure?
    1. Cardiac disease
    2. Hysterectomy
    3. Urinary infection
    4. Diabetes mellitus

28. The nurse has just inserted a nasogastric tube. The patient is coughing and gagging. The nurse takes a small amount of clear aspirated material and tests it with color-coded pH paper and the pH is 8. What would the nurse do **first**?
    1. Call the HCP to obtain an order for an x-ray to confirm placement.
    2. Ask the patient to speak his name and state his full address.
    3. Pull the tube out and tell the patient it was probably down his airway.
    4. Ask the RN to come and verify the tube placement before use.

29. Which patient is a candidate for the Purewick female external catheter?
    1. Patient is incontinent of bowel and bladder.
    2. Patient needs precise intake and output for 24 hours.
    3. Patient has urinary retention related to a new medication.
    4. Patient must be in supine position for 24 hours postprocedure.

30. Patient reports flatulence and a "bloated" feeling. Which intervention would the nurse try **first**?
    1. Obtain an order for rectal tube insertion.
    2. Assist the patient to get up and ambulate.
    3. Encourage the patient to drink more fluids.
    4. Help the patient select high-fiber foods for lunch.

31. An older patient reports that he frequently experiences constipation. Which areas will the nurse assess? **Select all that apply.**
    1. Toileting habits
    2. Activity and exercise
    3. Amount of fluid intake
    4. Daily hygiene routines
    5. Amount of dietary fiber
    6. Frequency of laxative use

CRITICAL THINKING ACTIVITIES

32. The nurse must insert an indwelling urinary catheter in a female patient who is very obese.

    a. Discuss the challenges of maintaining sterility while inserting a urinary catheter in obese female patients.

    _____

    _____

    _____

    _____

    _____

b. What steps can the nurse take to maintain sterility? _____

_____

_____

_____

_____

_____

33. The nurse sees that the HCP has ordered a straight catheter urine specimen from a patient who is transgender (male to female). What should the nurse assess before starting the procedure? (Note to student: If you are unsure about how to answer this question, have a discussion with your instructor and classmates.)

_____

_____

_____

_____

_____

_____

_____

_____

_____

NEXT-GENERATION NCLEX™ (NGN)

34. Matrix

Cognitive Skill: Take Action

Scenario: Following abdominal surgery, the patient develops abdominal distention with nausea and vomits a small amount of green bile emesis. The HCP orders nasogastric (NG) tube insertion for abdominal decompression. The RN inserts the tube and placement is confirmed by x-ray. The LPN/LVN is assigned to manage the care of the patient and the NG tube. Which essential actions are included in the patient's care?

Instructions: Use an X to indicate whether an action is essential, nonessential, or contraindicated.

Action	Essential	Nonessential	Contraindicated
Routinely measure and evaluate the contents of the suction canister.			
Instill 500 mL of normal saline and then siphon it out.			
Keep the head of the bed elevated at least 30 degrees at all times.			
Watch for signs and symptoms of dumping syndrome.			
Delegate oral and nasal hygiene to the UAP.			
If tube is not draining, turn the patient; this drains the stomach and may reposition the tube.			
Use 30 mL of normal saline or tap water to irrigate the pigtail.			
Secure tube to the nose with tape or nose guard; loop a rubber band around the end of tube and pin the band to the patient's gown.			

Care of Patients Experiencing Urgent Alterations in Health

chapter

16

Answer Key: A complete Answer Key is provided in your Additional Learning Resources on Evolve.

FIGURE

1. *Directions:* Refer to the figure and use the Rule of Nines to determine how much of the body surface is burned for an adult patient who has severe burns to the anterior and posterior thorax and both upper extremities. _____%

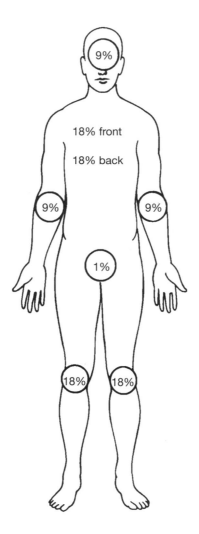

MULTIPLE CHOICE

Directions: Select the best answer(s) for each of the following questions.

2. The health care provider (HCP) directs the nurse to call Poison Control to get advice for a patient who comes to the health care facility for "feeling sick after spraying an enclosed area with insect spray." What information is necessary to report when calling Poison Control? **Select all that apply.**
   1. Patient is 20 years old.
   2. He weighs 160 lbs (72.6 kg).
   3. He is currently alert, nauseated, and has a mild headache (4/10).
   4. He started to feel dizzy and nauseated after spraying an enclosed area with insect spray.
   5. His symptoms started at 10 AM; this was several minutes after he started to use the spray.
   6. He was not using any personal protective equipment (PPE) when he applied the spray.
   7. He reports that his father used the same spray last week and had no problems.

3. The nurse is at a community event and several people are injured when a large tent structure is blown over by the wind. Which information is essential to convey when calling the emergency medical system (EMS) for help? **Select all that apply.**
   1. "I am a nurse; I work at a local hospital, and I have basic life support (BLS) certification."
   2. "One woman's legs are trapped under a heavy beam; she is alert and breathing."
   3. "Three children appear to have minor abrasions; one child's arm was splinted for possible fracture."
   4. "An older man with 'heart problems' is short of breath but has no external injuries."
   5. "A large tent structure in the city park has fallen and five people have been injured."
   6. "The parking lot is congested; the best access is on the south side of the park."

4. What would be included in a teaching plan for safety and response to an emergency in the home environment? **Select all that apply.**
   1. Keeping poisons locked away from children
   2. Maintaining a list of emergency phone numbers
   3. Keeping electrical cords in good repair with no fraying
   4. Teaching family members how to do cardiopulmonary resuscitation (CPR)
   5. Identifying and obtaining emergency first-aid supplies and instructions
   6. Reviewing use of handrails and removal of loose rugs or other obstacles

5. Which patient has the **best** chance to fully recover because of the nurse's actions?
   1. 4-year-old drowns; nurse starts CPR within 4 minutes of clinical death
   2. 32-year-old with brain death has a cardiac arrest; nurse starts CPR within 2 minutes
   3. 17-year-old with biologic death has a respiratory arrest; nurse immediately delivers rescue breaths
   4. 55-year-old is electrocuted; nurse starts CPR within 10 minutes of clinical death

6. Which patient has a condition that could resemble brain death?
   1. The patient has a blood alcohol level of 0.05%.
   2. The patient has a core temperature below 30° C (86° F).
   3. The patient has oliguria secondary to hypovolemic shock.
   4. The patient fainted and was unconscious for 5 minutes.

7. The nurse is teaching basic CPR to a new group of unlicensed assistive personnel (UAP). When would the nurse intervene?
   1. The UAP leans forward over the mannikin and creates pressure to depress the sternum at least 2 inches (5 cm).
   2. The UAP compresses at a rate of 100 to 120 compressions per minute without pausing between compressions.
   3. The UAP places the heel of one hand over the lower end of the sternum and places heel of the other hand on top.
   4. The UAP interlaces fingers to keep them off the chest and keeps hands in contact with the chest.

8. The nurse initiates CPR on a frail older woman who has cardiac arrest. During the compressions, the nurse hears and feels the cracking of the ribs. What would the nurse do?
   1. Change hand position and then continue compressions.
   2. Stop compressions and assess for crepitus or flail chest.
   3. Stop compressions but continue to deliver the rescue breaths.
   4. Verify correct hand position and continue compressions.

9. The nurse is caring for a patient who may have a cervical spine injury. The patient is lying flat and begins to vomit. What would the nurse do?
   1. Use an oral suction catheter to remove vomitus and direct the patient to hold breath during suctioning.
   2. Direct the patient to look straight ahead and not move his neck, then sit him upright using the bed mechanism.
   3. Direct several people, acting together as one unit, to help logroll the victim onto his side to allow drainage.
   4. Immediately report vomiting to the HCP and ask if cervical spine injuries have been ruled out.

10. The nurse notes heavy spurting of bright-red blood from the patient's groin area after he returns from an arteriogram procedure. The nurse dons clean gloves and applies gauze and direct pressure. The gauze is quickly saturated. What would the nurse do **first**?
    1. Increase the patient's IV fluid, take vital signs, monitor bleeding, and notify the HCP.
    2. Place an additional layer of gauze on top of the saturated dressing and continue to hold pressure.
    3. Elevate the hips and apply more pressure over the groin area; ask someone to check a distal pulse.
    4. Apply a pressure bandage and monitor distal pulses, sensation, and temperature of the skin.

11. The nurse arrives outside of the public library and finds a person lying on the ground. What is the **first** action to take?
    1. Check if the victim is unconscious.
    2. Check the carotid or brachial pulse.
    3. Move the victim to a flat, hard surface.
    4. Direct someone to call 911.

12. A patient is unresponsive to normal verbal stimuli and not breathing. How does the nurse assess for a carotid pulse?
    1. Assess the location of the pulse for a maximum of 5 seconds.
    2. Check strength of the pulse for 5 seconds and then compare it to the opposite side.
    3. Assess the pulse rate for 10 seconds and then check for 3-second capillary refill.
    4. Check the rate, rhythm, and strength of the pulse for a maximum of 10 seconds.

13. Which sign or symptom of a foreign body airway obstruction is of **greatest** concern?
    1. Patient says, "I think I swallowed something."
    2. Patient is coughing so hard that he can't speak.
    3. Patient makes a wheezing sound between coughs.
    4. Patient demonstrates a high-pitched inspiratory noise.

14. The person gives the universal sign for choking. How does the nurse prepare to perform abdominal thrusts?
    1. Instructs the person to lean over the back of a chair
    2. Places the fist over the sternum
    3. Places the fist slightly above the navel
    4. Puts the heel of the hand over the xiphoid process

15. For an unconscious adult victim with a foreign body airway obstruction, what would the nurse do?
    1. Apply a series of three quick chest thrusts.
    2. Repeat 10 abdominal thrusts and attempt to ventilate.
    3. Perform finger sweeps between abdominal thrusts.
    4. Visually look for object each time before providing a breath.

16. Which interventions are appropriate for a victim who is in hypovolemic shock at the scene of an accident? **Select all that apply.**
    1. Establish airway.
    2. Control bleeding.
    3. Keep the head elevated.
    4. Cover with a blanket or coat.
    5. Provide oral fluids, such as water.
    6. Administer over-the-counter analgesics.

17. During a camping trip, a person who is allergic to bee stings is stung by a bee. The nurse immediately scrapes the skin to remove the stinger. Which question would the nurse ask **first**?
    1. "What happens when you get stung by a bee?"
    2. "Do you want to go to the hospital?"
    3. "Where is your epinephrine pen?"
    4. "Do you have any diphenhydramine?"

18. The nurse finds a person lying at the bottom of a long staircase. The person is conscious but appears dazed and confused. There are no obvious injuries or signs of bleeding. What would the nurse do **first**?
    1. Assist the person to sit up and suggest that he rest on a step.
    2. Instruct the person to remain still and ask for permission to assist.
    3. Initiate spinal cord precautions and hold head and neck in alignment.
    4. Ask the person what happened and if he is having pain or distress.

19. Two nurses are shopping together in a mall and they witness a person collapse and become unresponsive. Based on assessment, they initiate two-rescuer CPR. Under which circumstances can the two nurses discontinue the CPR? **Select all that apply.**
    1. A relative of the unresponsive person tells them to stop.
    2. Mall personnel arrive with the automated external defibrillator (AED).
    3. The curious crowd pushes in and bystanders are loud and unruly.
    4. Trained medical personnel arrive and take over CPR.
    5. The person remains unconscious but spontaneous pulse and breathing occur.
    6. A layperson offers to take over the role of doing compressions.

20. The HCP informs a patient's wife that her husband has suffered brain death and is in an irreversible coma, even though his heart is still beating. Which comment indicates that the wife has understood what the HCP said?
    1. "His heart is still beating, so there is still a chance he'll recover."
    2. "He is in a coma, but do you think that he can hear what I say?"
    3. "I must notify the family so that everyone can come and say goodbye."
    4. "How long do you think he will have to stay in the intensive care unit?"

21. Which assessment finding confirms cardiac arrest?
    1. Absence of radial pulse
    2. Absence of carotid pulse
    3. Absence of spontaneous respirations
    4. Unresponsiveness to normal stimuli

22. The latest recommendation for CPR is to go "hard and fast" when performing chest compressions. What is the **best** rationale for maintaining the recommended 100-120 compressions/minute?
    1. The rescuer will become fatigued if compressions exceed 100/minute.
    2. Lacerations of the liver or spleen are more likely to occur if speed is excessive.
    3. Releasing external chest compression allows time for blood to flow back into the heart.
    4. A smooth motion is required to prevent rocking and rolling that decrease the force.

23. The nurse is performing CPR on an infant. What is the **most** common event that could occur?
    1. Fracture of the rib
    2. Gastric distention
    3. Aspiration of emesis
    4. Laceration of spleen

24. An infant is observed picking up something from the floor and putting it into his mouth before the mother can stop him. He demonstrates coughing, gagging, stridor, and respiratory distress. What would the nurse do **first**?
    1. Instruct the mother to hold the child and look into the mouth with a flashlight.
    2. Place the infant in a supine position and deliver five chest thrusts.
    3. Place two fingers just above the navel and deliver five abdominal thrusts.
    4. Hold the infant with the head lower than trunk and deliver five back blows.

25. The nurse is assessing a trauma patient who was treated for shock in the emergency department. Oliguria is noted and immediately reported to the HCP. Which complication is **most** related to this finding?
    1. Right-sided heart failure
    2. Kidney failure
    3. Paralytic ileus
    4. Electrolyte imbalance

26. The nurse hears a scream; a patient has slipped in the bathroom. There is bright-red blood spurting from her forearm. What would the nurse do **first**?
    1. Don sterile gloves and apply firm pressure using a sterile gauze pad.
    2. Use layers of sterile dressing material and wrap them snugly with an elastic bandage.
    3. Don clean gloves and use a clean towel to apply direct pressure; elevate the arm.
    4. Locate the brachial artery and use the heel of the hand to compress the artery.

27. Under what circumstances would the nurse use a tourniquet?
    1. The nurse is acting in good faith and conforms to Good Samaritan principles.
    2. The HCP gives a telephone order to apply a tourniquet.
    3. The victim tells the nurse to apply a tourniquet.
    4. Pressure and elevation have failed to control life-threatening bleeding.

28. An older patient comes to the clinic for epistaxis. It is readily controlled with steady pressure applied to the bridge of the nose. Which additional assessment is **most** important for this patient?
    1. Measuring the blood pressure
    2. Assess self-care and hygiene
    3. Ask about first-aid measures
    4. Checking an oral temperature

29. Which patient has the **greatest** risk for internal bleeding?
    1. A 20-month-old child who stumbled and struck his forehead on a coffee table
    2. A 70-year-old woman sustained a hip fracture and takes an anticoagulant
    3. A 25-year-old man who was punched and kicked in the stomach
    4. A 30-year-old woman who was admitted for postpartum hemorrhage

30. A young man, who is injured, is brought to the clinic by his friends. They are all very excited, but they are able to point out that he has a stick poking out of the anterior chest wall. Which symptoms indicate that the patient has a pneumothorax? **Select all that apply.**
    1. Pain worsens with inspiration and expiration efforts.
    2. Breathing is labored and difficult.
    3. A hissing sound is audible as air flows in and out of his chest.
    4. The patient is unconscious and unresponsive to normal stimuli.
    5. Pulse is weak, rapid, and thready.
    6. His chest does not expand on the side of injury during inspiration.

31. The home health nurse sees the patient lying on the floor. On entering the house, the nurse can smell a strong odor of gas and the house is extremely hot. What would the nurse do **first**?
    1. Step out of the house and call 911.
    2. Call Poison Control and describe situation.
    3. Establish responsiveness and start cooling measures.
    4. Open the windows and move the patient out of the house.

32. The nurse comes home and finds that her teenage son and his friends have been challenging each other to chug large shots of whiskey. Which adolescent needs to be taken to the hospital for serious alcohol intoxication?
    1. Face appears flushed and seems sleepy.
    2. Demonstrates slurred speech and continuously giggles.
    3. Is loudly singing and starting to remove clothes.
    4. Is incontinent of bowel and bladder and is hallucinating.

33. It's the Fourth of July and the nurse is working at a walk-in clinic. Several people who were viewing a parade come in and report abdominal cramps, headache, weakness, nausea, and diaphoresis. All are alert and oriented. Which intervention would the nurse use **first**?
    1. Establish peripheral intravenous sites on everyone.
    2. Give everyone several cool compresses.
    3. Assist everyone to remove constrictive clothing.
    4. Move everyone into a cool environment.

34. A person sustains full-thickness burns to both forearms while lighting an outdoor grill. The nurse would intervene if a bystander attempts to perform which action?
    1. Removes smoldering clothing
    2. Removes victim's wedding ring
    3. Applies an antiseptic cream to the burns
    4. Places forearms in cold water

35. Which patient is **most** likely to need a tetanus toxoid injection?
    1. Patient fell off a bike and has abrasions on the knee, last known tetanus shot was several years ago.
    2. Patient sustained a puncture wound from stepping on an old nail that went through his workboots.
    3. Patient was elbowed during a basketball game and has swelling and ecchymoses on right lateral chest.
    4. Patient sustained a deep cut on the hand while washing a drinking glass; there was extensive bleeding.

36. The patient has a sutured laceration on the palmar surface of the hand. When will the supervising nurse intervene?
    1. The student nurse positions the hand in the anatomical position before applying the bandage.
    2. The student nurse covers the entire wound with the dressing and roller gauze is applied uniformly.
    3. The student nurse applies roller gauze with a number of evenly spaced overlapping turns.
    4. The student nurse covers the tips of the fingers with the gauze bandage and secures roller gauze with tape.

37. The nurse is on a hiking trip and one of the children finds an injured bat and picks it up. The bat bites the child before any of the adults can intervene. What would the nurse do **first**?
    1. Monitor for shock and seek medical attention immediately.
    2. Capture the bat and observe for injury or signs and symptoms of disease.
    3. Immediately and thoroughly wash the bite area with soap and water.
    4. Assess for and control bleeding and apply a thick gauze bandage.

38. What are the signs and symptoms of hypothermia? **Select all that apply.**
    1. Bounding, rapid pulse
    2. Uncontrollable shivering
    3. Slow, slurred speech
    4. Disorientation and confusion
    5. Uncoordinated or decreased muscle control
    6. Mottled skin

39. For the unconscious victim with hypothermia, which intervention can be provided at the scene?
    1. Give small sips of warm liquid very slowly.
    2. Remove wet clothes and wrap in warm blankets.
    3. Submerge the victim in a warm tub of water.
    4. Gently rub extremities to stimulate circulation.

CRITICAL THINKING ACTIVITIES

40. The nurse comes upon the scene of a motor vehicle accident. Several people are standing around a woman who is lying on the ground in a supine position. She is crying and trying to sit up. The right sleeve of her blouse is torn and blood is pooling on the asphalt underneath her arm.

    a. How does the Good Samaritan law affect the nurse in the situation?_____

    _____

    _____

    b. What actions should the nurse take to help this victim? _____

    _____

    _____

    c. What assessments would lead the nurse to believe the victim is in shock? _____

    _____

    _____

    d. What interventions are appropriate for a victim in shock at the scene of an accident? _____

    _____

    _____

41. Review Box 16.2 and think about the events that necessitate CPR. Select one (or two) of the events that you are most likely to encounter because of your work or family/home situation and mentally "rehearse" how you would respond. Based on your mental rehearsal of the event, identify information, equipment, skills, or safety precautions that you want to have if the actual event happens.

    _____

    _____

    _____

    _____

    _____

    _____

    _____

NEXT-GENERATION NCLEX™ (NGN)

42. Enhanced Hot Spot

Cognitive Skill: Analyze Cues

Scenario: The nurse is hiking with a group of friends on a cool, windy autumn day. They come across a man who is sitting in the middle of the trail. He is alert but confused and his speech is slurred. His clothes are wet and muddy, and he is not wearing any shoes. Others in the group look around to see if they can find any additional clues about what happened to the man. The nurse starts to assess the man and notes that he is shivering and decides to assess him for additional signs of hypothermia.

What factors and observations support the nurse's decision to assess for additional signs and symptoms of hypothermia?

Instructions: Underline or highlight risk factors and assessment findings in the scenario that support the nurse's suspicion that the person is hypothermic.

Dosage Calculation and Medication Administration

Answer Key: A complete Answer Key is provided in your Additional Learning Resources on Evolve.

BASIC MATH REVIEW

Directions: Use basic math functions (e.g., addition, subtraction, conversion, rounding, etc.) to solve the review problems.

1. Change the improper fraction to a mixed number: $\frac{8}{5}$ = _____

2. Change the mixed number to an improper fraction: $7\frac{5}{8}$ = _____

3. Reduce the fraction to the lowest term: $\frac{25}{100}$ = _____

4. Add the fractions and reduce the sum to its lowest term: $2\frac{1}{3} + 5\frac{1}{4}$ = _____

5. Subtract the fractions and reduce the answer to its lowest term: $\frac{1}{2} - \frac{1}{3}$ = _____

6. Multiply the fractions and reduce the product to its lowest term: $\frac{1}{3} \times \frac{3}{12}$ = _____

7. Divide the fractions and reduce the answer to its lowest term: $\frac{3}{10} \div \frac{5}{25}$ = _____

8. Add the decimals: 57.629 + 14.22 = _____

9. Subtract the decimals: 0.089 − 0.0057 = _____

10. Round the decimal to hundredths and then to tenths: 5.753 = _____ _____

11. Multiply the decimals: 64.75 × 22.9 = _____

12. Divide the decimals and round to the nearest hundredth: 2.9 ÷ 0.218 = _____

13. Convert the fraction into a decimal: $\frac{1}{2}$ = _____

14. Convert the fraction into percent: $\frac{75}{100}$ = _____

15. Solve for X: 20 : 40 = X : 5   X = _____

TABLE ACTIVITY

16. *Directions:* In the table below, fill in the metric measures that are equivalent to the amount given as apothecary measures, according to the conversion information in your textbook.

Equivalents for Metric and Apothecary Measures

Metric	Apothecary
_____ milligrams	1 grain
_____ kilograms	1 pound
_____ kilograms	2.2 pounds
_____ milliliters	1 fluid ounce
_____ milliliters	1 pint
_____ milliliters	1 quart

Converting Equivalents

17. *Directions:* Convert and calculate the following equivalents using the equivalent measure information from your textbook for conversion.

    a. 30 mL = _____ ounces
    b. 1000 mL = _____ liters
    c. 1 L = _____ quarts
    d. 500 mL = _____ pints
    e. 60 mg = _____ grains
    f. 1 kg = _____ pounds
    g. 400 mL = _____ liters
    h. 2 mcg = _____ milligrams
    i. 4 mg = _____ grams
    j. 44 pounds = _____ kilograms (round to whole number)
    k. 5 mg = _____ micrograms
    l. 1 inch = _____ centimeters
    m. 25 inches = _____ centimeters
    n. 225 pounds = _____ kilograms (round to whole number)
    o. 8 ounces = _____ milliliters
    p. 24 ounces = _____ milliliters
    q. 250 mcg = _____ milligrams
    r. 3 teaspoons = _____ milliliters
    s. 2 tablespoons = _____ milliliters

CLINICAL APPLICATION OF MATH

Directions: Calculate the math problems using the equivalent measures from your text (i.e., 1 inch = 2.5 centimeters, 1 pound = 2.2 kilograms, 30 milliliters = 1 ounce, etc.).

18. The patient's height is 25 inches. What is the patient's height in centimeters? _____ centimeters

19. The patient's height is 36 inches. What is the patient's height in centimeters? _____ centimeters

20. The patient's abdominal girth is 38 inches. What is the patient's abdominal girth in centimeters? _____ centimeters

21. The patient weighs 158 pounds. What is the patient's weight in kilograms? _____ kilograms (round to whole number)

22. The patient weighs 57 pounds. What is the patient's weight in kilograms? _____ kilograms (round to whole number)

23. The patient weighs 12.2 kilograms. What is the patient's weight in pounds? _____ pounds (round to whole number)

24. Calculate the patient's total fluid intake for breakfast: 8 ounces of milk, 6 ounces of juice, and 10 ounces of coffee. _____ mL

25. Calculate the patient's total fluid intake for 24 hours: 16 ounces of milk, 10 ounces of coffee, 6 ounces of juice, 2 liters of water, 500 mL of IV fluid. _____ mL

26. Calculate the patient's total fluid intake and output for 24 hours: 6 ounces of milk, 16 ounces of coffee, 3 liters of water, 250 mL of IV fluid. Intake _____ mL
Urine 2950 mL, wound drainage 200 mL. Output _____ mL

27. The prescription is for carbamazepine 200 mg po tid. Available—carbamazepine 100-mg tablets. How many tablets should be given per dose? _____ tablets

28. The prescription is for methyldopa 250 mg po bid. Available—methyldopa 125-mg tablets. How many tablets should be given per dose? _____ tablets

29. The prescription is for penicillin suspension 500,000 units po. Available—penicillin suspension 200,000 units/5 mL. How much should be prepared? _____ mL

30. The prescription is for morphine 4 mg IM PRN for pain. Available—morphine 10 mg/mL. How much should be prepared? _____ mL

31. The prescription is for heparin 5000 units subQ. Available—heparin 10,000 units/mL. How much should be given? _____ mL

32. The prescription is for methylprednisolone sodium succinate 50 mg IV. Available—methylprednisolone sodium succinate 125 mg/2 mL. How much is prepared? _____ mL

33. Using Young's rule, identify the dose for a child who is 3 years old when the adult dose is 75 mg. _____ mg

34. Using Clark's rule, identify the dose for a child who weighs 30 pounds when the adult dose is 50 mg. _____ mg

35. Using Fried's rule, identify the dose for a child who is 10 months old when the adult dose is 100 mg. _____ mg

36. Using the body surface area calculation, identify the dose for a child with a body surface area of 1.1 when the adult dose is 10 mg. _____ mg

37. An IV is prescribed to infuse at 75 mL/hr. The drip factor is 10 gtt/mL. The rate of infusion should be _____ gtt/min.

38. An IV is prescribed to infuse at 125 mL/hr. The drip factor is 10 gtt/mL. The rate of infusion should be _____ gtt/min.

39. An IV is prescribed to infuse at 30 mL/hr with a microdrip set. The rate of infusion should be _____ gtt/min.

40. An IV of 1000 mL is to infuse over 6 hours. The drip factor is 15 gtt/mL. The rate of infusion should be _____ gtt/min.

41. An IV of 1000 mL is to infuse over 8 hours and the nurse will use an infusion pump that can be set to deliver fluid in mL/hour. What is the pump setting? _____ mL/hour

42. An IV of 250 mL contains potassium to be infused over 2 hours. The nurse will use an infusion pump that can be set to deliver fluid in mL/hour. What is the pump setting? _____ mL/hour

43. An IV of 100 mL contains an antibiotic to be infused over 30 minutes. The nurse will use an infusion pump that can be set to deliver fluid in mL/hour. What is the pump setting? _____ mL/hour

44. An IV of 250 mL contains an antibiotic to be infused over 1 hour and 30 minutes. The nurse will use an infusion pump that can be set to deliver fluid in mL/hour. What is the pump setting? _____ mL/hour

45. The health care provider (HCP) prescribes an IV infusion of dextrose 5% and normal saline to infuse at 125 mL/hour for 8 hours. The nurse uses an electronic infusion pump to alarm every 2 hours. How many mL should the patient receive in each 2-hour period? _____ mL

MULTIPLE CHOICE

Directions: Select the best answer(s) for each of the following questions.

46. The student nurse is administering the morning medications to the patient. When would the supervising nurse intervene?
    1. Student starts preparing the 9:00 AM medications at 08:45 AM and administers the medications by 9:15 AM.
    2. Student checks the label on the drug's container three times—before, during, and after preparation.
    3. Student asks, "Are you to Mr. Smith?" then hands medication and water to the patient.
    4. Student documents medications given at 9:15 AM immediately after leaving the patient's room.

47. When are the label checks for safe medication administration performed? **Select all that apply.**
    1. When removing the drug from where it has been stored
    2. When the pharmacy delivers a new batch of medications
    3. Before removing the medication from the container
    4. Before administering the drug to the patient
    5. At the end of every shift

48. A patient needs a PRN dose of pain medication. The HCP's prescription reads: 2 mg oral MS PRN for severe pain. The pharmacy sends magnesium sulfate. What would the nurse do **first**?
    1. Ask the patient if he has ever taken magnesium sulfate for relief of pain.
    2. Call the HCP and ask for clarification of the prescription.
    3. Use a drug reference and see if magnesium sulfate is a pain medication.
    4. Call the pharmacy and ask for clarification of what was sent.

49. A new nurse is working in a small rural long-term care facility. An older HCP routinely directs the care of the residents and he prefers to handwrite his notes and orders, rather than use a computer. What would the new nurse do **first** if the HCP's handwriting is illegible?
    1. Consult the director of nursing services about the HCP's behavior.
    2. Call the HCP for clarification whenever it is necessary.
    3. Ask the charge nurse for assistance in interpreting the handwriting.
    4. Gently offer to help the HCP learn how to use the computer.

50. Based on Joint Commission requirements, under what circumstances must the nurse perform medication reconciliation? **Select all that apply.**
    1. The patient has just been admitted to the medical-surgical unit.
    2. The HCP has just made morning rounds and several new medications are prescribed.
    3. The patient's daughter is taking her father home after a prolonged hospitalization.
    4. The patient is being transferred to a rehabilitation unit after having hip surgery.
    5. The patient has just finished a complete course of prescribed antibiotics.

51. The nurse is assigned to give routine immunizations to infants who are seen in the well-baby clinic. In addition to standard medication documentation, what must be recorded when giving immunizations?
    1. Duration and course of postinjection observation time
    2. Lot number of vial, manufacturer, and expiration date of vaccine
    3. Age of the child at time of any previous immunizations or vaccinations
    4. Informed consent with signatures from both parents or any guardians

52. The nurse is reviewing the prescriptions that the HCP wrote for several patients. Which one will the nurse attend to **first**?
    1. A prescription for a PRN stool softener
    2. A dose of antipyretic medication now
    3. A stat dose of IV epinephrine
    4. A one-time only dose of an anxiolytic

53. A prescription for codeine gr ½ is written for the patient. The medication is supplied in mg. How much would the nurse administer?
    1. 3 g
    2. 30 g
    3. 3 mg
    4. 30 mg

54. An IV of 500 mL D₅W is to infuse over 4 hours. The administration set is 15 gtt/mL. What is the correct number of gtt/min?
    1. 19 gtt/min
    2. 24 gtt/min
    3. 31 gtt/min
    4. 42 gtt/min

55. The nurse determines the location for an injection by identifying the greater trochanter of the femur, the anterosuperior iliac spine, and the iliac crest. Which injection site has the nurse located?
    1. Rectus femoris
    2. Ventrogluteal
    3. Dorsogluteal
    4. Vastus lateralis

56. Upon getting the assignment for the evening, the nurse notices that two patients on the unit have the same last name. What is the **best** way to prevent medication errors for these two patients?
    1. Ask the patients their names.
    2. Check the patients' identification bands.
    3. Ask another nurse about their identities.
    4. Verify their names with the family members.

57. The nurse is working in the newborn nursery and will be giving vitamin K injections to the babies. What is the preferred site for these injections?
    1. Deltoid
    2. Dorsogluteal
    3. Ventrogluteal
    4. Vastus lateralis

58. When preparing an opioid medication, the nurse drops the pill on the floor. What would the nurse do?
    1. Discard the medication in the biohazard container.
    2. Notify the pharmacy for a replacement dose.
    3. Wipe off the medication and administer it.
    4. Have another nurse witness the disposal of the pill.

59. When would the nurse use the Z-track technique?
    1. The patient is extremely obese.
    2. The child is younger than 5 years.
    3. The prescribed medication can irritate tissue.
    4. The prescribed dose of medication is very large.

60. A tuberculin skin test agent will be given to the patient. What site would the nurse select for this intradermal injection?
    1. Upper outer aspect of the arm
    2. Anterior aspect of the forearm
    3. Middle third of the anterior thigh
    4. A 2-inch diameter around the umbilicus

61. How does the nurse determine what the drip factor is for an IV set?
    1. Ask the charge nurse.
    2. Calculate the IV rate.
    3. Look in a reference book.
    4. Check the IV tubing box.

62. The nurse is observing the patient self-administer medication with a metered-dose inhaler (MDI). Which action by the patient requires correction and further instruction?
    1. Shakes canister to determine how much is left
    2. Inhales one puff with one inspiration
    3. Inhales medication slowly and deeply
    4. Waits 2-5 minutes between puffs

63. What types of medications cannot be crushed for ease of administration? **Select all that apply.**
    1. Extended-release capsules
    2. Tablets
    3. Sublingual tablets
    4. Enteric-coated tablets
    5. Sustained-release capsules

64. The nurse identifies that a patient is having an idiosyncratic reaction to a medication. Which patient's report is consistent with the nurse's analysis?
    1. Sedative medication causes him to be awake most of the night.
    2. Antianxiety medication seems to make the pain medication more effective.
    3. Previous dosage of pain medication does not seem to be working like it used to.
    4. Antibiotic medication seems to cause an uncomfortable, itchy rash.

65. Which route of drug administration will achieve the **fastest** onset of action?
    1. Intravenous
    2. Buccal
    3. Rectal
    4. Oral

66. The nurse has five stable patients, and each needs many medications. All of the medications are scheduled to be administered at 9:00 AM. What would the nurse do **first**?
    1. Inform the RN that some of the medications were given late, despite best efforts.
    2. Start at 08:30 AM and give medications to the most cooperative patients first.
    3. Administer as many medications at 9:00 AM as possible and then write an incident report.
    4. Ask the RN to change patient assignments so that medications are given on time.

67. An IV of 1000 mL 5% dextrose and 45% saline is to infuse over 8 hours. The IV fluid is started at 0800 hours. At 1400 hours, how much IV fluid has the patient received if the nurse correctly set the flow rate?
    1. 1000 mL
    2. 750 mL
    3. 625 mL
    4. 500 mL

68. The nurse hears in report that 1000 mL of normal saline was started at 3:00 AM to infuse at 125 mL per hour. At 7:30 AM, the nurse evaluates the patient and the IV infusion, which is running by gravity; the IV fluid bag shows that approximately 200 mL has been infused. What would the nurse do **first**?
    1. Calculate the amount of fluid that should have infused and then give it.
    2. Report the error to the charge nurse and write an incident report.
    3. Document the amount of fluid infused and the appearance of the site.
    4. Recalculate the drops/minute and reset the rate of flow to 125 mL/hour.

69. The HCP prescribes two medications and suggests to the nurse that they could be mixed together in the same syringe to prevent the patient from having to get two separate injections. The nurse mixes the drugs, but a precipitate forms in the syringe. What would the nurse do?
    1. Ask the HCP to verify the request to mix the drugs.
    2. Gently rotate the syringe between the palms of the hands to mix the solution.
    3. Discard the syringe and call the pharmacy for information about compatibilities.
    4. Administer the medications as prescribed and document the injection site.

70. The nurse is giving a patient the morning medications. The patient says, "I don't recognize this pill." What would the nurse say?
    1. "The medications that you will get in the hospital may be different than the ones you take at home."
    2. "Medications are made by different manufacturers. They can be chemically identical but have a different appearance."
    3. "Let me review the list of your home medications and I'll find out if anything new was prescribed for you."
    4. "I carefully checked all of your medications against the HCP's prescriptions and these are correct."

71. The patient reports having an anaphylactic reaction to an IV medication but cannot remember the name. The nurse informs the HCP and the HCP tells the nurse to go ahead and administer the prescribed medication. What would the nurse do?
    1. Refuse to administer the medication because the allergy history is not clarified.
    2. Take baseline vital signs and recheck the patient frequently during the infusion.
    3. Inform the charge nurse or RN about the potential for an adverse reaction.
    4. Call the pharmacy and see if they have any records of the patient's allergies.

72. The nurse has performed a medication calculation and has determined that to give the prescribed dose, 15 tablets would have to be administered to the patient. The nurse has asked two other nurses to recheck the calculations and the answer is always 15. What would the nurse do **first**?
    1. Give the 15 tablets because the calculations have been checked and rechecked.
    2. Call the pharmacy and ask if the medication comes in a different strength.
    3. Call the HCP and ask for verification of the prescription.
    4. Consult a reliable drug reference to see if the prescribed dose is within safe range.

73. Two nurses are standing in the medication area. Nurse A is preparing medication, but hears an alarm indicating that an unstable patient needs help right away. She hands the prepared medication to Nurse B and asks her to give it to the correct patient. What would Nurse B do **first**?
    1. Go ahead and give it because she witnessed all of the preparations that Nurse A made.
    2. Inform the charge nurse that Nurse A needs assistance because of a critical patient.
    3. Give the medication, but later indicate to Nurse A that she should do the documentation.
    4. Discard the prepared medication and prepare another dose and give it to the patient.

74. The nurse is supervising a nursing student who must give several medications. The nurse would intervene if the student performed which action?
    1. Puts a suppository in a uniform pocket
    2. Used aseptic technique to handle pills
    3. Looked at the meniscus when pouring a liquid
    4. Read the label of the bottle as she took it off the shelf

75. The patient has an order for a medication that is to be delivered via an MDI. Which chronic health condition is the patient **most** likely to have?
    1. Hypertension
    2. Chronic bronchitis
    3. Diabetes mellitus
    4. Arteriosclerotic heart disease

76. Which factor would be the **most** important in the nurse's decision to choose an 18-gauge needle?
    1. Viscosity of solution
    2. Age of patient
    3. Length of needle
    4. Weight of patient

77. The nurse is assessing an existing IV that seems to have stopped infusing. What would the nurse do **first**?
    1. Recalculate the drip rate and then count the number of drops per minute.
    2. Discontinue the IV and inform the RN or HCP.
    3. Check for infiltration and ask the patient about pain or discomfort.
    4. Try repositioning the patient's extremity or adjusting the height of the IV bag.

78. The nurse is performing an intradermal injection for an allergy test. He does not aspirate for this type of injection. What is the **best** rationale for the nurse's technique?
    1. This is standard procedure and he is following the procedure manual.
    2. Aspirating can cause bruising and the patient will receive many allergy tests.
    3. There are no major veins or arteries in the intradermal tissues.
    4. The needle is so fine and short that it is unlikely to cause tissue damage.

79. The nurse is assessing a patient who is receiving IV fluid and medication. Which finding is the **most** serious?
    1. The patient complains of pain at the insertion site.
    2. The patient is dyspneic and has a weak, thready pulse.
    3. The patient's arm is swollen and the skin is cool to the touch.
    4. The patient is very scared and upset because the IV bag is empty.

80. An older patient is receiving a medication that is potentially nephrotoxic. Which assessment is the **most** relevant to potential nephrotoxicity?
    1. Change of mental status
    2. Reduced urinary output
    3. Nausea and vomiting
    4. Increased blood pressure

81. Upon assessment of the IV insertion site, the nurse suspects that the patient has phlebitis. Which assessment finding supports the nurse's analysis?
    1. Edema at the site
    2. Erythema along the vein
    3. Cool skin around site
    4. Sluggish flow of IV fluid

82. The nurse is at home and her husband accidentally gets a caustic chemical splash in his eyes. What would the nurse do **first**?
    1. Drive him to the hospital and flush his eyes with sterile normal saline.
    2. Call Poison Control and ask for advice about the specific chemical.
    3. Gently flush his eyes with tap water for at least 15 minutes.
    4. Assess him for burning, changes in visual acuity, or pain.

83. Which patient is the **most** likely candidate for the use of a Morgan lens to flush the eye?
    1. Patient has allergic conjunctivitis in both eyes.
    2. Patient was sprayed in the eyes with pepper spray.
    3. Patient needs frequent eye irrigations at home.
    4. Patient has pain after prolonged use of contact lenses.

84. Which patient is **most** likely to need an ear irrigation?
    1. A child who inserted a dried pinto bean into the ear canal
    2. A toddler who has a severe ear infection with exudate
    3. A teenager who has bleeding from the ear after a fight
    4. An older patient who reports a crackling noise in ear

CRITICAL THINKING ACTIVITIES

85. Identify home health safety information that should be included in a teaching plan for medication administration.

_____

_____

_____

86. Look at the medication prescription below for patient John Smith and identify what parts of the prescription are missing.

    John Smith: BD 6/9/51
    Penicillin G potassium 1.2 million units
    Dr. James Jones

_____

_____

_____

87. The patient needs a medication; however, to deliver the correct dose, the nurse has to perform some calculations because the amount of medication in the vial exceeds the prescribed dose. It's a very busy day. The nurse is trying to train a new nurse, there is a call light on, an HCP wants to ask about a patient, the nurse left his calculator at home, and suddenly a patient falls on the floor. The nurse instructs the new nurse to perform the calculation and after a while they go to give the medication. The patient sustains no harm, but later the nurse thinks about his day and realizes that this situation could have harmed the patient. Analyze factors that could contribute to potential errors and discuss what the nurse should have done in this situation.

_____

_____

_____

_____

FIGURE

88. The HCP prescribes 0.07 mg of epinephrine. Epinephrine Injection, USP 1:1000 (1 mg/mL) is supplied in a 1-mL ampoule single-dose container. Indicate on the tuberculin syringe how many mL the nurse will draw up.

NEXT-GENERATION NCLEX™ (NGN)

89. Extended Multiple Response

Cognitive Skill: Take Action

Scenario: The nursing supervisor of the long-term care facility asks the night-shift nurse to stay and cover for the certified medication assistant (CMA) who will be 2-3 hours late. The duties include administering the scheduled routine medications to 60 residents. While the nurse is qualified to administer the medications, he has never taken on the role of CMA and recognizes that time and task management are essential.

What can the nurse do to prevent medication errors and maximize safety during medication administration?

Instructions: Place a check mark next to actions that the nurse would take to prevent medication errors and maximize safety while performing in the unfamiliar CMA role. **Check all that apply.**

_____   1.   Take medications that are readily available from medication dispensing systems.

_____   2.   Listen to residents' comments about their medications.

_____   3.   Leave drugs in their labeled packages.

_____   4.   Ask another nurse to help prepare the residents' doses.

_____   5.   Follow the six "rights" of medication administration.

_____   6.   Read labels at least three times.

_____   7.   Prepare all of the doses for the residents, then administer at the correct time.

_____   8.   Document all medications as soon as they are administered.

_____   9.   Quickly administer drugs to all of the cooperative residents.

_____   10.   Do not allow any other activity to interrupt the administration of medication to a patient.

Fluids and Electrolytes

chapter

18

Answer Key: A complete Answer Key is provided in your Additional Learning Resources on Evolve.

TABLE ACTIVITY

1. *Directions:* List the normal value range for the electrolytes.

Electrolyte	Normal Value Range
Sodium	a.
Potassium	b.
Chloride	c.
Magnesium	d.
Bicarbonate	e.

CLINICAL APPLICATION OF MATH AND CONVERSION

Directions: Calculate or make the necessary conversions for math problems encountered in performing skills for patients.

2. Diet and fluid restriction and medications have been administered to the patient to decrease excess fluid volume. On the first day, the patient's weight was 150 pounds. After therapy, the patient's weight is 145.5 pounds. Assuming that the weight change represents fluid loss, how much fluid did the patient lose? _____ L

3. A patient with chronic renal failure is having difficulty adhering to the dietary and fluid recommendations. At the last visit, the patient's weight was 205 pounds. Today, the patient's weight is 214 pounds. Assuming that the weight change represents fluid gain, how much fluid did the patient gain? _____ L

4. The nurse is totaling the intake and output (I&O) at the end of the 8-hour shift. Data from today is recorded on the flowsheet for the patient:

Intake	Output
0800: 8 ounces coffee, 6 ounces juice	0700: 300 mL urine
10:00: 300 mL water	0930: 450 mL urine
1200: 12 ounces of chicken broth, 5 ounces Jell-O	1400: 500 mL urine
1430: 200 mL water	1500: 250 mL urine

What is the total intake? _____ mL

What is the total output? _____ mL

5. The nurse is inserting a nasogastric tube into a patient for the purpose of decompressing the stomach. During the procedure, the patient vomits 500 mL of bile emesis. This is recorded on the flowsheet. Immediately after the tube placement is established and hooked to suction, 400 mL of green bile emesis flows through the tube into the collection canister. At the end of the shift, a total of 600 mL is noted in the canister, recorded on the flowsheet and then discarded. For the urinary drainage bag, at 0700: 300 mL was recorded and discarded; at 1200: 250 mL was recorded and discarded; and at 1500: 200 mL was recorded and discarded. What was the total output at the end of the shift? _____ mL

6. The health care provider (HCP) prescribes strict I&O on a postsurgical patient. The patient has an indwelling urinary catheter; the urinary drainage bag was emptied: 0800 for 400 mL, 1200 for 450 mL. At the end of the shift, there is 700 mL in the drainage bag. The patient had one episode of vomiting clear emesis of 300 mL. The patient also has a Jackson-Pratt drain with 15 mL at the end of the shift. The patient has an IV of normal saline that is infused at 125 mL/hour for the 8-hour shift. The patient is on a clear liquid diet and intake is shown below for the shift.

Intake
0800: 8 ounces diluted apple juice
1000: 200 mL water
1200: 6 ounces broth and 3 ounces diluted juice
1430: 400 mL water

What is the total intake for the 8-hour shift? _____ mL

What is the total output for the 8-hour shift? _____ mL

MULTIPLE CHOICE

Directions: Select the best answer(s) for each of the following questions.

7. The patient is experiencing hyperkalemia. What treatment does the nurse anticipate?
   1. Intravenous (IV) calcium
   2. Fluid restrictions
   3. Foods high in potassium
   4. Administration of loop diuretics

8. Following thyroid surgery, the patient reports nausea and a tingling sensation around nose, mouth, ears, fingers, and toes. The nurse observes muscle spasms in the patient's feet and hands. What is the **most** important sign/symptom for the nurse to observe for and report?
   1. Respiratory distress
   2. Altered mental status progressing to seizure
   3. Polyuria and excessive thirst
   4. Positive Chvostek's sign

9. Which patient has the **greatest** risk for dehydration?
   1. 30-year-old female with vomiting and diarrhea
   2. 72-year-old obese male with a fever and anorexia
   3. 2-year-old with an ear infection and vomiting
   4. 45-year-old underweight female with influenza

10. The nurse offers to take an older neighbor to the grocery store. As they are shopping, the neighbor tells the nurse that, "My doctor told me to watch my salt intake." Which items in the shopping cart would the nurse suggest they put back on the shelf? **Select all that apply.**
    1. Cheddar cheese
    2. Ketchup
    3. Oranges
    4. Pretzels
    5. Frozen TV dinner

11. The nurse sees that the patient is scheduled to have a potassium supplement. In addition to the last potassium level, what would the nurse assess before administering the potassium?
    1. Urinary output
    2. Blood pressure
    3. Respiratory rate
    4. Hematocrit level

12. The nurse notes that a resident who lives in a long-term care center has poor fluid intake and spends most of the day dozing in a chair. Based on this observation, which subjective report is the resident **most** likely to report?
    1. Shortness of breath
    2. Constipation
    3. Nausea
    4. Headache

13. A patient with diabetes reports nausea and headache and he appears lethargic. The nurse observes that he is breathing very deeply and rapidly. Based on the assessment findings and the laboratory results, what does the nurse suspect?

pH	7.30 (7.30)
Pa_{CO_2}	30 mm Hg (4 kPa)
Pa_{O_2}	70 mm Hg (9.33 kPa)
O_2 saturation	98%
HCO_3^-	18 mEq (18 mmol/L)
K^+	6.5 mEq/L (6.5 mmol/L)

    1. Metabolic alkalosis
    2. Metabolic acidosis
    3. Respiratory alkalosis
    4. Respiratory acidosis

14. The patient is encouraged by his doctor to eat foods that are rich in potassium. Which lunch tray would be the **best**?
    1. Seafood salad with crackers and strawberries with whipped cream
    2. Egg salad on whole grain bread with coffee and potato chips
    3. Grilled white toast with tomato soup and orange juice
    4. Pork cutlet with milk gravy and mushrooms and melon salad

15. The nurse is supervising a new nurse who will administer IV potassium to a patient. When would the supervising nurse intervene?
    1. New nurse delegates unlicensed assistive personnel (UAP) to obtain an infusion controller
    2. New nurse checks the HCP's prescription for the dose, route and time of medication
    3. New nurse draws dose with a sterile needle and syringe and scrubs the IV insertion port
    4. New nurse calls pharmacy to find out when the potassium infusion will be ready

16. Earlier in the shift a patient with severe diarrhea seemed irritable, anxious, and twitchy. The RN calls from the patient's room and asks that a vial of calcium gluconate be brought to the room immediately. In addition, to the calcium gluconate, which emergency equipment would the LPN/LVN try to quickly obtain for patient with a very low calcium?
    1. Chest tube insertion tray and oxygen mask
    2. IV pump and IV normal saline for bolus
    3. Automated external defibrillator
    4. Tracheotomy tray and a resuscitation bag

17. The nurse is assessing an older adult and observes dry mucous membranes, increased heart rate, decreased blood pressure, and poor skin turgor. The patient seems mildly confused and continuously asks for water. What would the nurse do **first**?
    1. Assess the patient for additional signs of dehydration.
    2. Offer the patient a glass of water and reassess in several hours.
    3. Count the respirations and assess for additional signs of respiratory acidosis.
    4. Call the supervising RN and the HCP and report assessment findings.

18. What is the **best** food source for calcium?
    1. Milk
    2. Meat
    3. Whole grains
    4. Green leafy vegetables

19. The patient has experienced a prolonged episode of diarrhea. Which clinical observation is consistent with the development of metabolic acidosis?
    1. Increased perspiration
    2. Increased respiratory rate
    3. Increased urinary output
    4. Decreased heart rate

20. The patient has had chronic obstructive pulmonary disease (COPD) for a number of years. Which set of arterial blood gas values indicates that the patient is in respiratory acidosis?
    1. pH 7.35, $Paco_2$ 40, O_2 saturation 96%
    2. pH 7.40, $Paco_2$ 45, O_2 saturation 95%
    3. pH 7.30, $Paco_2$ 50, O_2 saturation 93%
    4. pH 7.48, $Paco_2$ 55, O_2 saturation 98%

21. While in the delivery room with his wife, the father-to-be begins to develop an anxiety reaction and lightheadedness. Which intervention does the nurse use to prevent respiratory alkalosis?
    1. Coach panting respirations.
    2. Provide nasal oxygen.
    3. Have him breathe into a paper bag.
    4. Have him cough and deep-breathe.

22. A child has gotten into the medicine cabinet in the home and ingested the remaining contents of an aspirin (acetylsalicylic acid) bottle. Which acid-base imbalances does the nurse expect to observe as a result of excessive aspirin ingestion?
    1. Metabolic acidosis and respiratory alkalosis
    2. Metabolic alkalosis and respiratory acidosis
    3. Respiratory acidosis and metabolic acidosis
    4. Respiratory alkalosis and metabolic alkalosis

23. The patient has had continuous gastric suction. The nurse recognizes that acid-base imbalances can occur with this treatment. Which laboratory data confirms metabolic alkalosis?
    1. pH elevated, $Paco_2$ normal, and HCO_3^- elevated
    2. pH elevated, $Paco_2$ elevated, and HCO_3^- decreased
    3. pH decreased, $Paco_2$ decreased, and HCO_3^- decreased
    4. pH decreased, $Paco_2$ normal, and HCO_3^- decreased

24. What is the **best** way for the nurse to determine the patient's fluid balance?
    1. Assess vital signs.
    2. Weigh the patient daily.
    3. Monitor IV fluid intake.
    4. Check diagnostic test results.

25. The patient used excessive antacids, which resulted in a serum sodium level of 150 mEq/L (150 mmol/L). Why would the HCP instruct the nurse to give an IV hypotonic solution?
    1. To correct intracellular dehydration
    2. To correct intravascular volume
    3. To increase the sodium level
    4. To pull fluid from the cells

26. The nurse is caring for a postoperative patient. Which solution is the HCP **most** likely to prescribe to replace the fluid deficiency related to the patient's NPO (nothing by mouth) status in the pre- and postoperative period?
    1. Hypotonic solution
    2. Hypertonic solution
    3. Isotonic solution
    4. Parental nutrition

27. What purposes do the electrolytes serve in the body? **Select all that apply.**
    1. Maintenance of normal body metabolism
    2. Regulation of water balance in the body
    3. Regulation of water and electrolyte contents within cells
    4. Formation of hydrochloric acid in gastric juice
    5. Transportation of nutrients to cells and waste products from cells

28. The patient has been placed on a low-sodium diet to assist in the treatment of hypertension. Which patient statement indicates an understanding of the diet teaching?
    1. "Cheese is a good between-meal snack for me."
    2. "It is okay for me to eat at my favorite seafood restaurant."
    3. "In order for me to eat enough vegetables, I can prepare canned peas and corn."
    4. "I use a lot of fresh vegetables, although I should give up table salt."

29. Which patient has the **greatest** risk for developing hypokalemia?
    1. Has a small bowel obstruction
    2. Has renal failure
    3. Consumes excessive alcohol
    4. Takes prescribed loop diuretic

30. The nurse is monitoring an older patient who is receiving a fluid bolus for dehydration. The nurse notices that the patient suddenly has a slight cough and seems a little short of breath. The patient reports, "I'm okay." What would the nurse do **first**?
    1. Notify the RN and the HCP.
    2. Auscultate the lungs and assess for fluid overload.
    3. Stop the bolus infusion and establish a saline lock.
    4. Weigh the patient and compare to baseline.

31. The nurse receives notification from the laboratory that a patient's potassium level is 6 mEq/L (6 mmol/L). The nurse has paged the HCP and is awaiting a call back. What would the nurse do **first**?
    1. Attach the patient to a cardiac monitor.
    2. Encourage foods and fluids that contain potassium.
    3. Prepare a dose of intravenous calcium gluconate.
    4. Check medications that could affect potassium levels.

32. The nurse is checking the laboratory data of a woman who is at risk for osteoporosis. Which electrolyte value is **most** relevant to this condition?
    1. Sodium level
    2. Calcium level
    3. Potassium level
    4. Phosphorus level

33. The nurse hears in report that the patient has been receiving aluminum hydroxide to correct an electrolyte imbalance. Which electrolyte level would the nurse check to evaluate the efficacy of the medication?
    1. Phosphorus level
    2. Magnesium level
    3. Bicarbonate level
    4. Calcium level

34. The nurse is caring for a patient who had surgery on the parathyroid glands. Which electrolyte level in the low-normal range is the **greatest** concern?
    1. Calcium
    2. Sodium
    3. Potassium
    4. Magnesium

35. The patient has a medical diagnosis of diabetic ketoacidosis. Which clinical manifestation indicates that the blood buffer system is exhausted?
    1. Urinary output is decreased.
    2. Respiratory rate is increased.
    3. Heart rate is decreased.
    4. pH is increased.

36. The patient is on mechanical ventilation. The arterial blood gas results indicate that the patient has respiratory alkalosis. What would the nurse do **first**?
    1. Suction the airway for excessive secretions or a mucus plug.
    2. Notify the RN or the HCP.
    3. Check the ventilator settings and compare to the orders.
    4. Deliver breaths using a bag-valve-mask with high-flow oxygen.

37. The patient needs to have accurate intake and output recorded for every shift. Which sensible fluid losses must be included in the output? **Select all that apply.**
    1. Diarrhea stools
    2. Hemovac drainage
    3. Contents from an ileostomy bag
    4. Secretions from nasogastric suction
    5. Drainage from indwelling urinary catheter bag
    6. Water in the water-seal chamber of the chest tube

38. The nurse is supervising a nursing student who is inserting an intravenous (IV) catheter. Which action prompts the supervising nurse to intervene?
    1. Student looks for vein in the forearm distal to a dialysis shunt
    2. Student palpates a vein by pressing to feel a soft, bouncy resistance.
    3. Student removes the tourniquet after 30 seconds of looking for a vein
    4. Student looks for a vein in the most distal area of the nondominant arm.

39. The RN initiates a blood transfusion and then the LPN/LVN is assigned to monitor patient. An hour after the transfusion is started, the patient reports nausea, "not feeling right" and demonstrates wheezing. What would the LPN/LVN do **first**?
    1. Notify the RN who started the transfusion.
    2. Take vital signs and auscultate lung sounds.
    3. Stop the transfusion and keep vein open with normal saline.
    4. Slow the transfusion and observe for other signs of distress.

40. The patient has an IV infusion of normal saline. The patient reports mild discomfort at the insertion site and the nurse observes the skin is pale, edematous, feels cool to the touch, and the flow rate is sluggish. What would the nurse do?
    1. Reposition the arm.
    2. Increase the flow rate.
    3. Call the HCP.
    4. Discontinue the IV.

41. The nurse meets resistance while attempting to flush an intermittent saline lock with 10 mL of saline. Which action would the nurse take **first**?
    1. Reposition arm and increase the force.
    2. Assess for kinks or clamped tubing.
    3. Remove the saline lock and reestablish.
    4. Flush with low-dose heparin solution

CRITICAL THINKING ACTIVITIES

42. The nurse is caring for an older patient who was brought to the hospital for confusion. The family reports that the patient lives alone and is usually alert and independent, but recently complained of stomach cramps, vomiting, and diarrhea. The nurse notes that home medications include a diuretic and blood pressure medication. Mucous membranes are dry. Laboratory results show potassium 3.4 mEq/L (3.4 mmol/L) and serum sodium 127 mEq/L (127 mmol/L).

    a. Identify at least two considerations for the older adult patient regarding fluid, electrolyte, and acid-base balance.

    _____

    _____

    b. What is the clinical significance of a serum potassium of 3.4 mEq/L (3.4 mmol/L)?_____

    _____

    _____

    c. For this patient, what factors are likely to be contributing to the current serum potassium value?

    _____

    _____

d. What are the most common signs/symptoms associated with hypokalemia, and what are the nursing interventions for the imbalance?

_____

_____

e. What is the clinical significance of a serum sodium of 127 mEq/L (127 mmol/L)? _____

_____

_____

f. Identify the **most** common signs and symptoms of hyponatremia, and nursing interventions for the imbalance.

_____

_____

g. The nurse is monitoring the patient's I&O. What would be counted as part of the output?

_____

_____

43. The nurse is caring for a patient with pneumonia. The patient is having dyspnea. The following laboratory data are available for review.

pH	7.30 (7.30)
$Paco_2$	50 mm Hg (6.67 kPa)
Pao_2	70 mm Hg (9.33 kPa)
O_2 saturation	90%
HCO_3^-	22 mEq (22 mmol/L)

a. What do these laboratory values suggest for this patient? _____

_____

b. What signs and symptoms are likely to be associated with the laboratory values? _____

_____

_____

_____

c. What treatment does the nurse anticipate will be ordered for this patient?_____

_____

_____

_____

NEXT-GENERATION NCLEX™ (NGN)

44. Matrix

Cognitive Skill: Take Action

Scenario: The patient has chronic kidney disease and has trouble adhering to dietary recommendations and managing medications. Consequently, the patient has had frequent episodes where his serum potassium level was greater than 5 mEq/L (5 mmol/L). Currently, his potassium level is 5.5 mEq/L (5.5 mmol/L). He was referred to home health for close monitoring of potassium level and assistance with diet and medications.

Which HCP prescriptions and nursing interventions will the nurse use?

Instructions: Use an X to indicate which HCP prescriptions and nursing interventions are essential, nonessential, or contraindicated.

HCP Prescriptions and Nursing Interventions	Essential	Nonessential	Contraindicated
Monitor I&O.			
Administer sodium polystyrene sulfonate.			
Encourage intake of foods such as bananas, dried fruits, peanut butter.			
Be alert for stridor, dyspnea, or crowing.			
Monitor bowel sounds, as well as number and character of bowel movements.			
Administer potassium chloride (KCl) supplement.			
Assess vital signs.			
Monitor serum potassium level.			

Nutritional Concepts and Related Therapies

chapter

19

Answer Key: A complete Answer Key is provided in your Additional Learning Resources on Evolve.

SHORT ANSWER

Directions: Using your own words, answer each question in the space provided.

1. Identify the six classes of nutrients and their general function. _____

   _____

   _____

2. For each vitamin, identify a food source, its function in the body, and signs and symptoms of deficiency and toxicity (if applicable).

   a. Vitamin A: _____

   _____

   b. Vitamin D: _____

   _____

   c. Vitamin K: _____

   _____

3. For each mineral, identify a food source, its function in the body, and signs and symptoms of deficiency and toxicity (if applicable).

   a. Calcium: _____

   _____

   b. Potassium: _____

   _____

   c. Sodium: _____

   _____

CLINICAL APPLICATION OF MATH AND CONVERSION

Directions: Calculate or make the necessary conversions for math problems encountered in performing skills for patients.

4. The health care provider (HCP) prescribes an enteral feeding to infuse at 30 mL/hour for 3 hours and then to check the residual and notify with the results. How many mL will the patient receive in 3 hours? _____ mL

5. The patient was directed by the HCP to consume 1500 kcal/day to achieve weight-loss goals. If the patient consumes 60% carbohydrates, 20% protein, and 20% fats, calculate the total number of grams/day for carbohydrates _____ g; fats _____ g; and protein _____ g. (Recall that carbohydrates and protein will provide 4 kcal/g. Fats provide 9 kcal/g.)

6. According to the dietary reference intake (DRI), the protein requirement for healthy adults is 0.8 g/kg of body weight per day. How many grams of protein does a man require if he weighs 185 pounds? _____ g

7. According to the DRI, the carbohydrate requirement for healthy adults should be between 45% and 65% of daily kilocalories per day. For a person who is consuming 1500 kilocalories per day, what is the range of kilocalories that should come from carbohydrates? _____ kcal to _____ kcal

8. The nutrition label on a jar of peanut butter indicates that there are 16 g of total fat, 8 g of carbohydrates, and 7 g of protein per serving. Based on information from the textbook (carbohydrates and protein will provide 4 kcal/g and fats provide 9 kcal/g), calculate how many kilocalories are in a serving of peanut butter. _____ kcal

9. Calculate your own body mass index (BMI). _____

10. A patient with end-stage renal disease has the following urinary output from the past 24 hours: 15 mL at 0700, 20 mL at 1200, 30 mL at 1700, 10 mL at 2100, and 5 mL at 0400. The HCP's prescription for fluid restriction is 750 mL + urine output from previous 24 hours. How much fluid is the patient allowed to have? _____ mL

11. The patient is receiving enteral feedings per nasogastric (NG) tube. The provider prescribes water to infuse at 100 mL/hr every 6 hours. How much water per NG tube should the patient receive every 24 hours? _____ mL

TABLE ACTIVITY

12. *Directions:* Complete the table below with the missing numerical value or the interpretation of the numerical value. The first block is done for you.

Numerical Value	Interpretation of Numerical Value
LDL Cholesterol	
<100	Optimal
100-129	
	Borderline high
160-189	
	Very high
Total Cholesterol	
	Desirable
200-239	
≥240	
HDL Cholesterol	
<40 men; <50 women	

FIGURE LABELING

13. *Directions:* Label the figure with the correct tube feeding sites.

MULTIPLE CHOICE

Directions: Select the best answer(s) for each of the following questions.

14. The nurse is teaching a patient who has heart failure to read nutrition labels on food products. Which nutritional fact is the **most** important for this patient to pay attention to?
    1. The total number of kilocalories of fat per serving
    2. The % daily value of fiber provided in a serving
    3. The number of milligrams of sodium per serving
    4. The number of grams of protein per serving

15. The patient has risk for osteoporosis. Which foods is the nurse **most** likely to suggest?
    1. Eggs, raw fruits and vegetables
    2. Whole-grain breads and pasta, and poultry
    3. Green leafy vegetables and citrus fruits
    4. Sardines, tofu, cheese, and broccoli

16. Which laboratory result is the nurse **most** likely to examine to determine if the treatment for iron deficiency anemia is effective?
    1. Hemoglobin level
    2. Electrolyte values
    3. Blood clotting factors
    4. Albumin level

17. Which patient is **most** likely to benefit from an increase in dietary fiber?
    1. Has chronic obstructive pulmonary disease
    2. Has a high risk for metabolic syndrome
    3. Has a high risk for osteoporosis
    4. Has a recent diagnosis of hepatitis

18. A parent tells the nurse, "The school nutritionist advised parents to send packed lunches that include complete proteins, but I'm not exactly sure what that means." Which is the **best** response?
    1. "What would you normally send in a packed lunch?"
    2. "Just pack a variety of foods that you know your child will eat."
    3. "Complete proteins are generally of animal origin, like eggs or meat, but a complete protein can also be made of a combination of plant-based foods."
    4. "Does your child have any dietary restrictions or food allergies?"

19. A patient is interested in adding antioxidants to the diet. What is the **best** advice?
    1. Take vitamin supplements, especially A, C, and E.
    2. Eat a wide variety of fruits and vegetables.
    3. Eat dairy products such as cheese, yogurt, and milk.
    4. Take a multi-vitamin and mineral supplement.

20. According to the National Institute of Health's Office of Dietary Supplements, which patient would be advised to have an additional 35 mg/day of vitamin C beyond the usual recommended adult dose?
    1. A patient who was recently diagnosed with cancer.
    2. A patient who has recent onset of cold symptoms.
    3. A patient who drinks alcohol daily.
    4. A patient who smokes cigarettes every day.

21. The patient is interested in lowering his cholesterol levels and reducing the risk of cardiovascular disease. Which breakfast tray offers the **most** water-soluble fiber to help the patient meet his goals?
    1. Half a grapefruit with hard-boiled egg
    2. Hash-browned potatoes with sausage patty
    3. Yogurt with honey, granola, and fresh strawberries
    4. Oatmeal topped with cinnamon and raw apple slices

22. Which patients have conditions that would prompt the nurse to monitor serum sodium levels? **Select all that apply.**
    1. The patient is having a prolonged high fever.
    2. The patient has severe diarrhea and vomiting.
    3. The patient has iron deficiency anemia.
    4. The patient has chronic kidney disease.
    5. The patient has cystic fibrosis.

23. The home health nurse sees that the patient's potassium level is 3.6 mmol/L. There is nothing in the patient's medication or health history that should affect the potassium levels. What will the nurse do?
    1. Tell the patient to make an appointment to see the HCP as soon as possible.
    2. Suggest that the patient eat sweet potatoes, fruits, vegetables, fresh meat, legumes, and milk.
    3. Take vital signs and assess the patient for signs/symptoms of hyperkalemia.
    4. Instruct the patient to have a potassium test repeated every 12-18 months.

24. The nurse is assessing an older resident at a long-term care center. The resident appears flushed, skin turgor is poor, mucous membranes are dry, and resident seems unusually irritable. What would the nurse do **first**?
    1. Test for gag reflex; then offer oral fluids.
    2. Obtain an order for electrolyte values.
    3. Take vital signs and check urine specific gravity.
    4. Check blood sugar and offer a popsicle.

25. A woman is in the first trimester of pregnancy. She reports several episodes of nausea and vomiting, a headache, and irritability. The nurse observes shallow breathing and perspiration, and the woman appears shaky and nervous. What would the nurse do **first**?
    1. Check blood glucose level.
    2. Take the temperature.
    3. Check pulse oximeter reading.
    4. Attach electrocardiogram monitor.

26. The patient is going to be discharged with a prescription for an anticoagulant medication. Which question would the nurse ask?
    1. "How many servings of leafy green vegetables would you normally eat in a week?"
    2. "Do you drink at least 8 glasses of fluid every day?"
    3. "What would you typically eat for breakfast every morning?"
    4. "Are you having any problems with constipation or adequate fiber intake?"

27. The patient reports noticing that his gums bleed very easily. If the bleeding is caused by a nutritional deficiency, which types of food will correct the problem?
    1. Milk, egg yolks, and liver
    2. Broccoli, peppers, and tomatoes
    3. Cereals, legumes, and nuts
    4. Poultry, fish, and brown rice

28. Which patient is at risk for pernicious anemia and is **most** likely to be prescribed a vitamin B_{12} supplement?
    1. Frequently tries different weight-loss plans
    2. Eats small amounts of a variety of foods
    3. Prefers meat and potatoes, with very few vegetables
    4. Adheres to a strict vegan diet

29. The nurse is working with a patient who requires an increase in complete proteins in the diet. Which foods will the nurse recommend? **Select all that apply.**
    1. Soy
    2. Eggs
    3. Peanuts
    4. Beans
    5. Fish
    6. Yogurt

30. A patient reports routinely taking high doses of vitamin supplements. Which vitamin has the **greatest** potential for toxic effects related to high dosage?
    1. A
    2. B_1 (thiamine)
    3. B_2 (riboflavin)
    4. C

31. A patient with ascites has fluid restrictions of 1000 mL/24 hours. The nurse observes that the patient frequently asks visitors and staff to give him extra fluids. What would the nurse do **first** to improve the patient's compliance?
    1. Assess the patient's understanding of the fluid restrictions.
    2. Offer suggestions to decrease sensation of thirst (e.g., chew gum).
    3. Post a sign over the bed that indicates fluid limits.
    4. Instruct family, friends, and staff that fluids are limited and measured.

32. Which item is allowed on a clear liquid diet?
    1. Orange juice
    2. Gelatin
    3. Sherbet
    4. Cream soup

33. Which patient is **most** likely to be prescribed a carbohydrate-modified diet?
    1. Has heart failure
    2. Has hypertension
    3. Has cirrhosis of the liver
    4. Has diabetes mellitus

34. An Asian American patient reports experiencing nausea, a bloated feeling, and flatulence after eating. Which question is the **most** relevant?
    1. "Do you have any food allergies?"
    2. "Are you following the MyPlate guidelines?"
    3. "What did you eat just before the onset of the symptoms?"
    4. "Is anyone who ate the same food having the same symptoms?"

35. Patients with nasogastric (NG) tubes may develop otitis media. What will the nurse do to prevent this occurrence?
    1. Increase fluid intake.
    2. Remove and reinsert the tube every 24 hours.
    3. Suction the nose and mouth.
    4. Turn the patient side to side every 2 hours.

36. The nurse is evaluating the performance of an unlicensed assistive personnel (UAP) who is feeding a patient. Which action indicates a need for correction?
    1. Offering the patient the bedpan before the meal.
    2. Placing the patient in a recumbent position.
    3. Providing opportunity for hand hygiene before the meal.
    4. Talking with the patient during the feeding.

37. Which admission assessments would be performed for long-term care residents in relation to potential nutritional problems? **Select all that apply.**
    1. Problems with fine motor movements
    2. Ability to chew and swallow different textures of foods
    3. Typical daily fluid intake
    4. Ability to obtain and prepare own food
    5. Dietary restrictions related to chronic health problems
    6. Food preferences or rituals related to cultural background

38. The nurse sees an order for "clear liquid diet, advance as tolerated to regular diet." What does the nurse do to get the **best** food selection for the patient?
    1. Contact the HCP for clarification of the order.
    2. Ask the patient if he is hungry and what he prefers to eat.
    3. Assess the patient's overall response to the clear liquid diet.
    4. Call the nutritionist and ask for an individualized diet plan.

39. The mother asks the nurse about giving strained fruits to her infant. When would this food be introduced?
    1. 2 months
    2. 5 months
    3. 8 months
    4. 12 months

40. The patient is taking a diuretic medication every day. Which electrolyte value is the **most** important to monitor?
    1. Chloride
    2. Sodium
    3. Phosphorus
    4. Potassium

41. What are nursing responsibilities in promoting nutrition for patients? **Select all that apply.**
    1. Assisting patients to eat or drink
    2. Designing diet plans for patients with chronic health problems
    3. Recording the patient's fluid and food intake
    4. Observing the patient for signs of poor nutrition
    5. Communicating dietary concerns to other members of the health care team
    6. Monitoring laboratory values that are related to nutritional intake

42. The patient has just ordered lunch at a restaurant. According to the USDA MyPlate recommendations, which food item would the patient plan to divide and take a portion home in a carry-out box?
    1. 10 ounces grilled skinless chicken breast
    2. 1 cup of steamed vegetables
    3. ¾ cup of mixed fruit salad
    4. ¾ cup of brown rice pilaf

43. The patient is trying to understand the difference between dietary reference intakes (DRIs) and recommended dietary allowances (RDAs). Which patient statement **best** indicates an understanding of DRIs?
    1. "DRIs replace the RDAs but are similar, so I could use either one to monitor my cholesterol."
    2. "Using DRIs, I could decrease my risk for diabetes and monitor my sugar consumption."
    3. "RDAs apply to healthy adult Americans; but I should rely on DRIs because I am overweight. "
    4. "DRIs are based on disease states; so I can use them as a guideline to control my thyroid problem."

44. Following bariatric surgery, a patient experiences nausea, cramping, diarrhea, sweating, lightheadedness, and palpitations after eating. What is the **most** important self-care measure for the nurse to reinforce?
    1. Immediately report the symptoms to the surgeon; surgical intervention may be necessary.
    2. Be patient and live with the symptoms; they are expected and temporary.
    3. Avoid concentrated sweets and drink fluids 30-60 minutes before and after meals.
    4. When symptoms occur, replace the next meal with extra fluids such as diluted juices.

45. The patient has sustained severe injuries in an accident. Which food sources supply the nutrient that plays the **biggest** role in helping the patient to build and repair injured tissue?
    1. Green vegetables and bright-colored fruits
    2. Pasta and breads made from whole grains
    3. Beans, legumes, and soy products
    4. Lean meats, poultry, and fish

46. The nurse routinely participates in long distance endurance sports, such as running, swimming, and cycling. Which foods would the nurse eat to have energy over a longer period of time?
    1. Corn and potatoes
    2. Milk and citrus fruits
    3. Honey and table sugar
    4. Chocolate and electrolyte drinks

47. The nurse is talking to a patient who has high cholesterol and a family history of cardiovascular disease. Which foods are **most** likely to counteract the high cholesterol?
    1. Wheat bran and celery
    2. Orange juice and white rice
    3. Lettuce and pears
    4. Oats and barley

48. The patient reports sensations of bloating, gas, and constipation after adding lots of fruits, vegetables, and whole grains to her diet. So she has decided to go back to her former dietary pattern and exclude these foods. What is the **best** advice that the nurse can give the patient?
    1. "Resume former dietary patterns and contact your HCP."
    2. "Slowly increase intake of fiber foods and drink at least 8 glasses of water each day."
    3. "Start with a fiber supplement instead of fruits, vegetables, and whole grains."
    4. "Excessive fiber intake can lead to osteoporosis and anemia in women."

49. The patient expresses a strong preference for beef that is marbled with fat at every meal, because of the flavor and the feeling of fullness and satisfaction. Nurse would advise that this eating habit is likely to increase risk for which health condition?
    1. Osteoporosis
    2. Cirrhosis of the liver
    3. Diabetes mellitus
    4. Atherosclerosis

50. The patient tells the nurse that he has problems with his cholesterol so a friend told him to eat avocadoes. What is the **best** response?
    1. "Avocadoes are very high in fat so the total cholesterol will increase."
    2. "Avocadoes are a source of monounsaturated fats, which are thought to lower bad cholesterol."
    3. "Avocadoes are yellow fruits, and fruits generally do not affect cholesterol levels."
    4. "Avocadoes are a source of trans-fatty acids, which will increase the good cholesterol."

51. The patient was advised by the HCP to "watch intake of cholesterol." Which question is the **most** useful in assessing the likelihood of the patient's adherence to the provider's advice?
    1. "Do you understand what 'watch your intake of cholesterol' means?"
    2. "How do you plan to manage your intake of cholesterol?"
    3. "Would you like a list of foods that contain high amounts of cholesterol?"
    4. "What do you normally eat in a 24-hour period?"

52. Which laboratory value would the nurse check to evaluate the protein status of a patient who has been receiving medical nutrition therapy?
    1. Hemoglobin
    2. Albumin
    3. White blood cell count
    4. Electrolyte values

53. A patient has symptoms of steatorrhea and flatulence. Which diet is the HCP **most** likely to recommend?
    1. Carbohydrate-modified diet
    2. Protein-restricted diet
    3. Sodium-restricted diet
    4. Fat-controlled diet

54. The nurse is talking to a 17-year-old female whose parents have reluctantly allowed her to start a vegan diet if she agrees to talk to an HCP before beginning the diet. The HCP is **most** likely to monitor her for which nutrition-related condition?
    1. Anorexia nervosa
    2. Rickets
    3. Iron deficiency anemia
    4. Marasmus

55. Which patient is at the **greatest** risk for a negative nitrogen balance that will lead to atrophy of muscles?
    1. The patient gets nothing by mouth for several days due to intractable nausea and vomiting.
    2. The patient is in the first trimester of a normal pregnancy.
    3. The patient sustained severe burns to 50% of the body surface.
    4. The patient has been fasting for several days for a religious ritual.

56. During a trip to a developing country, the nurse observes that many of the toddlers appear very fat with enlarged abdomens and swollen extremities. Which nutritional deficiency is associated with these symptoms?
    1. Carbohydrates
    2. Fats
    3. Vitamins
    4. Protein

57. The patient reports a habit of smoking at least one pack of cigarettes every day. Which foods would the nurse encourage the patient to eat, because of the heavy smoking habit?
    1. Fish and poultry
    2. Milk products
    3. Citrus fruits
    4. Whole grains

58. A 69-year-old patient reports frequently taking antacids. Why does this patient have an increased risk for developing pernicious anemia?
    1. Low stomach acidity blocks the absorption of vitamin B_{12} from foods.
    2. Antacids interfere with the body's ability to use heme iron.
    3. Older people who take antacids are less likely to produce intrinsic factor.
    4. Antacids inhibit the digestion of foods that supply vitamin C.

59. The mother reports that her child took a few extra chewable vitamins, because he thought they were gummy candies. Which question is the **most** important to assess for potential toxicity?
    1. "Does the product contain vitamin C?"
    2. "How much does the child weigh?"
    3. "Is iron listed as one of the ingredients?"
    4. "Did you induce vomiting?"

60. Which patient would not be offered low-fat milk?
    1. 15-year-old female with type 1 diabetes
    2. 26-year-old female who is in the third trimester of pregnancy
    3. 68-year-old female who has hip fracture related to osteoporosis
    4. 18-month-old female who is transitioning to cow's milk

61. Which parental action encourages good dietary habits in the child?
    1. Allow the child to eat whenever he is hungry and skip meals if he is not hungry.
    2. Give the child whatever the rest of the family is eating; do not cater to special requests.
    3. Encourage the child to help with food preparation and create a positive environment.
    4. Give everyone the same serving size and quietly remove leftover food.

62. The nurse is talking to an adolescent girl about nutrition, but the girl seems bored, uninterested, and unlikely to try any of the nurse's suggestions. What would the nurse do?
    1. Delay the discussion until the girl initiates interest.
    2. Explain the science of physiology and nutrition.
    3. Assess the girl's interest in other health topics.
    4. Describe how nutrition improves skin and facial appearance.

63. The UAP brings holiday cupcakes to the long-term care center and passes them out to all of the residents before checking with the nurse. What would the nurse do **first**?
    1. Ask the UAP to collect the cupcakes and then determine who is allowed to have one.
    2. Praise the UAP for bringing seasonally appropriate good cheer to the residents.
    3. Remind the UAP that not all residents should have too much sugar, so next time, ask first.
    4. Sit with the residents, enjoy the cupcakes, and make the food into a social occasion.

64. A patient is on fluid restrictions because of renal failure. Which interventions would the nurse use? **Select all that apply.**
    1. Encourage the patient to drink most of the fluid allowance in the morning.
    2. Explain the various sources of fluid such as IV fluids, gelatin, and fluids taken with medications.
    3. Suggest chewing gum and sucking on breath mints.
    4. Explain the rationale for fluid restrictions.
    5. Show the volume of fluid that is allowed for the shift.
    6. Post a sign in the room so that visitors are aware of fluid restrictions.

65. The patient is trying to lose weight because he is obese and has been told that he has a high risk for diabetes, coronary heart disease, and stroke. What is the **most** important point that the nurse would emphasize?
    1. Strictly adhere to 1500 kcal/day, but eat a variety of foods.
    2. Take a multivitamin and mineral supplement while dieting.
    3. Exercise 60-90 minutes most days of the week.
    4. A weight loss of 5% to 15% can reduce health-related risks.

66. Which patient is **most** likely to be a candidate for bariatric surgery?
    1. Body mass index of 40 or higher
    2. Body mass index of 35 or higher
    3. Body mass index of 23 with severe cardiovascular disease
    4. Body mass index of 17 with diabetes

67. The patient is newly diagnosed with type 2 diabetes. In talking to the patient about diet management, what would the nurse suggest?
    1. Suggest the patient follow a standardized preprinted menu for each meal.
    2. Indicate that two or more servings of fried fish would be beneficial.
    3. Closely monitor and control intake of table sugar and desserts.
    4. Emphasize consistent mealtimes; approximately every 4-5 hours.

68. A patient who is a known diabetic presents with weakness, diaphoresis, and disorientation. What would the nurse do **first**?
    1. Encourage the patient to drink a lot of water.
    2. Give the patient a glass of milk.
    3. Establish intravenous access and give glucose.
    4. Have the patient suck on a hard candy.

69. What is the best way for the nurse to assess for proper nasogastric tube placement prior to administering a tube feeding?
    1. Observe the patient's comfort while in sitting position.
    2. Auscultate for a gurgling sound over the epigastric region after pushing air through the nasogastric tube.
    3. Give a test dose of a small amount of water and observe the patient's reaction.
    4. Aspirate gastric fluid and check pH.

70. Which dietary alterations would be recommended to the patient experiencing poor wound healing?
    1. Increase protein and vitamin C.
    2. Increase fluid intake and avoid fructose.
    3. Restrict intake of carbohydrate and concentrated sweets.
    4. Increase calories and reduce sodium intake.

71. Which instructions would the nurse give to the patient who has been prescribed an iron supplement? **Select all that apply.**
    1. Take the iron with orange juice.
    2. Drink a glass of milk after the iron supplement if needed to settle the stomach.
    3. Keep the iron supplement in a high cabinet out of reach of children.
    4. Take fiber supplement and iron together to avoid constipation.
    5. Chew calcium antacid tablet after iron to avoid feelings of reflux.
    6. Limit iron in the diet while taking iron supplement.

CRITICAL THINKING ACTIVITIES

72. The nurse is working on a medical-surgical unit and has identified several patients who may need enteral feeding.

    a. What are the indications for the use of enteral feeding? _____

    _____

    _____

    b. Identify the nursing assessments and interventions for enteral feeding in the following situations.

        i. Patient assessment before feeding: _____

        _____

        ii. Assessment of gastric aspirate: _____

        _____

        iii. Gastric residual based on provider's parameters: _____

        _____

        iv. Formula is cold: _____

        _____

        v. Occlusion of the tubing is suspected: _____

        _____

      vi. After feeding is given: _____

            _____

      vii. Documentation: _____

            _____

  c. What are the possible complications or problems associated with enteral feeding? _____

     _____

     _____

     _____

73. The nurse is talking to a 25-year-old woman who is approximately 10 pounds underweight for her age and height, but is otherwise in good health. She would like some information about healthy diet and lifestyle, because she and her husband are thinking about trying to have a baby.

  a. Explain to this young woman why there is an increased need for nutrients during pregnancy.

     _____

     _____

  b. Which vitamins would be recommended for the pregnant patient and what is the function of these vitamin supplements? What are the food sources for each vitamin?

     _____

     _____

     _____

  c. What can the nurse tell the patient about her current weight in relation to getting pregnant?

     _____

     _____

  d. What can the nurse tell the patient about foods and lifestyle activities that should be avoided?

     _____

     _____

74. In your own words, explain what you would tell a patient about "bad" cholesterol and "good" cholesterol.

     _____

     _____

     _____

NEXT-GENERATION NCLEX™ (NGN)

75. Extended Multiple Response

Cognitive Skill: Analyze Cues

Scenario: The patient has recently undergone bariatric surgery. The patient is motivated to learn and understands the need to make many changes to the way he used to eat. Which of the following activities would be recommended for this patient?

Instructions: Place an X next to the activities which would be recommended after bariatric surgery.

_____	1.	Eating three meals daily
_____	2.	Sitting upright after a meal
_____	3.	Drinking fluids 30 minutes after a meal
_____	4.	Eating raisins with a meal
_____	5.	Eating unsweetened oatmeal for breakfast
_____	6.	Consuming an egg
_____	7.	Eating a piece of avocado with the meal
_____	8.	Including a glass of wine with the meal
_____	9.	Drinking a glass of water with each meal

Complementary, Integrative, and Alternative Therapies

Answer Key: A complete Answer Key is provided in your Additional Learning Resources on Evolve.

MULTIPLE CHOICE

Directions: Select the best answer(s) for each of the following questions.

1. All patients should be advised to discuss use of complementary, integrative, and alternative therapies with their health care provider (HCP); however, which patient needs extra encouragement to check with the HCP before trying reflexology?
   1. Has type 2 diabetes
   2. Is in the first trimester of pregnancy
   3. Has chronic pulmonary disease
   4. Had fractured ankle in childhood

2. The patient says, "I take an anticoagulant because I have atrial fibrillation and I like to use ginseng because I heard it can prevent diabetes." Based on the patient's comments, what is the **most** important data set for the nurse to follow up?
   1. Look at the patient's current and previous blood glucose levels.
   2. Put the patient on the cardiac monitor and compare to previous tracings.
   3. Check the patient's current and previous clotting times.
   4. Take a full set of vital signs and compare current values to previous.

3. Which outcome statement indicates that valerian is being used appropriately and is a successful therapy for the patient?
   1. The patient reports that his upper respiratory infection resolved much faster than expected.
   2. The patient states he feels more alert and has better mental concentration after several doses.
   3. The patient reports that the nausea is relieved, and the abdominal pain has subsided.
   4. The patient feels that he is sleeping more soundly, and quality of sleep seems much better.

4. The patient has a bone infection in the lower leg. Which patient education brochure is the nurse **most** likely to prepare for the patient?
   1. Antibiotic Therapy and Surgery for Osteomyelitis
   2. How to Effectively Use Tea Tree Oil for Infections
   3. Risks and Benefits of Chiropractic Therapy
   4. Advantages and Disadvantages of Energy Field Therapy

5. Which nurse is correctly using a complementary, integrative, and alternative therapy to assist older residents in a long-term care center to evoke memories of past Christmas holidays?
   1. Nurse A puts up strings of red, white, and green lights to create a positive energy field.
   2. Nurse B uses biofeedback and monitors respiratory rate as people listen to Christmas music.
   3. Nurse C applies animal-assisted therapy by showing a movie about Santa's reindeer.
   4. Nurse D uses an aromatic infuser filled with pine scent and the residents decorate a tree.

6. For most patients, magnet therapy has neither beneficial nor detrimental effects; however, for which patient would magnet therapy be contraindicated?
   1. The patient has rheumatoid arthritis.
   2. The patient has a pacemaker.
   3. The patient had knee replacement surgery.
   4. The patient has terminal ovarian cancer.

7. Currently, which patients are **most** likely to be prescribed and benefit from tetrahydrocannabinol (THC)?
   1. Patients with fibromyalgia or chronic fatigue syndrome
   2. Patients with clinical depression or anxiety disorders
   3. Patients with addictions to alcohol or opioid analgesics
   4. Patients with cancer or acquired immunodeficiency syndrome

8. Which outcome statement indicates that the prescribed dronabinol is a successful therapy for a patient with cancer?
   1. The tumor is reduced in size and pressure on surrounding tissues is reduced.
   2. The patient reports decreased nausea and an improvement in appetite.
   3. The patient reports sleeping longer and resting more comfortably.
   4. Fever and pain are reduced, and white cell count is improving.

9. What is the **most** common element of relaxation strategies?
   1. Rhythmic breathing
   2. Control of muscle groups
   3. Awareness of environment
   4. Meditation

10. The patient suffered a traumatic event as a child; however, the event is not something the patient ever thinks or talks about. Which therapy would be **most** likely to trigger a memory that would require psychological intervention?
    1. Biofeedback
    2. Reflexology
    3. Yoga
    4. Accupressure

11. The nurse is collecting data for the health history of a new patient. What is the **best** rationale for directly asking the patient about the use of complementary, integrative, and alternative medicine therapies?
    1. Many patients use unconventional therapies but hesitate to tell the HCP.
    2. A complete health history is essential for every patient.
    3. Alternative therapies must be listed for insurance coverage.
    4. Nurses should be advocates for holistic care for patients.

12. The nurse is seeking evidence-based practice information related to complementary, integrative, and alternative therapies for cancer patients. What would be the **best** source of this information?
    1. Consult an updated comprehensive medical-surgical nursing textbook.
    2. Use the Internet to search for "cancer" and "alternative therapies."
    3. Access National Center for Complementary and Integrative Health (NCCIH) website.
    4. Talk to the local chapter of the American Cancer Society.

13. Why do herbal products have the potential to cause problems for consumers? **Select all that apply.**
    1. Do not have the same rigorous study as pharmaceuticals
    2. Reduced level of accountability for the manufacturers
    3. Not required by law to demonstrate safety, efficacy, or quality of products
    4. Wide variations in potency, quality, and chemical content
    5. No standardized dosages have been established for most herbs
    6. More potent than pharmaceuticals because the whole plant is used

14. Which patient statement indicates a correct understanding of the patient teaching information about using herbal preparations?
    1. "Herbal preparations are made from plants and are natural and safe."
    2. "These are over-the-counter products so they don't have dangerous side effects."
    3. "If I follow the package instructions on dosage, I'll be okay."
    4. "The herbs should be discontinued at least 2 weeks before any surgery."

15. The patient has heart failure and takes digoxin. He tells the nurse that he is thinking about taking *Ginkgo biloba* because it is supposed to improve memory by increasing circulation to the brain. What is the **best** response?
    1. "You sound like you might be worried about memory loss."
    2. "Digoxin has a lot of herb-drug and drug-drug interactions."
    3. "Let me contact your HCP so you can discuss this with him."
    4. "I will get you some additional information about *Ginkgo biloba*."

16. A 42-year-old female patient has a family history of osteoporosis and would like advice about the use of complementary, integrative, and alternative therapies for prevention of osteoporosis. Which brochure would the nurse prepare for the patient?
    1. "Medical Uses of Acupuncture"
    2. "Benefits of Chiropractic Therapy"
    3. "Understanding Reflexology"
    4. "Learning About T'ai chi"

17. Which patient statement indicates understanding of a therapy that could help with smoking cessation?
    1. "I could consult an herbalist and smoke herbal leaf instead of tobacco."
    2. "Acupuncture stimulates accupoints and has been used to treat addictions."
    3. "Inhalation of lavender oil relieves stress and decreases craving for a cigarette."
    4. "Biofeedback would increase my awareness about my physiologic cravings."

18. Which patient would **not** be a candidate for therapeutic massage?
    1. A pregnant woman who would like to have a foot massage
    2. A postsurgical patient who wants the legs massaged to relieve cramping
    3. An older patient who has an ache in the upper back after prolonged sitting
    4. A school-age child who has been confined to bed for several days

19. The older patient disrobes to take a shower. The young nursing student who is assigned to assist with hygiene is shocked and repulsed by the appearance and condition of the patient's skin. What should the student do?
    1. Quickly excuse herself and step out into the hall to recover composure.
    2. Smile and avoid looking at the patient directly, but continue to assist with care.
    3. Apologize to the patient and then seek out the instructor for advice.
    4. Make eye contact, smile, and assist the patient to maintain safety in the shower.

20. The nurse is working in a long-term care center and recognizes that older residents are at risk for "skin hunger." What would the nurse do to address this problem?
    1. Ensure that herbal lotion enriched with vitamins and protein is applied after bathing.
    2. Identify residents who are comfortable with hugging and touching by staff members.
    3. Consult with a holistic nutritionist to design meals that supply nutrition for the skin.
    4. Apply herbal sunscreens to protect the skin and take residents into the sun.

21. Which patient should be cautioned that inhalation of essential oils could exacerbate symptoms?
    1. Takes as-needed (PRN) medication for asthma
    2. Recently diagnosed with major depression
    3. Currently experiences excessive stress related to work
    4. Underwent chiropractic treatments for back pain

22. The nursing student has severe test anxiety. She is using guided imagery to help reduce anxiety just before the beginning of each test. What is the desired outcome of this type of therapy?
    1. Controls response to stimuli by regulating expectations and perceptions
    2. Learns to deep-breathe and include all senses during times of stress
    3. Visualizes warmth entering the body on inspiration and tension leaving on expiration
    4. Creates an image of self successfully passing the exam

23. What are the advantages of animal-assisted therapy? **Select all that apply.**
    1. Research indicates that animals have a calming effect.
    2. Animals can stimulate mental activity through interaction.
    3. Most families have a pet that will be familiar to the patients.
    4. Everyone likes animals because they decrease loneliness.
    5. Patients who like animals are usually not allergic to them.
    6. Being around an animal can reduce blood pressure and anxiety.

24. The NCCIH funds research that relates to complementary and integrative therapies. Which criteria are considered when studies are selected for funding? **Select all that apply.**
    1. Current evidence supports further research.
    2. Goals of research are attainable if the study is correctly designed.
    3. Study outcomes will change patient health practices.
    4. Manufacturers will profit if research supports product efficacy.
    5. Study addresses an important need for information.
    6. Consumers trust products that have been investigated by research.

25. In 2018, the Food and Drug Administration approved Epidiolex (cannabidiol). Which patient is the **most** likely candidate to get a prescription for this new drug?
    1. Patient has cancer and experiences severe nausea and vomiting after chemotherapy.
    2. Patient has a severe form of epilepsy that has not responded to other medications.
    3. Patient has severe pain and desires to avoid the addictive properties related to opioids.
    4. Patient has choice of treatment for marijuana abuse as an alternative to incarceration.

26. A university student says, "Me and some of my friends have occasionally been vaping THC, just for fun. It's safer than then getting drunk and it's legal on the campus." Which action would the nurse take **first**?
    1. Offer the student a brochure on safety issues of vaping and e-cigarettes.
    2. Tell the student that he should talk to his parents about this behavior.
    3. Ask the student about what he knows about THC and vaping.
    4. Notify the supervising RN and HCP about the student's comment.

CRITICAL THINKING ACTIVITIES

27. Consider the cognitive skills of focusing, passivity, and receptivity, and discuss the use of relaxation therapy with the following patients.

    a. A 77-year-old woman with advanced dementia is frequently restless. She will pace and demonstrate nonpurposeful movements. Her family has asked the nurse to help her to be calmer and relax.

        _____

        _____

        _____

    b. A 23-year-old college student is extremely anxious about doing well. At times, he has studied to the point of exhaustion. He reports taking "uppers" so that he can stay awake and study. Currently, it appears that he is under the influence of stimulants because he is talking very fast about a math problem that he is working on and he appears jittery and nervous.

        _____

        _____

        _____

    c. A 62-year-old retired military officer appears very tense, but he tells the nurse that he doesn't have any problems with anxiety, tension, or stress. Furthermore, he informs the nurse that if he did have any problems, he would control them on his own. His wife tries to tell the nurse that he does need some help to relax, but he cuts her off abruptly.

        _____

        _____

        _____

28. A neighbor tells the nurse that he is no longer seeing an HCP and that he has discontinued his prescribed medications in favor of herbs and other types of complementary, integrative, or alternative therapies for his health problems, which include diabetes, high blood pressure, and heart problems. What should the nurse do?

    _____

    _____

    _____

NEXT-GENERATION NCLEX™ (NGN)

29. Extended Multiple Response

Cognitive Skill: Analyze Cues

Scenario: The nurse is working at a long-term care facility. An older resident from an Asian culture has hypertension, diabetes, and atrial fibrillation. She takes an antihypertensive medication, insulin, and an anticoagulant. The resident requests some ginseng tea and there is a bottle of goldenseal root capsules on the bedside table. The nurse recognizes that there are cultural considerations in relation to complementary, integrative, and alternative therapies, but is also concerned because of the resident's health conditions and prescribed medications.

Which actions would the nurse take?

Instructions: Place a check mark next to actions that demonstrate that the nurse is considering the resident's cultural beliefs and safety. **Check all that apply.**

_____	1.	Respect the resident's beliefs and look for ways to combine therapies if possible.
_____	2.	Instruct the family to take the goldenseal and store it at home.
_____	3.	Tell the resident that ginseng is not available and offer an alternative tea.
_____	4.	Advise the resident to stop using herbs because of drug-herb interactions.
_____	5.	Collect data about frequency, route, and strength of herbs that the resident uses.
_____	6.	Alert the supervising nurse and the HCP about assessment findings.
_____	7.	Ask the resident to describe the benefits of the ginseng and goldenseal.

Pain Management, Comfort, Rest, and Sleep

Answer Key: A complete Answer Key is provided in your Additional Learning Resources on Evolve.

MULTIPLE CHOICE

Directions: Select the best answer(s) for each of the following questions.

1. Which nursing action empowers the patient to become an active partner in managing pain?
   1. Administers prescribed pain medication in a timely fashion
   2. Acknowledges the patient as expert in his own experience of pain
   3. Advocates for therapies that provide sufficient relief of pain
   4. Assesses the pain before and after giving pain medication

2. The nurse identifies that the patient with coronary insufficiency is having referred pain. Which finding substantiates the nurse's interpretation?
   1. Patient reports she is having pain in her left jaw.
   2. Patient demonstrates grimacing when pain starts.
   3. Patient reports that chest hurts during exercise.
   4. Patient reports that symptoms are relieved with rest.

3. The patient reports lower back pain that is dull and intermittent. Which description **most** strongly suggests that the patient is having chronic pain?
   1. Sometimes the pain interferes with sleep or work.
   2. The pain has been off and on for about 11 months.
   3. Over-the-counter medications give temporary relief.
   4. Prolonged sitting seems to make the pain worse.

4. What is an expected assessment finding that demonstrates the action of epinephrine on the body during an episode of acute pain?
   1. Blood glucose is lower than normal.
   2. Description of pain is disproportionate.
   3. Pain medication quickly relieves the pain.
   4. Pulse and respiratory rates are increased.

5. The patient reports that pain medication used to help, but now is less effective. The patient also reports fatigue, sleep disturbance, and depression. The nurse suspects a synergistic effect. Based on the nurse's interpretation of the data, which intervention would the nurse try **first**?
   1. Advocate for a change of medication or an increase of dose.
   2. Tell the patient that this is an expected side effect that will pass.
   3. Assess sleep patterns and control environment to facilitate rest.
   4. Ask the health care provider (HCP) to prescribe an antidepressant medication.

6. Although placebos are rarely used, what is the **best** physiologic explanation for how they relieve pain?
   1. Action of a placebo mimics "fight or flight," which is triggered by epinephrine.
   2. Placebos partially close the "gate," so the passage of pain impulses is blocked.
   3. Chemically, placebos inhibit the synthesis of prostaglandins that mediate pain.
   4. Placebos cause the release of endorphins, which attach to opioid receptor sites.

7. For a patient who is having an acute myocardial infarction, the nurse anticipates that the HCP will order morphine to relieve pain. Which harmful physical effect of unrelieved pain is the **greatest** concern for this patient?
   1. Increased oxygen demand
   2. Decreased gastric motility
   3. Depressed immune response
   4. Increased mental confusion

8. It is now 2300 and the patient is requesting a PRN (as needed) dose of pain medication. The nurse checks the medication administration record and sees that the patient has received:

0400	2 tablets 500 mg acetaminophen
0900	2 tablets oxycodone 5 mg and 325 mg acetaminophen
1300	2 tablets 500 mg acetaminophen
1800	2 tablets 500 mg acetaminophen

What would the nurse do **first**?

   1. Give two tablets of oxycodone 5 mg and acetaminophen 325 mg.
   2. Wait 2 hours, and then give two tablets 500 mg of acetaminophen.
   3. Call the HCP and report the overdose of acetaminophen.
   4. Use a drug reference to verify recommended dosage of acetaminophen/24 hours.

9. What is the **greatest** concern with patient-controlled analgesia (PCA) by proxy?
   1. It's more difficult for the nurse to monitor dosage and assess response.
   2. There is a greater chance of oversedation and opioid toxicity.
   3. The patient becomes a passive recipient in the pain management process.
   4. The patient's pain is more likely to be unrelieved or undertreated.

10. A patient tells the nurse that he has been sleeping in a recliner chair for the past several months because "It is easier to fall asleep and stay asleep." What is the nurse **most** likely to suspect and assess for?
   1. Back or spinal problems
   2. Problems with breathing
   3. Headaches with visual problems
   4. Restless leg syndrome

11. The patient had a surgical procedure this morning and is requesting pain medication. The nurse assesses the patient's vital signs and decides to withhold opioid medication. Which finding supports this decision?
   1. Pulse = 90/min
   2. Respirations = 10/min
   3. Blood pressure = 130/80 mm Hg
   4. Temperature = 99° F (37.2° C) rectally

12. The nurse is caring for a patient who has arthritis. Which medication does the nurse anticipate the HCP will prescribe?
    1. Naloxone
    2. Gabapentin
    3. Aspirin
    4. Morphine

13. The patient is receiving an epidural opioid. What is a complication of this treatment?
    1. Diarrhea
    2. Hypertension
    3. Urinary retention
    4. Tachycardia

14. An older adult patient who has osteoarthritis suffers from chronic pain. Based on the patient's age and medical condition, which pain medications is the nurse **most** likely to query if they are prescribed for the patient? **Select all that apply.**
    1. Meperidine
    2. Acetaminophen
    3. Morphine sulfate
    4. Nonsteroidal antiinflammatory drugs
    5. Combinations of opioid drugs

15. Which nursing intervention demonstrates the application of the gate control theory of pain?
    1. Performs a back massage using warmed lotion
    2. Administers acetaminophen as needed
    3. Elevates a patient's sprained ankle to prevent swelling
    4. Repositions the patient every 2 hours

16. Which nursing action demonstrates that the nurse is complying with the Joint Commission standards of pain management?
    1. Documents that medication is given after the patient receives it
    2. Incorporates knowledge of the patient's culture in pain management
    3. Assesses the patient's pain and reassesses pain after interventions
    4. Stays current with the latest information about pain therapies

17. The nursing student reports to the nurse that a postoperative patient is asking for pain medication. What is the **most** important question that the nurse will ask the student to answer?
    1. "Can you give the medication yourself?"
    2. "What did the patient tell you about his pain?"
    3. "Did you try any nonpharmacologic interventions?"
    4. "What do you know about the prescribed medication?"

18. The patient agrees to try guided imagery as a noninvasive method of pain relief. Before they begin the therapy, which instruction is the nurse **most** likely to give?
    1. "I'll use a combination of firm and light strokes during the therapy."
    2. "The skin will be stimulated with a mild electric current that reduces pain."
    3. "Tell me about a place and time where you felt relaxed and peaceful."
    4. "We have to use specialized equipment to identify your biologic responses."

19. What is the **greatest** advantage of using nonpharmacologic pain management techniques as an adjunct to pain medication?
    1. Inexpensive and easy to perform
    2. Based on the gate control theory
    3. Low risk and few side effects
    4. Gives patients some control over pain

20. The nurse is talking to a patient who wants to try transcutaneous electric nerve stimulation. Which condition is **most** important to bring to the attention of the HCP?
    1. The patient has a cardiac pacemaker device.
    2. The patient uses an older model of hearing aid.
    3. The patient has a metallic hip joint.
    4. The patient has a history of a broken back.

21. The HCP prescribes 1000 mg acetaminophen every 4 hours as needed for pain. What would the nurse do?
    1. Assess the patient every 4 hours and give the medication as needed.
    2. Give the medication as needed during the daytime hours only.
    3. Call the HCP and ask for clarification of the order.
    4. Call the pharmacy and ask if the medication comes in 1000-mg tablets.

22. The nurse is caring for several patients who are receiving morphine. Which patient is **most** likely to have problems with respiratory depression?
    1. A patient with a history of chronic back pain who is receiving epidural morphine for an acute exacerbation
    2. An older patient who is postoperative for a fractured hip and is receiving patient-controlled analgesia
    3. A child who received an intramuscular injection prior to having fracture reduction of the forearm
    4. An older patient with end-stage uterine cancer who is receiving an oral form of morphine

23. What is the physiologic rationale for avoiding use of meperidine for patients with sickle cell disease?
    1. There is a direct action that causes sickling of blood cells.
    2. Renal insufficiency will be present to some degree.
    3. Underlying respiratory distress results in respiratory depression.
    4. Patients with sickle cell disease are more prone to seizures.

24. The home health nurse sees an order for meperidine for a 63-year-old patient with cancer who requires long-term opioid treatment. What is the **best** rationale for the nurse to question this medication order?
    1. Meperidine is an older drug that is now rarely prescribed for any condition.
    2. The patient cannot be continuously monitored for adverse effects in the home setting.
    3. The patient is not young nor healthy and is therefore more likely to suffer side effects.
    4. Repeated administration of meperidine increases the risk of accumulation.

25. The nurse hears in report that the patient with diabetes has reported a tingling, burning sensation in the lower extremities. Which drug is the nurse **most** likely to administer for this type of discomfort?
    1. Ketorolac tromethamine
    2. Tramadol
    3. Acetaminophen
    4. Duloxetine

26. The patient reports that the prescribed opioid dose does not seem to provide the same relief for his acute pain compared to 4 weeks ago. Based on the nurse's knowledge of pharmacology, what does the nurse recognize?
    1. The patient has developed a physical tolerance.
    2. The patient has a psychological dependence.
    3. The patient probably has an addiction.
    4. The patient is experiencing chronic pain.

27. The nurse is talking to a patient who reports feeling tired and not getting enough sleep. Which question related to the patient's medication is **most** relevant to designing interventions for the patient's problem?
    1. "Which antiinflammatory medication has the HCP suggested?"
    2. "Has there been a recent increase in the dosage of your opioid medication?"
    3. "What time of the day do you usually take your diuretic medication?"
    4. "Are you taking your antiemetic medication before or after meals?"

28. The student nurse is looking at nursing jobs to consider after graduation. Which shift is **most** likely to cause sleep-wake cycle disruption?
    1. Straight night shift
    2. Rotating day to night shift
    3. Weekends-only evening shift
    4. Monday to Friday day shift

29. The HCP has ordered blood pressure, pulse, and respirations every 2 hours for 12 hours. It is currently 8:00 PM and the nurse knows that the patient has been having a lot of problems sleeping in the hospital. Which strategy would the nurse try **first**?
    1. Clarify the necessity of the order with the HCP.
    2. Explain to the patient that vital signs will only be taken every 2 hours for 12 hours.
    3. Tell the unlicensed assistive personnel (UAP) to quietly take vital signs every 2 hours.
    4. Apply an automatic blood pressure cuff that can programmed for every 2 hours.

30. The nurse enters the patient's room at 3:00 AM and finds that the patient is awake and sitting up in a chair. The patient tells the nurse that she is not able to sleep. What would the nurse do **first**?
    1. Obtain a prescription for a hypnotic.
    2. Instruct the patient to return to bed.
    3. Provide a glass of warm milk with honey.
    4. Ask about methods that have helped her sleep.

31. Which patient is the **most** likely candidate to be prescribed an analgesic that would be considered an abuse deterrent medication?
    1. Has history of alcohol abuse and needs postoperative pain management
    2. Has a history of substance abuse and needs immediate relief for traumatic amputation
    3. Has cognitive problems that effect self-administration of pain medications
    4. Has a history of opioid abuse and has an acute exacerbation of chronic pain

32. Which type of opioid would be prescribed to manage episodes of acute breakthrough pain?
    1. Patient-controlled analgesia
    2. Short-acting
    3. Long-acting
    4. Extended-release

33. During the night shift, the UAP reports the vital signs to the experienced nurse who recognizes that various stages of sleep affect vital signs. Which patient needs follow-up assessment for an unexpected finding?
    1. Patient in stage 1 sleep: vital signs are significantly lower than during waking hours.
    2. Patient in stage 2 sleep: gradual and progressive fall in vital signs.
    3. Patient in stage 3 sleep: vital signs decline but remain regular.
    4. Patient in rapid eye movement (REM) sleep: increased or fluctuating blood pressure.

CRITICAL THINKING ACTIVITIES

34. The patient is experiencing difficulty sleeping while in the hospital. She reports this is the first time she has been in the hospital and the sounds and smells seem very strange. In addition, she reports feeling mildly anxious because "so many people come in and out of the room at all hours of the day and night." She looks tired and seems mildly irritable. Identify nursing interventions that may be implemented to promote sleep.

    _____

    _____

    _____

35. a. Think about the patients whom you have cared for during your clinical experiences and identify at least five possible causes for the discomfort that your patients were experiencing.

    _____

    _____

    _____

    b. Describe what you did to relieve your patients' discomfort. _____

    _____

    _____

    _____

36. The increased incidence of opioid addiction has been in the news. Discuss with your classmates and instructor how the potential for opioid abuse could affect your nursing practice.

_____

_____

_____

_____

NEXT-GENERATION NCLEX™ (NGN)

37. Cloze

Cognitive Skill: Analyze Cues

Scenario: The nurse works in a long-term care facility. Many of the residents have chronic health conditions such as diabetes, musculoskeletal disorders, chronic obstructive pulmonary disease (COPD), heart failure, and arthritis that cause pain and discomfort. In addition, some of the residents have cognitive impairments and others are prone to low self-esteem, anxiety, and depression. The nurse must apply knowledge of changes related to aging and pain management in caring for these residents.

Instructions: Choose the most likely options to complete the statement below.

Residents with arthritis or chronic musculoskeletal disorders are likely to be prescribed NSAIDs, which create an increased risk for ___1___. Patients with ___2___ experience changes in peripheral vascular function and skin that affect pain sensation. For severe chronic pain, some residents may receive opioid medications and older adults are susceptible to side effects of opioids because of changes in ___3___ and a reduction in cardiac output.

Options for 1	Options for 2	Options for 3
gastric and renal toxicity	arthritis	serum proteins and liver and renal function
urinary retention and constipation	diabetes	ability to swallow and decreased gag reflex
memory loss and confusion	COPD	food and fluid intake
hormonal and metabolism changes	depression	ability to accurately report pain
respiratory depression and acidosis	cognitive impairment	allergic and immune response

Surgical Wound Care

Answer Key: A complete Answer Key is provided in your Additional Learning Resources on Evolve.

MULTIPLE CHOICE

Directions: Select the best answer(s) for each of the following questions.

1. What does the nurse observe during the first phase of healing if fibrin is functioning correctly?
   1. Erythema, heat, edema, and pain occur.
   2. There is an overgrowth of whitish collagen.
   3. Wound looks irregular, raised, and purplish.
   4. Clot begins to form and bleeding subsides.

2. To address the signs and symptoms of the inflammatory phase, which action would the nurse perform?
   1. Cover the wound with clean gauze and apply direct pressure.
   2. Elevate the injured part and apply an ice pack as ordered.
   3. Observe for purulent exudate and cleanse the wound.
   4. Observe for granulation tissue and keep the wound moist.

3. During the reconstruction or proliferation phase of healing, what is the **most** serious complication?
   1. Keloid formation
   2. Granulation tissue
   3. Wound dehiscence
   4. Phagocytosis

4. On the first day post-surgery, how often does the nurse inspect the surgical dressings and what does he or she expect to see?
   1. Inspects every hour for the first 24 hours and expects to see serous and serosanguineous fluid.
   2. Inspects every 2-4 hours for the first 24 hours and expects to see sanguineous and serosanguineous fluid.
   3. Inspects once every 8 hours for the first 24 hours and expects to see sanguineous and serosanguineous fluid.
   4. Inspects every 5 minutes for the first hour and expects to see serous and sanguineous fluid.

5. Which type of dressing prevents air impurities and oxygen from passing to the wound ?
   1. Wet-to-dry dressing
   2. Dry dressing
   3. Transparent dressing
   4. Occlusive dressing

6. The nurse observes that the dressing over the wound has exudate that has a strong, pungent odor. Which action is the **most** important?
   1. Weigh the soiled dressing.
   2. Cleanse the wound with an antiseptic.
   3. Perform a wound culture.
   4. Circle and date the drainage on the dressing.

7. What is an important nursing responsibility associated with a Penrose drain?
   1. Drainage in bulb should be observed and measured, suction should be reestablished.
   2. Ensure that the irrigation pressure does not exceed 4-15 psi.
   3. Drain should be observed for patency and flushed as needed.
   4. Drainage on dressing should be observed, position of safety pin is noted.

8. With appropriate instruction and supervision, which tasks related to wound care can be delegated to unlicensed assistive personnel (UAP)? **Select all that apply.**
   1. Emptying a closed drainage container
   2. Removing sutures or staples
   3. Applying an abdominal binder
   4. Assessing breathing with a breast binder in place
   5. Measuring intake and output

9. The nurse sees that the patient takes steroids for a respiratory condition. What would be an expected affect of steroids on wound healing?
   1. Decreased inflammatory response
   2. Prolonged bleeding times
   3. Decreased keloid formation
   4. Impaired formation of granulation tissue

10. The nurse is applying a dressing over the insertion site of a peripheral intravenous catheter. Which dressing is the **best** choice?
    1. Sterile tape with dry gauze
    2. Steri-Strips and transparent dressing
    3. Transparent dressing
    4. Sterile pad with chevron taping

11. After abdominal surgery, a patient is at risk for wound stress related to coughing and moving. Which equipment does the nurse need to teach the patient the self-care measure of splinting?
    1. An abdominal binder
    2. A pillow or rolled blanket
    3. A large triangular bandage
    4. Several wide elastic bandages

12. Which lunch tray is **best** for providing protein, vitamins A and C, and zinc, the nutrients required for wound healing?
    1. A peanut butter sandwich with a glass of milk
    2. A bowl of bean soup with crackers and iced tea
    3. Broiled seafood with spinach salad and tomato juice
    4. Stir-fried mixed vegetables with rice and hot tea

13. The patient has no contraindications for fluid intake. Over a 24-hour period, he drank 16 ounces of decaffeinated coffee, 10 ounces of juice, 6 ounces of milk, and a half a liter of soda. Which instructions would the nurse give about fluid intake to promote wound healing?
    1. Instructs the patient to continue drinking the same amount as he drank today
    2. Tells the patient that tomorrow he should try to drink twice as much as today
    3. Advises the patient that drinking excessive fluid is likely to decrease appetite for food
    4. Suggests that he drink 2-3 additional 8-ounce servings of his favorite fluid every day

14. The nurse is caring for a patient who has a large abdominal incision. The patient tells the nurse that she is afraid to sit up or even move because of the pain and the strain on the incision site. Which instructions would the nurse give to the patient?
    1. "Rest in bed until the incision site is less tender and healing has progressed."
    2. "Roll to one side, use your elbow as a lever, and push to a sitting position."
    3. "Hold a pillow next to your abdomen and roll forward into a sitting position."
    4. "Call for assistance whenever needed and someone will help you sit up."

15. A patient has just returned from surgery. Which initial assessments would the nurse make related to the surgical site? **Select all that apply.**
    1. Inspect the protective dressing that was placed by the surgical team.
    2. Look at the area around the dressing and record observations.
    3. Check under the patient to make sure that exudate is not pooling.
    4. Carefully remove the dressing and inspect the suture line for intactness.
    5. Expect and note amount of serous drainage that is coming from the wound.

16. A patient had surgery 4 days ago and now reports an increase in pain and has a temperature of 101.6° (38.7° C). The incision site looks red compared to yesterday and a small amount of purulent drainage is seeping around the suture line. Which laboratory result will the nurse check before contacting the surgeon?
    1. Hemoglobin and hematocrit
    2. White blood cell count
    3. Platelet count
    4. Blood glucose level

17. Which patient is **most** likely to benefit from the application of a triangular binder?
    1. Has a chronic pressure injury on the sacral area
    2. Has a possible fracture in the forearm
    3. Has venous stasis ulcer on left ankle
    4. Has a surgical wound on the lateral chest area

18. The nurse is preparing to remove the patient's staples, but after assessment, the nurse decides that the staples should not be removed. Which finding supports this decision?
    1. The wound edges were partially separated.
    2. Dried serous drainage was noted around the staples.
    3. The patient was anxious about staple removal.
    4. Early keloid formation was observed.

19. The nurse is preparing to change the patient's dry sterile dressing. Upon attempting the removal of the old dressing, it adheres to the site. What would the nurse do?
    1. Notify the surgeon.
    2. Leave the dressing alone.
    3. Pull the dressing off quickly.
    4. Moisten the dressing with saline.

20. The patient returned to the unit 3 hours ago after having surgery on the abdomen, and the dressing is now saturated with red, watery drainage. What would the nurse do **first**?
    1. Notify the charge nurse and the surgeon.
    2. Take the patient's vital signs and assess for pain.
    3. Securely reinforce the dressing with layers of gauze.
    4. Remove the dressing and observe the wound site.

21. After a total abdominal hysterectomy, a postoperative patient develops a wound evisceration. What would the nurse do **first**?
    1. Check patency of the intravenous (IV) site for delivery of fluids.
    2. Place the patient in low Fowler's position to reduce strain on the wound.
    3. Prepare the patient for surgery and contact the surgeon.
    4. Cover the wound with a sterile dressing moistened with saline.

22. A postoperative patient who was happy and cheerful earlier now demonstrates restlessness and anxiety. He reports feeling "a little lightheaded." He is mildly diaphoretic and his pulse feels thready. What assessments does the nurse perform to identify a suspected complication?
    1. Checks the pulse rate, blood pressure, and assesses for pain
    2. Assesses for localized warmth or redness with tenderness
    3. Observes the incision site for wound edge approximation
    4. Takes the temperature and checks for purulent drainage

23. The patient has a T-tube in place following an abdominal cholecystectomy. What is the expected output of bile in the first 24 hours?
    1. 30 mL per hour
    2. 250-500 mL
    3. 10-50 mL
    4. 1-2 L

24. The nurse is observing a new staff member perform a sterile dry dressing change. The nurse would intervene if the staff member performed which action?
    1. Loosens tape and gently pulls toward the incision
    2. Uses sterile gloves to remove the old dressing
    3. Cleanses wound by starting at incision moving outward
    4. Allows antiseptic cleansing solution to air-dry

25. A nurse is supervising a nursing student who is doing a wet-to-dry dressing change. What does the nurse do when the student applies a dry dressing over the wet gauze?
    1. Directs the student to moisten all of the layers.
    2. Hands the student an occlusive dressing.
    3. Tells the patient that the student is doing a great job.
    4. Suggests removal of all layers and starting over.

26. The nurse is assessing the amount of drainage that the patient has from a surgical wound and finds that 650 mL has drained from 9:00 AM until now, 11:40 PM. What would the nurse do **first**?
    1. Record the amount and appearance of the drainage and continue to observe.
    2. Take the patient's vital signs, assess for other symptoms, and inform the surgeon.
    3. Make sure that the patient's linens are clean and dry and empty the drainage receptacle.
    4. Apply a pressure dressing and place the patient in a supine position.

27. The patient needs a breast binder. What is the **most** important consideration when implementing this application?
    1. Respiratory function must not be restricted.
    2. Vomiting and nausea are a contraindication.
    3. Binders cannot be used for patients who are obese.
    4. Older patients have difficulty tolerating the binder.

28. The nurse hears in report that the patient is "uncooperative" and complains and weeps during the dressing change. Which action would the nurse take **first**?
    1. Describe procedure, give pain medication, and explain that waiting 30 minutes reduces pain.
    2. Assess the patient's understanding and perception of the dressing change procedure.
    3. Demonstrate the dressing change to the patient and supervise while he/she does the procedure.
    4. Pour 30 mL of normal saline over the dressing and wait 30 minutes for the exudate to soften.

29. The nurse is assessing the skin of an older patient and notices a small skin tear on the patient's forearm. Which type of dressing is preferred for this type of wound?
    1. Hydrogel dressing
    2. Impregnated gauze dressing
    3. Transparent dressing
    4. Hydrocolloid dressings

30. If tape must be applied to the skin to secure a dressing on a patient with fragile skin, which type of tape is preferred?
    1. Adhesive tape
    2. Hypoallergenic tape
    3. Twill tape
    4. Paper tape

CRITICAL THINKING ACTIVITIES

31. The nurse is caring for a 72-year-old patient who is being treated for a chronic ulcer on the right lower leg. The patient lives alone. He is diabetic and reports poor vision. The nurse notes that the patient has trouble with fine motor control. He reports that he does his own meal preparation, although he admits that he doesn't make the effort to prepare fresh produce. He is 15 pounds underweight and he has "cut down on his smoking."

    a. Identify factors that may impair wound healing for this patient. _____

    _____

    _____

    b. Discuss how the nurse applies knowledge about older adults to help this patient achieve wound healing.

    _____

    _____

    _____

    _____

    _____

    _____

32. The student nurse is preparing to perform wound irrigation for a patient. The nursing instructor asks the student to answer the following questions before starting the procedure.

    a. What is the purpose of wound irrigation? _____

    _____

    b. What equipment is needed for irrigation at the patient's bedside? _____

    _____

    c. How is the syringe positioned for the irrigation? _____

    _____

    d. What is the direction of cleansing? _____

    _____

    e. What findings should be immediately reported to the health care provider (HCP)? _____

    _____

33. Discuss some of the difficulties that a homeless patient could have performing wound care after being discharged from the hospital. What strategies could the nurse use to help a homeless patient achieve wound care and prevent complications?

_____

_____

_____

_____

_____

_____

NEXT-GENERATION NCLEX™ (NGN)

34. Extended Drag and Drop

Cognitive Skill: Take Action

Scenario: The nurse works on a medical-surgical unit in an acute care hospital. Many of the patients are older and have chronic health conditions such as diabetes. The nurse uses knowledge of factors that impair wound healing to anticipate problems and initiate interventions.

Instructions: In the left column are factors that impair wound healing. Nursing interventions are listed in the right column. In the space provided, write the number for the best nursing intervention to address each factor. Each intervention will be used only once.

Factors that Impair Wound Healing	Nursing Interventions
_____ 1. Tension and stress on sutures have potential for disruption of wound incision.	a. Encourage adequate amounts of calories and fluids.
_____ 2. Fatty tissue lacks adequate blood supply.	b. Carefully observe; signs of inflammation are not always obvious.
_____ 3. Hyperglycemia supports overgrowth of fungal and yeast infections.	c. Wound care is needed for a longer period.
_____ 4. Steroids reduce inflammatory response.	d. Control blood sugar to reduce the physiologic changes associated with diabetes.
_____ 5. Aging causes vascular changes that impair circulation.	e. Instruct to splint abdominal wound during coughing.
_____ 6. Stress from severe trauma increases nutritional requirements.	f. Observe obese patients for wound infection, dehiscence, and evisceration.

Specimen Collection and Diagnostic Testing

chapter
23

Answer Key: A complete Answer Key is provided in your Additional Learning Resources on Evolve.

MATCHING

Directions: Match the suffix on the left to the correct definition on the right and give an example for each.

Suffix	Definition
_____ 1. -oscopy	a. Procedure involving puncture of a body cavity
_____ 2. -ogram	Example _____
_____ 3. -ography	b. Procedure in which an image is produced
_____ 4. -centesis	Example _____
	c. Actual image or results of a test
	Example _____
	d. Procedure in which body structures are visualized
	Example _____

FIGURE LABELING

5. *Directions:* Label the veins of the arms and hands on the figure.

Basilic vein

Cephalic vein

Median cubital vein

Radial vein

Median vein of forearm

Superficial dorsal vein

Dorsal venous arch

FIGURE LABELING

6. *Directions:* Label the placement of the chest (precordial) leads on the figure.

V_1—Fourth intercostal space (ICS) at right sternal border
V_2—Fourth ICS at left sternal border
V_3—Midway between V_2 and V_4
V_4—Fifth ICS at midclavicular line
V_5—Left anterior axillary line at level of V_4 horizontally
V_6—Left midaxillary line at level of V_4 horizontally

DELEGATION

7. Which specimen collections are usually possible to delegate to unlicensed assistive personnel (UAP)?

    Directions: Indicate yes or no in the space provided.

    _____   a.   Urine by midstream collection
    _____   b.   Gastric secretion from nasogastric tube
    _____   c.   Blood sample by venipuncture
    _____   d.   Sputum specimen by suctioning
    _____   e.   Blood sample for glucose
    _____   f.   Wound cultures
    _____   g.   Stool for ova and parasites
    _____   h.   Throat culture

    _____   i.   Sputum specimen by expectoration
    _____   j.   Nasal culture
    _____   k.   Emesis
    _____   l.   Nasopharyngeal culture
    _____   m.   Cerebrospinal fluid
    _____   n.   Stool for hemoccult
    _____   o.   Stool from colostomy

MULTIPLE CHOICE

Directions: Select the best answer(s) for each of the following questions.

8. Which laboratory blood test is **most** likely to require written informed consent?
   1. Complete blood count
   2. Human immunodeficiency virus test
   3. Platelet count
   4. Blood glucose testing

9. The patient reports seeing black, tarry stool. Which question is the nurse **most** likely to ask?
   1. "Are you straining or noticing discomfort with bowel movements?"
   2. "Have you eaten a lot of red meat in the past few days?"
   3. "Are you having any pain or discomfort in the upper mid-abdomen?"
   4. "Have you ever had a problem with hemorrhoids?

10. The clinic nurse sees that the health care provider (HCP) has ordered a sputum specimen for acid-fast bacillus. Which action is the nurse **most** likely to clarify with the HCP?
    1. "Shall I instruct the patient to collect the specimen in the early morning?"
    2. "If the patient cannot expectorate a specimen, is nasotracheal suction allowed?"
    3. "Is the patient allowed to smoke, drink, and eat after the sputum is collected?"
    4. "Should the patient be placed in a negative pressure isolation room?"

11. The postsurgical patient has chills, fever, and malaise. The HCP has instructed the nurse to report the laboratory results as soon as they are available. Which laboratory result is definitive for confirmation of infection and effective treatment?
    1. White blood cell count
    2. Wound culture and sensitivity
    3. Red blood cell count
    4. Electrolyte levels

12. According to the blood-borne pathogen standards of Occupational Safety and Health Administration, health care facilities are required to make a written exposure control plan. Which health care worker has sustained a major significant exposure?
    1. Nursing student injures self while recapping a needle used to draw up the patient's insulin.
    2. UAP picks up blood-stained linen without donning gloves.
    3. Nurse sustains a deep cut with profuse bleeding while trying to raise a patient's side rails.
    4. Phlebotomist sustains a deep puncture caused by a needle used to collect blood.

13. What is the **best** rationale for drawing at least two blood cultures from two different sites?
    1. This is the standard method used to detect bacteremia.
    2. If only one culture shows bacteria, technician error is assumed.
    3. If both cultures show an infecting agent, bacteremia is confirmed.
    4. If both cultures show different infecting agents, skin contamination is assumed.

14. The nurse is planning care for several patients who will need postprocedural care. Which patient will require serial neurovascular assessments on bilateral extremities?
    1. Patient having cardiac catheterization
    2. Patient having a bone scan
    3. Patient having electrocardiography
    4. Patient having paracentesis

15. The nurse is interviewing a patient who needs to be scheduled for colonoscopy. Which patient comment would cause the nurse to contact the HCP before giving instructions for the usual oral bowel preparation?
    1. "I take insulin for my diabetes."
    2. "I have heard the bowel prep is awful."
    3. "I think I might have acute diverticulitis."
    4. "My father died of colon cancer."

16. The patient had a colonoscopy 2 hours ago and reports that abdominal pain seems to be increasing. Which assessments would the nurse perform if colon perforation is suspected? **Select all that apply.**
    1. Take vital signs and compare with baseline.
    2. Gently palpate abdomen for tenderness and distention.
    3. Perform digital rectal examination to check for blood.
    4. Observe for tolerance of clear oral fluids.
    5. Observe stools for bleeding and note color and amount.

17. Shortly after the patient returns from having a liver biopsy, he reports chest pain and trouble breathing. He seems restless and anxious. The RN says that he might have a pneumothorax. What will the nurses do before calling the HCP? **Select all that apply.**
    1. Assess rate, rhythm, and depth of respirations.
    2. Check pulse oximeter reading.
    3. Assess blood coagulation profile.
    4. Listen to breath sounds.
    5. Apply oxygen if needed.

18. The postoperative patient demonstrates some mild dizziness and mild shortness of breath when moving from sitting to standing position. Which laboratory value would the nurse check **first**?
    1. Red blood cell count
    2. White blood cell count
    3. Blood urea nitrogen
    4. Creatinine level

19. Prior to a paracentesis, which assessments would be performed? **Select all that apply.**
    1. Weight
    2. Height
    3. Abdominal girth
    4. Baseline vital signs
    5. Peripheral pulses

20. The nurse needs to perform venipuncture on an older patient whose veins are very fragile. What is the **best** strategy for the nurse to use?
    1. Gently tap over the vein.
    2. Apply a warm compress.
    3. Use a Vacutainer.
    4. Use a small-gauge needle.

21. The nurse is using a commercially prepared tube for the collection of an aerobic wound specimen for culture. After collecting the specimen with the swab, what would the nurse do?
    1. Place the swab into the collection tube, close it tightly, and keep the specimen warm.
    2. Take the swab and mix it with the special color-changing reagent in the collection tube.
    3. Place the swab into the collection tube and add the liquid culture medium.
    4. Crush the ampule at the end of the tube and put the tip of the swab into the solution.

22. Following a lumbar puncture, what does the nurse do to prevent a postpuncture spinal headache?
    1. Reduces the patient's fluid intake
    2. Places the patient in a high-Fowler's position
    3. Informs the HCP if a headache develops
    4. Instructs the patient to lie in the supine position

23. The patient is to have a thoracentesis performed. The nurse assists the patient to which position for this test?
    1. Dorsal recumbent
    2. Supine with the arms held above the head
    3. Sitting up and leaning over a table
    4. Side-lying with the knees drawn up

24. The patient requests information about a scheduled magnetic resonance imaging study. What would the nurse tell the patient to expect?
    1. "You shouldn't eat or drink for 4 hours before the test."
    2. "You will hear humming and loud thumping sounds."
    3. "You will have minor discomfort in the area being tested."
    4. "You will be assisted to make frequent position changes."

25. The nurse is teaching the patient how to collect a specimen for blood glucose monitoring at home. Which patient action demonstrates correct technique?
    1. Allows the blood specimen to drop onto the test strip
    2. Uses the center of the finger for the puncture
    3. Holds the finger upright after puncture
    4. Vigorously squeezes the fingertip after puncture

26. What is included in the instructions to the patient for collection of a midstream urine sample?
    1. Use a clean specimen cup and try not to touch the inside of the cup.
    2. Collect at least 200 mL of urine into the specimen cup.
    3. Void into the toilet, stop urinating, and then urinate into the cup.
    4. Bathe or shower the perineal area before collection.

27. The student nurse is obtaining a urine specimen from a patient with an existing indwelling catheter. When would the supervising nurse intervene?
    1. Performs hand hygiene and applies clean gloves for the procedure.
    2. Clamps the drainage tubing for 30 minutes before specimen collection begins.
    3. Disconnects the catheter from the drainage tubing and collects the urine in a specimen cup.
    4. Unclamps the drainage tube after collection and observes for urine flow.

28. The patient will be catheterized for residual urine. What is the correct technique for this procedure?
    1. Catheterize the patient when the bladder is full.
    2. Obtain an order for an indwelling catheter.
    3. Catheterize the patient within 10 minutes of voiding.
    4. Use clean technique to obtain the sample.

29. A patient requires venipuncture to obtain a blood sample for diagnostic testing. Which laboratory result is the **greatest** concern related to the venipuncture?
    1. High blood glucose level
    2. Low platelet count
    3. Elevated blood urea nitrogen
    4. Low sodium level

30. How does the nurse properly use a tourniquet when performing a venipuncture?
    1. Ties it into a single knot
    2. Leaves it in place for no more than 1-2 minutes
    3. Places it 6-8 inches above the selected site
    4. Ties it tight enough to occlude the distal pulse

31. The patient is suspected of having a urinary tract infection (UTI). The HCP has ordered a urine specimen for culture and sensitivity testing. The patient asks, "Can't I just get a prescription for antibiotics?" What is the **best** response?
    1. "This is just a routine test for any patient suspected of having a UTI."
    2. "Your HCP feels this test is necessary in determining your diagnosis."
    3. "I can contact your HCP if you would like to ask for a prescription."
    4. "Different bacteria can cause a UTI and the test results will indicate the best antibiotic."

32. When performing a Hemoccult slide test to determine the presence of occult blood in a stool specimen, which action is correct?
    1. Use two separate areas of the stool when obtaining the specimen.
    2. Obtain the specimen from the toilet bowl.
    3. Perform the test control before obtaining the specimen.
    4. Take the specimen immediately to the laboratory to prevent hemolysis.

33. An older patient had a bronchoscopy several hours ago and now seems restless and confused compared to baseline behavior. Which assessment is the **most** important?
    1. Orientation to person, place, and time
    2. Pulse oximeter reading and respiratory rate
    3. Time and dosage of antianxiety medications
    4. Time of last food and fluid ingestion

34. An older female patient needs diagnostic testing that requires nothing by mouth (NPO) for 12 hours prior to the test and a bowel preparation. The test has been cancelled twice; once for retained stool and once for equipment problems. Which intervention is the **priority**?
    1. Explain the cancellations to the patient using terms that she can easily understand.
    2. Call the diagnostic technician to ensure that the test gets done.
    3. Assess the patient for dehydration and fluid and electrolyte imbalances.
    4. Call the HCP and ask if the test can be postponed for a few days.

35. The nurse has just informed the patient that he should collect a sputum specimen in the morning. Which additional instruction will the nurse give?
    1. "Brush your teeth and use mouthwash just prior to collecting the specimen."
    2. "Drink extra water the day before collection to decrease the thickness of mucus."
    3. "Inhale and cough deeply and then spit the clear saliva into the sterile cup."
    4. "Do not eat any red meat or drink any caffeinated beverages."

36. The nurse has just received laboratory results for an unfamiliar test, so he is unsure if the results are within normal limits. What would the nurse do **first**?
    1. Call the HCP and read the results exactly as they are shown.
    2. Ask the patient if he is having any unusual symptoms or complaints.
    3. Call the laboratory technician and ask for an explanation of the results.
    4. Check the facility's laboratory manual for information about the test.

37. The nurse has orders for voided midstream urine specimens for several patients. Which patient is **most** likely to require an order for a straight catheterized specimen rather than a voided midstream specimen?
    1. A 25-year-old female who finished her menstrual period yesterday
    2. A 55-year-old female diabetic patient who is very overweight
    3. A 63-year-old male who has difficulty with urination due to prostate problems
    4. An 18-year-old male who has a Glasgow coma score of 4 after a head injury

38. Several patients require stool specimens for diagnostic testing. Which patient's stool specimen must be taken immediately to the laboratory after it has been obtained?
    1. Patient traveled to a foreign country and reports abdominal cramping with diarrhea.
    2. Patient saw very dark black stool several days ago, but now stool seems normal.
    3. Patient (small child) is suspected of swallowing a plastic marble 3 days ago.
    4. Patient saw stool floating in toilet and there was an oily film in the water.

39. The nurse is suctioning the patient to obtain a sputum specimen. During the 10 seconds of suctioning, the cardiac monitor shows bradycardia and the patient becomes very diaphoretic. What is the **best** explanation for this occurrence?
    1. Patient demonstrated anxiety due to the procedure.
    2. Nurse caused hypoxia by suctioning for a prolonged time.
    3. Cardiac changes are unrelated to the procedure.
    4. Catheter caused direct stimulation of vagal nerve fibers.

40. The nurse notes purulent drainage from a wound and decides to obtain an order for a wound culture. Prior to contacting the surgeon, which additional data will the nurse obtain? **Select all that apply.**
    1. Check oral temperature.
    2. Look at trends of white blood cell count.
    3. Ask about subjective symptoms such as chills or fatigue.
    4. Assess for pain at the wound site.
    5. Review the previous documentation about the wound.

41. A patient is newly admitted for pneumonia with possible early sepsis. The nurse is reviewing the admission orders. Which order would be done **first**?
    1. Intravenous antibiotics
    2. Blood cultures from two sites
    3. Chest x-ray
    4. Blood chemistries

42. The nurse is supervising a nursing student who will perform venipuncture to obtain a blood sample for blood chemistries. The nurse will intervene if the student performs which action?
    1. Applies a warm compress to the arm on the side of a mastectomy
    2. Obtains a Vacutainer and different colors of collection tubes
    3. Applies a tourniquet 3 inches above elbow and palpates the antecubital space
    4. Releases the tourniquet after 2 minutes of trying to locate a vein

43. A patient had a diagnostic study with a contrast medium 4 hours ago. Now he has swelling and itching around the eyes, a rapid pulse, and mild dyspnea. What would the nurse do **first**?
    1. Administer an as-needed (PRN) dose of diphenhydramine and call the HCP.
    2. Call the Rapid Response Team and bring resuscitation equipment to the bedside.
    3. Contact the health care team member who administered the contrast medium.
    4. Apply a cool compress to reduce the swelling and instruct the patient to rest.

44. The UAP reports two unsuccessful attempts to get enough blood to adequately cover the test strip to check the blood glucose. Which factors could interfere with getting an adequate drop of blood? **Select all that apply.**
    1. Environmental temperature of the room
    2. Technique used to obtain the sample
    3. Position of the patient's arm
    4. Improper calibration of the glucometer
    5. Problems with peripheral circulation
    6. Condition of the skin on hands and fingers

45. The nurse is supervising a new nurse who must collect gastric secretions from a nasogastric (NG) tube. When would the supervising nurse intervene?
    1. New nurse uses an alcohol swab to scrub the NG tube prior to inserting a sterile needle.
    2. New nurse assists the patient to a high-Fowler's position and places a towel underneath the NG tube.
    3. New nurse disconnects the NG tube from the suction or the gravity drainage.
    4. New nurse verifies NG tube placement to ensure aspiration of gastric contents.

46. The nurse is suctioning a patient to obtain a sputum specimen. Which occurrence is expected?
    1. As the suction catheter is inserted into the tracheostomy, there is resistance.
    2. As the suction catheter is inserted into the trachea, the patient begins to cough.
    3. As suction is applied, oxygen saturation drops below normal for several minutes.
    4. As the suction catheter is withdrawn, the patient begins to exhale very deeply.

47. The nurse has tried several times to obtain a throat culture on a patient, but the patient has gagged, moved, and contaminated the tip of the swab during each attempt. What would the nurse do **first**?
    1. Have the patient look in the mirror, give him the swab, and coach him through the procedure.
    2. Inform the HCP that several unsuccessful attempts have been made.
    3. Instruct the patient to open mouth and say a very long "ahhhhh" and avoid using a tongue blade.
    4. Obtain an order for a mild local anesthetic that will temporarily suppress the gag reflex.

48. The nurse needs to perform venipuncture to obtain a blood sample for blood chemistries. Which factors influence the nurse's choice of sterile needles? **Select all that apply.**
    1. Age of patient
    2. Condition of veins
    3. Nurse's familiarity with product
    4. Syringe method versus vacuum tube method
    5. Type of blood chemistry test ordered
    6. Color of the collection tube

49. Nurse A is aware that Nurse B, who is not very skilled at venipuncture, is sticking her patients more than the recommended two times as stated by hospital policy. What would Nurse A do **first**?
    1. Report Nurse B to the nurse manager for violating hospital policy.
    2. Watch Nurse B and offer to perform venipunctures after two attempts.
    3. Assess Nurse B's understanding and skill in performing venipuncture.
    4. Ask the charge nurse to assess Nurse B's understanding of hospital policy.

50. As the nurse is performing an electrocardio-
    gram (ECG), the patient reports very mild left
    anterior chest pain. What would the nurse do
    first?
    1. Stop the procedure and obtain the crash
       cart and other emergency equipment.
    2. Continue the procedure and tell the patient
       to relax and not to worry.
    3. Stop the procedure and obtain an order for
       pain medication.
    4. Continue procedure and make notation of
       pain on the request slip or ECG strip.

CRITICAL THINKING ACTIVITIES

51. The nurse is caring for a patient who is scheduled to have a thoracentesis.

    a. What assessments should be performed prior to the procedure? _____

    _____

    _____

    _____

    _____

    b. Why would it be particularly important to assess this patient's lung sounds and presence of cough
       before the procedure?

    _____

    _____

    _____

    _____

    c. Describe the nursing responsibilities related to the care of the patient before and during the
       thoracentesis.

    _____

    _____

    _____

    _____

    d. Describe the assessments and care that the nurse should perform after the thoracentesis procedure.

    _____

    _____

    _____

    _____

NEXT-GENERATION NCLEX™ (NGN)

52. Extended Multiple Response

Cognitive Skill: Take Action

Scenario: The nurse is caring for a 78-year-old woman who is scheduled to have a urinalysis, blood chemistries, and an abdominal scan with contrast media. The patient is alert and cooperative. She is thin and reports a poor appetite and fluid intake. The patient demonstrates some trouble with fine motor movements of the hands and some mobility issues related to arthritis, but she is able to independently perform most activities of daily living.

Which nursing interventions would the nurse use for the older patient?

Instructions: Place a check mark next to the interventions the nurse would use. **Check all that apply.**

_____ 1. Assess patient's ability to collect a midstream urine specimen.

_____ 2. Obtain an order for a catheterized urine specimen if needed.

_____ 3. Use an 18-gauge needle for venipuncture for blood specimens.

_____ 4. For venipuncture, loosely apply the rubber tourniquet.

_____ 5. Assess for allergies to contrast media prior to the abdominal scan.

_____ 6. Assess for dehydration before and after the abdominal scan.

_____ 7. Administer pain medication prior to abdominal scan.

_____ 8. Monitor for dyspnea, wheezing, or hemoptysis after the abdominal scan.

_____ 9. Monitor for bleeding or swelling at the catheter insertion site after the abdominal scan.

_____ 10. Monitor for delayed reaction to contrast media (i.e., dyspnea, rashes, tachycardia, urticaria).

_____ 11. Encourage oral fluids after the abdominal scan.

Lifespan Development

Answer Key: A complete Answer Key is provided in your Additional Learning Resources on Evolve.

TABLE ACTIVITY

1. *Directions:* Insert the expected values of vital signs for different age groups.

Age Group	Temperature	Pulse	Respirations (at Rest)	Blood Pressure
Infants, 12 months				
Toddler, 1-3 years				
School-age, 6-12 years				
Adolescent, 12-19 years				

MULTIPLE CHOICE

Directions: Select the best answer(s) for each of the following questions.

2. Which nursing action addresses the gradual decline in life expectancy and the increase in death rates among young and middle-aged adults in the United States?
   1. Cares for young adult patients who have been accidently injured or disabled
   2. Offers brochures that encourage cancer screening for vulnerable groups
   3. Reports signs and symptoms of substance abuse to the health care provider (HCP)
   4. Administers prescribed medications to assigned patients in a timely manner

3. Which behaviors exemplify the qualities of functional families? **Select all that apply.**
   1. Mother tells daughter that being homecoming queen is an expected family tradition.
   2. Parents encourage children to try after-school activities to meet new friends.
   3. Family attends a ceremony that honors the youngest son's contribution to the community.
   4. During family dinnertime, children are encouraged to talk about activities and interests.
   5. Older sibling shows younger brother several methods to solve math problems.
   6. Parents buy their children clothes, computers, cell phones, and other trendy items.

4. Which type of family is **most** likely to seek the services of the health care team for a child with a physical or mental disability?
   1. Grandfamily
   2. Adoptive family
   3. Extended family
   4. Nuclear family

5. Which nursing actions contribute to accomplishing the *Healthy People 2020* Health Indicators? **Select all that apply.**
   1. Administers medication using the six rights
   2. Reinforces the need for preventive dental care
   3. Encourages patients to routinely exercise
   4. Assists patients to locate smoking cessation literature
   5. Shows respect and courtesy to older patients
   6. Teaches patients how to limit fats and sugar in the diet

6. The nurse is interviewing a woman who is from a different culture than the nurse's. The nurse directs the questions to the woman, but the woman consistently looks toward her husband and he answers. What would the nurse do **first**?
   1. Ask the husband to leave the room and continue the interview with the wife.
   2. Continue the interview and observe for additional nonverbal behaviors.
   3. Direct the questions to the husband, because the wife is deferring to him.
   4. Discontinue the interview and seek advice about how to interact with this couple.

7. The nurse determines that the family is primarily autocratic. Which observation supports the nurse's analysis?
   1. Mother assumes dominance in decision-making.
   2. Parents implement strict rules and expectations.
   3. Uncle controls the finances.
   4. Children participate in negotiations.

8. Which patient needs to get both pneumococcal and influenza vaccines?
   1. 68-year-old resident in an assisted living facility
   2. 3-year-old who goes to daycare every weekday
   3. 21-year-old who lives in a college dorm
   4. 30-year-old pregnant woman in the first trimester

9. Which patient group is the nurse **most** likely to assess for possible exposure to teratogens?
   1. A group of preschoolers who attend a day-care setting
   2. Residents who live at a long-term care center
   3. A group of young women who are planning pregnancy
   4. A group of adolescents who are at risk for substance abuse

10. The nurse is assessing a 6-month-old infant, who was 21 inches (53 cm) long at birth. Based on expected growth patterns, what height would the nurse expect on measuring this healthy baby?
    1. 22 inches (56 cm)
    2. 27 inches (69 cm)
    3. 30 inches (76 cm)
    4. 31 inches (79 cm)

11. The nurse is assessing a 1-year-old child who weighed 9 lbs (4 kg) at birth. Based on expected growth patterns, how much should this healthy child weigh? _____ lbs (kg)

12. Most of the weight gain in the first months of life is in the form of fat. What is the **best** physiologic explanation for this gain of fat?
    1. Fat provides insulation and a source of nourishment if teething or other problems decrease food intake for a few days.
    2. In cephalocaudal growth, fat must be deposited in areas of the trunk and abdomen before growth in extremities can occur.
    3. Breast milk or prepared formulas are high in nutrients that are more readily converted to fat than to muscle or bone tissue.
    4. Muscle and bone require more protein and calcium, so development of these tissues is concurrent with intake of solid foods.

13. The mother of a 5-month-old infant reports the child is irritable; gums are red and edematous, and he demonstrates excessive drooling. What would the nurse recommend?
    1. Advise the mother to contact the HCP for treatment of infection.
    2. Suggest the mother wipe and massage the gums and offer sips of clear water.
    3. Teach the mother to brush the gums with a soft brush and fluoride toothpaste.
    4. Advise the mother to give an infant dose of acetaminophen for discomfort.

14. Under which circumstance would the nurse advise the parents to contact the HCP about their 1-year-old infant?
    1. Child seems restless and makes little noises during short napping periods.
    2. Baby cries persistently during usual sleep periods and is inconsolable.
    3. Infant sleeps 12 hours a night and takes one nap during the day.
    4. Child frequently kicks and stretches when in the supine position.

15. Which infant behavior is consistent with Piaget's theory that infants are in the sensorimotor stage of cognitive development?
    1. Clings to the parent and protests any separation
    2. Reaches for objects and puts them into mouth
    3. Demonstrates shoulder control prior to hand control
    4. Frequently says, "me" and "no"

16. The working mother has an 8-month-old child who has to go to daycare while she works. How can the nurse **best** help the mother prepare for the first day of daycare?
    1. Explain the likelihood of separation anxiety as a normal behavior.
    2. Emphasize that the child is likely to sleep most of the day, so he won't miss her.
    3. Describe the benefits of parallel play for cognitive development.
    4. Validate the mother's feelings of guilt and reassure that daycare is beneficial.

17. The HCP tells the first-time parents how to introduce new foods to the infant. Which information would be reinforced? **Select all that apply.**
    1. Citrus fruits may be given before the infant is 6 months of age.
    2. Foods should be mixed together to improve intake of nutrients.
    3. Cereals should be started before vegetables and meats.
    4. New foods should be introduced one at a time.
    5. Several days should pass between introducing new foods.

18. The nurse is watching a group of mothers interact with their young children. Which behavior by a mother **most** strongly suggests that additional assessment for potential child abuse might be required?
    1. Retrieves toddler whenever he tries to run or jump or perform active movements
    2. Allows toddler to climb on a table space that is meant for snacks and drinks
    3. Berates and shames her toddler for refusing to share toys with other children
    4. Talks to other mothers and allows the toddler to fuss without comforting him

19. The nurse is interviewing the parents of a toddler who must be admitted for 23-hour observation for a febrile illness. What is the **most** important question to ask about the child's bedtime?
    1. "Would you prefer that he gets milk or juice in a night bottle?"
    2. "What do you usually do when you put him to bed?"
    3. "How many hours does he usually sleep?"
    4. "What would you like me to tell him about sleeping away from home?"

20. The mother is ordering lunch for her toddler. The nurse would intervene if the mother selected which food for the toddler?
    1. Milk
    2. Peanut butter sandwich
    3. Carrot sticks
    4. Small banana

21. The parents report that their 3-year-old child has not started talking, but he seems happy and active and engaged with the world in non-verbal ways. What would the nurse advise the parents to do?
    1. Advise the parents to read to the child and ask him to name familiar objects.
    2. Suggest expanding opportunities for parallel play, such as at daycare or play groups.
    3. Reassure parents that children grow and develop at their own individual pace.
    4. Suggest consultation with the HCP for possible hearing or speech problems.

22. The HCP asks the nurse to please watch the 4-year-old child because she needs to talk privately to the mother. What is the **best** way for the nurse to interact with the child?
    1. Take the child to the cafeteria and buy him a snack.
    2. Give him some crayons and paper and ask him to draw a picture.
    3. Ask him to "help" by sorting a bag of rubber bands by size and color.
    4. Explain why he has to wait and give him a book to read.

23. The school nurse notices that an 8-year-old boy comes to the nursing office during recess for a "tummyache" which seems to disappear as soon as recess is over. What would the nurse do **first?**
    1. Call the parents and review symptoms that warrant an appointment with the HCP.
    2. Ask the teachers if there are any unusual classroom behaviors going on.
    3. Alert the principal that there may be some bullying or rough play during recess.
    4. Contact the parents and discuss the pattern of stomachache and recess time.

24. A mother reports that her child occasionally complains of pain in the legs particularly at night. Which question would the nurse ask to determine if this is an expected symptom?
    1. "Has the child been running?"
    2. "How old is your child?"
    3. "Has your child appeared anxious?"
    4. "How much does your child weigh?"

25. The nurse must give the school-age child an immunization. Based on the nurse's awareness that the child is in the concrete operational stage, what would the nurse do prior to giving the child the injection?
    1. Ask a helper to hold the child to prevent movement.
    2. Suggest that the child pretend that she is getting a fairy's kiss.
    3. Tell the child that it hurts a bit, but prevents sickness.
    4. Make extra efforts to protect modesty and privacy.

26. Which routine check-ups or screenings are recommended for school-age children? **Select all that apply.**
    1. Vision testing
    2. Dental examination every 6 months
    3. Hearing testing
    4. Scoliosis screening
    5. Cancer screening
    6. Human immunodeficiency virus testing

27. The nurse must perform a dressing change on a 7-year-old child. The nurse explains that the procedure will not be painful, but the child appears apprehensive. What is the **best** approach for the nurse to use?
    1. Demonstrate the procedure on a doll and answer questions.
    2. Ask the child to hold the tape and give praise for cooperation.
    3. Premedicate with a mild anxiolytic medication and explain.
    4. Coach the parent through the procedure and stand back.

28. The school nurse is talking to a child who sustained an abrasion and bruise during recess. When the nurse asks the child what happened, he begins to cry, shakes his head, and refuses to answer. What would the nurse do **first?**
    1. Tell him that all information is confidential, so he doesn't have to feel embarrassed or afraid.
    2. Call the parents and inform them that the child is emotionally overwhelmed and can't talk.
    3. Consult the school principal to see if something unusual happened on the playground.
    4. Talk to him while treating the wounds and give encouragement to establish rapport.

29. A parent expresses concern because her healthy, active 11-year-old son seems very short. She reports that all men on both sides of the family are tall. What is the **best** information that the nurse can give to the mother about growth and development? **Select all that apply.**
    1. During the school-age period, the growth pattern is usually gradual and subtle.
    2. A second period of rapid growth is expected during adolescence.
    3. From ages 6-12, height increases by about 2 inches (5 cm).
    4. He is probably lacking essential nutrients that contribute to height and weight.
    5. Distant genetic factors are likely to predispose him to a shorter height.

30. Which parent is doing the **best** job of using good parenting tips in dealing with an adolescent child?
    1. Parent permits 17-year-old son to set own curfew time on weekends.
    2. Parent gives up smoking cigarettes and encourages 18-year-old to quit too.
    3. Parent respects 15-year-old daughter's privacy by not asking questions about friends.
    4. Parent allows 13-year-old unlimited computer time if grades are maintained.

31. The parent reports that her 15-year-old daughter seems more moody than usual and she is concerned because there was a teenager in the neighborhood who recently committed suicide. What is the **most** important question that the nurse would ask to determine if the daughter has a high risk for suicide?
    1. "Has she had a change in appetite?"
    2. "Is there a change in her ability to concentrate?"
    3. "Is she preoccupied with thoughts of death?"
    4. "Has she talked about ways to commit suicide?"

32. The nurse is working with a group of parents of high school students. During the discussion, the following statements are made by the parents. Based on an understanding of the needs of adolescents, which statement requires follow-up by the nurse?
    1. "We try to set reasonable limits on dating and are encouraging group activities."
    2. "Teenagers who participate in social activities should be home by 9:00 PM on school nights."
    3. "We are generally not in favor of allowing sex education to be taught at school."
    4. "There are numerous after-school activities, so we suggest focusing on two or three."

33. Which behaviors indicate that the young adult is achieving the developmental tasks of early adulthood? **Select all that apply.**
    1. Lives at home with parents, but is saving for an apartment deposit.
    2. Accepts that sister's decision to have a big family is okay.
    3. Establishes a permanent relationship with a same-sex partner.
    4. Decides to postpone marriage and focus on career.
    5. Identifies with and seeks out gay and lesbian peer groups.

34. Which behavior demonstrates that a 60-year-old adult is meeting his developmental task of generativity?
    1. Ruminates over fears and lifetime failures
    2. Reorganizes personal belongings and assets
    3. Gives advice to nephew about succeeding in life
    4. Reviews will for distribution of worldly goods

35. A 53-year-old woman tells the nurse that she has been experiencing flushing, mood swings, night sweats, and breast tenderness for the past several months. Based on knowledge of lifespan development, which question is the nurse **most** likely to ask?
    1. "Do you have a personal or family history of breast cancer?"
    2. "When was your last normal menstrual period?"
    3. "Have you experienced a change in libido?"
    4. "Have you ever been told that you have osteoporosis?"

36. The nurse is assessing the vision of an older adult patient. Which finding requires follow-up?
    1. Presbyopia
    2. Visualization of half of the field
    3. Decreased depth perception
    4. Slowed accommodation

37. The nurse is working in a long-term care facility. Which activity will help the residents meet the developmental task of ego integrity as described by Erikson?
    1. Taking the residents out to lunch at a restaurant
    2. Reminiscing about past important events
    3. Assisting residents to maintain personal hygiene
    4. Leading the residents in an arts and crafts project

38. The home health nurse is visiting an older patient who lives alone. She is underweight and the kitchen is unusable because of dirt and clutter. What would the nurse do **first**?
    1. Contact a local organization that will deliver meals to the house.
    2. Notify supervising RN to determine if elder neglect is an issue.
    3. Assess for additional factors that are contributing to the malnutrition.
    4. Weigh the patient and calculate the body mass index.

39. Based on knowledge of normal changes of the cardiovascular system, which recommendation would the nurse make to an older adult?
    1. Maintain a low-fat, low-sodium diet.
    2. Obtain streptococcal pneumonia vaccine.
    3. Encourage coughing and deep-breathing.
    4. Change position frequently.

40. Which behavior **most** strongly indicates that the older adult is successfully aging?
    1. Spends a lot of time with adult children trying to make up for lost time
    2. Studies Latin and combines subject matter with previous interest in literature
    3. Tries various complementary and alternative therapies to improve appearance
    4. Works through a "bucket list" with an uncharacteristic enthusiasm

41. Which health care worker is demonstrating ageism?
    1. Physical therapist accompanies a resident who lives in a long-term care facility to go outside for a walk
    2. Phlebotomist examines an older patient's veins and tells the nurse that successful blood draw is unlikely
    3. HCP tells an older woman that it would be best if her husband was in hospice care
    4. Nurse continuously smiles and nods as an older patient sharply criticizes the nursing care

42. Which activity would the nurse encourage for an older adult who wanted to improve his/her memory?
    1. Independently completing activities of daily living (ADLs)
    2. Watching television programs that are relaxing
    3. Engaging in activities such as puzzles, reading, and hobbies
    4. Spending time reflecting on past accomplishments

43. Which health promotion point is **most** important to prevent onset or reduce problems related to coronary artery disease, hypertension, osteoarthritis, osteoporosis, diabetes, obesity, and chronic obstructive pulmonary disease?
    1. Low-fat and low-carbohydrate diet
    2. Regular, paced exercise routine
    3. Eight hours of sleep or short daytime naps
    4. Medication compliance as prescribed

CRITICAL THINKING ACTIVITIES

44. Visit the home of friend, family member, or classmate who has an infant or very young child or visit a daycare center that offers care for infants or very young children. Observe the setting, the way that the child interacts with the environment and other family members/people, and then review the safety rules for infants and children. Identify which rules that the family/daycare center already has in place and identify areas where safety could be improved.

_____

_____

_____

_____

45. A young mother expresses frustration because she is having trouble toilet training her 18-month-old child. She reports that the child shows no interest in learning to use the "potty chair." She tells you that she has tried to sit the child on the potty chair and instructed the child to "urinate." She says that her child frequently has temper tantrums when she places him on the chair.

   a. What can you tell the mother about physiologic development related to toilet training? _____

   _____

   _____

   _____

   _____

   b. Use Erikson's stages of psychosocial development to explain how the mother can respond to the child during toilet training.

   _____

   _____

   _____

   c. What can you tell the mother about the child's temper tantrums? _____

   _____

   _____

   _____

   _____

46. Recall a recent interaction with an older person (patient, family member, neighbor, friend) and select one of the theories of aging that helps you understand an aspect of aging for that person. Describe what you saw and then explain how the selected theory supports your understanding.

_____

_____

_____

_____

NEXT-GENERATION NCLEX™ (NGN)

47. Extended Drag and Drop

Cognitive Skill: Take Action

Scenario: The nurse works in an assisted living facility. The residents are older but maintain various levels of independence in ADLs; however, many need some assistance because of changes related to aging. The nurse uses interventions that address the expected changes in aging.

Instructions: In the left column are normal changes associated with aging. Nursing interventions are listed in the right column. In the space provided, write the letter for the best nursing intervention to address normal changes. Each intervention will be used only once.

Normal Changes	**Suggested Nursing Interventions**
_____ 1. Bones are more porous; joint stiffness decreases range of motion, mobility, and agility	a. Encourage regular, paced exercise with adequate rest periods. Maintain low-fat, low-sodium diet.
_____ 2. Presbyopia, slowing of accommodation, narrowing of visual field and decrease in depth perception	b. Observe for signs of urinary tract infections. Observe closely for adverse drug reactions.
_____ 3. Presbycusis, degenerative changes within ear structure; increase in buildup of wax production	c. Inspect skin for impairment or signs of pressure. Change position frequently.
_____ 4. Respiratory muscles weaken, maximum breathing capacity reduced; decreased cough reflex action; more susceptible to respiratory infection	d. Assess for indigestion. Offer five or six small daily meals. Encourage regular toileting habits.
_____ 5. Loss of elasticity and narrowing of blood vessels, with an increase in blood pressure; decreased cardiac output	e. Maintain mobility. Encourage passive and active exercises. Use assistive aids when indicated.
_____ 6. Skin is paler, thinner, more fragile, and prone to injury; decreased moisture, elasticity, and loss of subcutaneous fat	f. Face individual. Speak slowly, clearly, and in lower tones. Do not shout. Control background noise.
_____ 7. Decreased renal blood flow; less effective filtration; decreased bladder elasticity and capacity; need for more frequent voiding	g. Encourage annual eye examinations. Place articles within visual field. Use night-lights.
_____ 8. Decreased chewing efficiency, esophageal motility, and gastric enzyme secretion; less absorption of nutrients; slowing of peristalsis	h. Encourage coughing and deep-breathing. Administer pneumococcal vaccine. Discourage smoking.

Loss, Grief, Dying, and Death

chapter

25

Answer Key: A complete Answer Key is provided in your Additional Learning Resources on Evolve.

MULTIPLE CHOICE

Directions: Select the best answer(s) for each of the following questions.

1. Which nursing action represents one of the eight domains established by the National Consensus Project for Quality Palliative Care?
   1. Assists the provider to intubate a patient who is in respiratory arrest
   2. Teaches the patient self-care measures to resume independent life at home
   3. Helps the patient to identify previously used coping strategies and develop new ones
   4. Assists the patient to maintain hope for a successful recovery and return to function

2. Which action is the **best** indicator that an older widow is moving through grief towards closure?
   1. Shuts the door of her husband's study so that his belongings are out of sight
   2. Tells her son to throw out all of her husband's belongings so that she won't have to look at them
   3. Sorts through her husband's belongings and saves some items for grandchildren and donates the rest
   4. Sits in the study every evening and handles items that represent shared memories

3. For which patient would the nurse design and implement interventions to facilitate anticipatory grief?
   1. Woman reports fatigue and depression after death of a child and subsequent divorce.
   2. Young athlete is informed that he needs a below-the-knee amputation due to osteosarcoma.
   3. Reluctant older adult is brought by daughter-in-law to live in an assisted living center.
   4. Young woman who never knew her father continues to grieve over the missing relationship.

4. The nurse has a good relationship with an older man who was recently placed on hospice care. He speaks fondly about his adult children but admits to being very rough on them while they were growing up. What would the nurse do **first** to facilitate anticipatory grieving for the man and his family?
   1. Call the children and suggest that their father would like to see them.
   2. Ask the health care provider (HCP) if the prognosis was explained to the family.
   3. Invite the family in and observe the interaction and relationship between the members.
   4. Talk to the man about his perception of his current relationship with his children.

5. The home health nurse is visiting an older patient who had an exacerbation of chronic obstructive pulmonary disease (COPD). Which finding **best** supports the nurse's analysis of dysfunctional grieving?
   1. In addition to COPD, the patient has multiple other chronic health problems.
   2. Patient ruminates over loss of health and vigor that started years ago.
   3. Nurse observes pictures of family and friends and fun times from past years.
   4. Patient lives alone and appears to have limited social or familial support.

6. The nurse is caring for a hospice patient who is frequently experiencing episodes of pain and dyspnea. The family is devoted and frequently visits, but today the patient is difficult to arouse, and they accuse the nurse of overmedicating the patient. What would the nurse do **first**?
   1. Listen to their concerns and clarify their goals for the patient.
   2. Explain that the medication was administered as prescribed.
   3. Call the HCP and ask that the medication be discontinued.
   4. Contact the RN so that the care plan can be adjusted.

7. The nurse enters the room and the family is standing around the dying patient loudly praying and chanting. The wife invites the nurse to join in. What would the nurse do **first**?
   1. Instruct them to quietly pray and chant.
   2. Decline to join but allow them to continue.
   3. Politely set a time limit on the chanting.
   4. Assess effects of the activity on the patient.

8. The nurse is teaching the entire family, which includes a preschooler and a school-aged child, about how to care and interact with an older member of the family who is dying and being cared for at home. Which activities would be **best** to suggest to the preschooler and school-aged child, respectively?
   1. Listen to music with grandma and help her brush her teeth.
   2. Eat breakfast with grandma and help her swallow liquids.
   3. Watch television with grandma and help her to the bathroom.
   4. Draw a picture for grandma and organize her photo album.

9. Which outcome statement **best** indicates that one of the primary goals of palliative care has been met?
   1. Patient reports relief from pain and nausea.
   2. Patient verbalizes a wish to die as soon as possible.
   3. Patient was not alone at the time of death.
   4. Patient had personal affairs arranged before death.

10. In the care of the dying patient, which tasks can be delegated to the unlicensed assistive personnel (UAP)? **Select all that apply.**
    1. Recognize grief and communicate therapeutically.
    2. Assist the patient into a position of comfort.
    3. Assist the patient with taking oral fluids.
    4. Ensure that patient is clean and dry, and linens are changed as needed.
    5. Support the family when patient's condition changes.

11. Which person is **most** likely to suffer from a maturational loss?
    1. A woman married to a police officer who is informed that he has been shot and killed.
    2. A college student who has never been away from home goes to Europe to study.
    3. A school-aged child who witnesses the family pet being killed by a speeding car.
    4. A middle-aged woman who was married for 30 years and is being divorced by her husband.

12. A student who normally gets "A" grades receives a "C" on her project and experiences a loss of confidence. Which behavior **best** indicates that the student is achieving growth because of this situational loss?
    1. Does the project over and over again until the teacher gives her an "A."
    2. Tells her parents to go to see the teacher and advocate for a grade change.
    3. Asks another teacher to look at the project and give an opinion about the grade.
    4. Requests a review of the project's strengths and weaknesses against the criteria.

13. Following the death of her husband, a wife feels that he is still with her. She also reports having dreams and vivid memories of him. Which question would the nurse ask to assess the sense of presence that the wife has described?
    1. "Do you think he is trying to tell you something?"
    2. "What are your religious beliefs about life after death?"
    3. "How do you feel about these dreams and experiences?"
    4. "Would you like to see a doctor about these symptoms?"

14. On seeing the body of his little brother who just died from cancer, a 10-year-old sibling screams, "I won't go to the funeral! I won't go!" The mother is sobbing and the father begins to yell. What would the nurse do **first**?
    1. Take the child aside and quietly talk to him about his feelings about death.
    2. Encourage the father to stop yelling because it is not helpful.
    3. Ask the mother to hold her child so that he can be supported and comforted.
    4. Calmly close the door and stay with the family while they express themselves.

15. A nurse is talking to a 63-year-old woman who underwent grief therapy for unresolved grief related to the death of her husband. Which behavior **best** indicates that the therapy is helping?
    1. She frequently visits his gravesite.
    2. She invites his old friends to dinner.
    3. She talks about things they used to enjoy.
    4. She cooks and serves his favorite foods.

16. As the nurse is performing medication teaching, the older woman begins to cry. "My grandson got into my pills and overdosed. He didn't die, but my daughter won't even speak to me." Which is the **most** therapeutic response?
    1. "Well, thank goodness he is okay. She should be happy about that."
    2. "I'm sure everything will work out. She'll get over it; give her time."
    3. "You feel like you were to blame for this, but accidents do happen."
    4. "Every time you look at your medicine, you think about that incident."

17. The hospice nurse is visiting a family of a deceased patient. During the visit, the son displays symptoms of a grief attack. Which intervention would the nurse use?
    1. Ensure that other members of the household do not get attacked.
    2. Reassure the son that he is safe and that no one will attack him.
    3. Help the son recognize that the attack is a type of grief response.
    4. Report the symptoms of the attack to the HCP.

18. The UAP tells the nurse that the dying patient's family keeps calling for assistance with minor tasks that they could easily do for the patient. What would the nurse do?
    1. Tell the UAP to do whatever the family or patient wants him/her to do.
    2. Encourage the family to participate in care to increase feelings of control.
    3. Ask the UAP to clarify what he/she means by "assistance with minor tasks."
    4. Assess the family's desire and ability to participate in the care of the patient.

19. Which statement by the family member of a dying patient **best** indicates a healthy retention of hope?
    1. "We are planning to take our father on one last trip to Europe next year."
    2. "My sister is coming from California next week; I know he wants to see her."
    3. "He really loves to golf and is looking forward to playing again this summer."
    4. "We know a man from our church who beat his cancer; Dad can do the same."

20. The patient is sobbing. When the nurse tries to find out what is wrong, the patient angrily says, "I'm dying! I have pain! My children are losing their mother! We are in debt up to our eyeballs! And God seems to be on a coffee break!" What does the nurse do **first** to identify and prioritize the patient's problems?
    1. Use Maslow's Hierarchy and first address the physical issue of pain.
    2. Ask the RN to assume care because of multiple complex problems.
    3. Collect additional data about each concern and consult with the RN.
    4. Review the plan of care and determine if these are old or new issues.

21. Which signs and symptoms would the nurse expect to observe in the patient who is nearing death? **Select all that apply.**
    1. Lowered blood pressure
    2. Rapid, bounding pulse
    3. Irregular respiratory pattern
    4. Mouth-breathing with dry mucous membranes
    5. Rapid, anxious eye movements

22. The terminally ill patient has been experiencing severe pain and requested that the HCP assist her to end her suffering. What would the nurse do if the HCP prescribes a morphine dosage that could cause respiratory depression and respiratory arrest?
    1. Administer the medication as prescribed.
    2. Refuse to give the prescribed dose.
    3. Tell the HCP to administer the dose.
    4. Consult the nursing supervisor for advice.

23. On assessing the dying patient, the nurse notes that the pulse rate is 30/min, the respiratory rate is 8/min, and the systolic blood pressure is palpated at 60. The patient has a Do Not Resuscitate (DNR) order. What would the nurse do **first**?
    1. Call the family to the bedside.
    2. Make the patient comfortable.
    3. Call for help and get the crash cart.
    4. Start an IV and give a fluid bolus.

24. Which nursing action demonstrates that the nurse is performing his/her responsibilities according to the National Organ Transplantation Act (Public Law 98-507, 10-14, 1984) and the Uniform Anatomical Gift Act?
    1. Assists the HCP who certified death to remove suitable organs.
    2. Ensures that the clinical signs of death are present before death is certified.
    3. Explains the process of organ donation and transplant to the family.
    4. Contacts a qualified health care professional to ask family about organ donation.

25. Which actions indicate that the health care team is fulfilling the Dying Person's Bill of Rights? **Select all that apply.**
    1. Nurse assesses pain and administers pain medication accordingly.
    2. Patient's choice of spiritual leader is contacted and rituals are allowed.
    3. Family is allowed to decide how much information is given to patient.
    4. Health care team creates a living will and advance directives for the patient.
    5. Nurse gives comfort measures and talks to a patient who is in a coma.
    6. Patient is allowed to make decisions, even though she seems indecisive.

26. Which nursing action is **most** likely to be affected by the patient's advance directives?
    1. Instructing UAP on how to perform post-mortem care
    2. Advising the HCP that the pain medication is not working
    3. Assisting the HCP to intubate for respiratory arrest
    4. Contacting the family if the patient dies unexpectedly during the night

27. The nurse is working in a pediatric outpatient clinic. There is an 8-year-old child whose grandfather has just died. Based on the developmental level of the child, what type of response would the nurse anticipate?
    1. "Grandpa will come back soon. He just went to see Grandma."
    2. "Grandpa was old and supposed to die. My cat was old; he died too."
    3. "I was bad at school and talked back to Mom. That's why Grandpa died."
    4. "It was better that Grandpa died quickly and didn't have to suffer a long time."

28. The patient tells the nurse that he has a durable power of attorney for health care and medical treatment. Which is the **most** important information to obtain from the patient?
    1. The name and phone number of the person who will make health care decisions
    2. The name and phone numbers of the family member who is next of kin
    3. The patient's written permission to disclose information to the attorney
    4. The patient's wishes about his or her care when death is near

29. What is **most** likely to be included in postmortem care? **Select all that apply.**
    1. Remove all tubings, dressings, and drains.
    2. Wash hands and don gloves.
    3. Care for valuables and personal belongings.
    4. Close patient's eyes and mouth if needed.
    5. Place patient supine with arms at the sides.

30. The nurse has been working throughout a pandemic and witnessed an unprecedented number of deaths. Which of the following would be healthy coping strategies? **Select all that apply**
    1. Develop an after-work decompression routine to use before leaving the workplace.
    2. Reflect on the nurse's vital role of saving or rescuing patients from the pandemic.
    3. Request a leave of absence before the pressure builds too much.
    4. Request support from colleagues during difficult days.
    5. Take a few moments during a break to call and laugh with a child at home.
    6. Conceal feelings of stress from supervising RN who is also experiencing excessive pressure during the pandemic.

31. A 68-year-old man has a diagnosis of terminal cancer and is in hospice care. Which phase of Kübler-Ross' stages of dying is **most likely** represented by his withdrawal from interactions with his family and the hospice nurse?
    1. Acceptance
    2. Denial
    3. Depression
    4. Anger
    5. Bargaining

32. Which statement would be normal for a 4-year-old whose father has just died?
    1. "I shouldn't have talked back to my father."
    2. "My father is with God and in peace now."
    3. "My father will come back when he feels better."
    4. "I will die like my father one day."

CRITICAL THINKING ACTIVITIES

33. The patient's husband died in an automobile accident a year ago. She is still experiencing insomnia and feelings of worthlessness and anger, and she continues to avoid family and social functions.

    a. What physical assessments will the nurse perform on this patient? _____

    _____

    _____

    _____

    b. Discuss how physical and social aspects of human functioning influence the grieving process.

    _____

    _____

34. Nurse A is a new nurse who recently started working on the unit. Nurse A likes and respects Nurse B, an experienced nurse who has been caring for terminal patients for a long time. Nurse A notices that Nurse B is efficiently caring for patients, but seems progressively cold, uncaring, and indifferent about everyone's feelings. Nurse B is particularly critical of one family because of how they act toward the staff and the dying family member.

   a.   Discuss what could be happening to Nurse B. _____

   _____

   _____

   _____

   _____

   _____

   b.   What can Nurse A do to help Nurse B? _____

   _____

   _____

   _____

   _____

   _____

35. The older patient who is receiving palliative care verbalizes the "wish to die." What would the nurse do to differentiate whether the patient is experiencing acceptance or depression?

   _____

   _____

   _____

   _____

   _____

NEXT-GENERATION NCLEX™ (NGN)

36. Extended Multiple Response

Cognitive Skill: Analyzes Cues

Scenario: The patient has a diagnosis of COVID-19 and has failed to improve after 3 weeks on a ventilator. The patient, family, and HCP, through shared decision-making, have discontinued the ventilator and the patient has been placed in hospice care. In accordance with institutional policy during the pandemic, visitors have not been allowed. But now, for end-of-life care, two visitors are allowed to be with the patient. The patient's wife and son have arrived and are crying and eager to be with their loved one. The patient's current vital signs are T 98.6° F, BP 60/40, pulse 40 and thready, respirations 8 and irregular. The patient is sleepy but can be roused.

Instructions: Place an X in front of each action that the nurse would take in this scenario.

_____ 1. Assist patient up to a chair for visiting.
_____ 2. Assist visitors to don personal protective equipment (PPE).
_____ 3. Inform visitors of risk of contracting COVID-19.
_____ 4. Offer to set up video communication for other family members to virtually visit.
_____ 5. Request a qualified health care professional to offer the option of organ donation.
_____ 6. Provide oral care to the patient every shift.
_____ 7. Leave the room as the family members arrive to allow privacy.
_____ 8. Remove all tubing and catheters from the patient.
_____ 9. Tell visitors to discard PPE in the trash after visiting.
_____ 10. Give oxygen via nasal cannula per protocol for dyspnea.
_____ 11. Provide skin care with gentle cleansing and lubrication of skin.

Health Promotion and Pregnancy

Answer Key: A complete Answer Key is provided in your Additional Learning Resources on Evolve.

TABLE ACTIVITY

1. *Directions:* For the parameters on the left, enter the expected change on the right.

Cardiovascular Changes in Pregnancy

Parameter	Change
Heart rate	
Blood pressure	
Blood volume	
Red blood cell mass	
Hemoglobin	
Hematocrit	
White blood cell count	
Cardiac output	

MULTIPLE CHOICE

Directions: Select the best answer(s) for each of the following questions.

2. What would the nurse expect the patient to report as presumptive signs of pregnancy? **Select all that apply.**
   1. Amenorrhea
   2. Nausea and vomiting
   3. Breast changes
   4. Positive home pregnancy test
   5. Urinary frequency

3. The woman is in the first trimester of pregnancy and tells the nurse that she has morning sickness almost every day. Which intervention would the nurse suggest **first?**
   1. Taking an over-the-counter antacid
   2. Keeping a daily symptom diary
   3. Drinking a tea made of ginger root
   4. Nibbling a few soda crackers before rising

4. While there are many variations that the nurse might see, what would be the **most** likely behaviors that a man would demonstrate during paternal adaptation?
   1. Establishes a relationship with the unborn child, and prepares for the birth experience
   2. Prepares for the paternal role accompanied by fantasy, pleasure, and intense learning
   3. Experiences the *couvade syndrome* with nausea, other gastrointestinal issues, and fatigue
   4. Views pregnancy as proof of masculinity and dominant role within the family

5. The woman is in the third trimester of pregnancy and the nurse observes that the woman's feet and ankles are unusually swollen. What is the **most** important assessment for the nurse to make?
   1. Ask the woman if she has been resting and elevating her legs.
   2. Assess the peripheral pulses and movement of the ankle joints.
   3. Assess for edema of the face, presacral area, or fingers.
   4. Ask the woman how much fluid she typical drinks in a day.

6. The health care provider (HCP) tells the nurse that a couple expecting their first child is considering testing to detect chromosomal abnormalities. Which informational pamphlets is the nurse **most** likely to prepare? **Select all that apply.**
   1. "Amniocentesis Can Reveal Information About Genetic Factors"
   2. "What an Ultrasound Shows About the Health of Your Baby"
   3. "Chorionic Villus Sampling to Detect Genetic Disorders of the Fetus"
   4. "Quadruple Marker Screening: A Low-Risk Test"
   5. "The Biophysical Profile of You and Your Baby"
   6. "Nuchal Translucency Screening to Assess for Potential Down Syndrome"

7. The pregnant woman reports blurring and double vision. Which assessment would the nurse **immediately** perform?
   1. Check the patient's blood pressure.
   2. Assess the patient's visual acuity.
   3. Auscultate the lungs and count respirations.
   4. Assess balance and coordination.

8. The woman has entered her 16th week of pregnancy and asks the nurse, "How is the baby growing?" What would the nurse tell the mother?
   1. "Your baby has developed head hair."
   2. "Your baby weighs about 27 ounces."
   3. "Your baby has settled into a favorite position."
   4. "Your baby has formed all organs and structures."

9. What would the nurse tell the patient who has noted facial swelling in the third trimester of pregnancy?
   1. "This is a temporary condition caused by increased blood flow resulting from high estrogen levels."
   2. "An increased blood volume results in increased water retention, but the swelling should go away."
   3. "Facial swelling is something that has to be reported to your HCP for follow-up care and evaluation."
   4. "This should be reported to your provider because swelling signals an increased amount of melanocyte-stimulating hormone."

10. The nurse notes in the HCP's documentation that the patient is experiencing ptyalism. What would the nurse instruct the patient to do?
    1. Eat small, frequent meals.
    2. Suck on hard candy.
    3. Sit up after eating.
    4. Avoid eating spicy foods.

11. Which exercise would the pregnant woman be taught to avoid?
    1. Water exercise due to risk of pool water entering vagina
    2. Prenatal yoga due to risk of overheating
    3. Ice hockey due to risk of injury
    4. Cycling on a stationary bicycle due to risk of falling

12. The pregnant patient has been instructed to count fetal movements (kick count). Which statement demonstrates that the patient understands the procedure?
    1. "I should count all movements during a 24-hour period."
    2. "I should choose a time of day after I have done my own exercises."
    3. "My baby should move at least 10 times in a 1- to 2-hour period."
    4. "I should feel the baby move at least four times after I have eaten a meal."

13. Which patient response indicates that she understands how to perform Kegel exercises?
    1. "The exercises are most beneficial if they are done 10 times in a row, at least three times a day."
    2. "If I could perform the exercises 100 times in a row, I will only have to do them once a day."
    3. "I will perform the exercises whenever I have time to sit and concentrate for at least 20 minutes."
    4. "The exercises are most beneficial if I start performing them right after I deliver my baby."

14. After delivery, the nurse is examining the placenta. Which is the **most** important observation that the nurse would note and document?
    1. Weight of the placenta
    2. Presence of the placental barrier
    3. Appearance of the "Shiny Schultz"
    4. Intactness of the placenta

15. The nurse is examining the umbilical cord immediately after delivery. Which finding would be reported to the HCP for further investigation of fetal anomalies?
    1. The cord has two vessels—one artery and one vein.
    2. The cord contains a significant amount of Wharton's jelly.
    3. The cord is 50 cm long and 2.5 cm in diameter.
    4. The cord has a pale white, ropelike appearance.

16. The nurse is assessing fetal heart tones on a woman who is 12 weeks pregnant. Which is the correct method for this procedure?
    1. Use an amplified stethoscope and listen at the midline of the abdomen.
    2. Place the Doppler just above the symphysis pubis and apply firm pressure.
    3. Instruct the patient to drink a quart of water prior to abdominal ultrasound.
    4. Insert the transvaginal ultrasound probe into the vagina.

17. The nursing student is preparing to measure fundal height. At which step would the supervising nurse intervene?
    1. Reviews the established protocol to measure this specific patient
    2. Verifies the patient's identity by asking name and birthdate
    3. Obtains a disposable paper tape measuring device
    4. Instructs the patient to lie on the examination table

18. The nurse is comparing today's fundal height measurement with the previous recording taken 5 weeks ago. What is the significance of a stable or decreased measurement?
    1. Possible intrauterine growth restriction
    2. Possible multifetal gestation
    3. Possible excessive amniotic fluid
    4. Expected normal finding

19. The patient is at risk for a miscarriage. Which diagnostic test result is consistent with a miscarriage?
    1. Elevated levels of maternal serum alpha-fetoprotein
    2. Declining levels of quantitative human chorionic gonadotropin
    3. Increasing levels of amniotic fluid
    4. Positive findings for chorionic villus sampling

20. The nurse is helping the woman prepare for an abdominal ultrasound. Which information is correct?
    1. "You will have to drink several cups of water after the procedure to flush the bladder."
    2. "We will help you assume the lithotomy position for the examination."
    3. "The procedure is a little uncomfortable; just signal if you need to take a break."
    4. "You and your partner can watch the images on the screen if you would like to."

21. The mother has diabetes and is at risk for placental insufficiency. The results of the nonstress test shows three fetal movements accompanied by two increases of 15 bpm in a 20-minute period. On hearing the results, she starts crying. What would the nurse be prepared to do for the patient?
    1. Encourage the mother to express feelings of anxiety or uncertainty.
    2. Prepare the mother for additional testing, such as the contraction stress test.
    3. Reassure the mother that crying with relief and joy is an understandable response.
    4. Support the mother through a repeat of the nonstress test for validation.

22. The mother is in her second trimester and reports "premilk" is leaking from her breasts. What would the nurse tell the mother?
    1. "Any discharge from the nipples should be considered abnormal and evaluated by the HCP."
    2. "Premilk or colostrum is not supposed to start until immediately after delivery."
    3. "Premilk will be pumped and discarded in order to stimulate the true breast milk."
    4. "If excessive leakage is a problem, breast pads can be useful."

23. The nurse is interviewing a woman who has just found out that she is pregnant. From a nursing standpoint, which is the **best** rationale for asking about insurance coverage for maternity and newborn care?
    1. Information is used to determine the frequency of the prenatal visits.
    2. Admission to the hospital is based on the type of insurance coverage.
    3. Family will have additional stress related to finances if there is no insurance coverage.
    4. Number and frequency of diagnostic tests can be altered if there is no coverage.

24. The nurse is taking a health history and the information is likely to be used later during genetic counseling. Which question is the **most** appropriate in the initial data collection?
    1. "How do you feel about undergoing genetic testing?"
    2. "What would you do if an abnormality is detected?"
    3. "Is there a family history of genetic diseases in the family? "
    4. "Would you like information about genetic defects?"

25. The patient had her last menstrual period (LMP) on August 18, 2021. Using Nägele's rule, when is the estimated date of birth (EDB)?
    _____

26. Define the parity of the pregnant woman using the GTPAL system: She has been pregnant four times, delivered three full-term infants, had no abortions or preterm deliveries, and has three living children. _____

27. The pregnant woman reports frequently feeling ill in the morning with bouts of nausea throughout the day. Which question is **most** important to differentiate between morning sickness and the more serious condition of hyperemesis gravidarum?
    1. "How much and how frequently are you eating meals?"
    2. "Do you notice that you are salivating more than usual?"
    3. "Have you been vomiting? If yes, how frequently?"
    4. "Are you experiencing heartburn? If yes, when does it occur?"

28. The pregnant woman is a heavy smoker and she feels that it is unlikely that she will be able to quit. Because of the oxygen deprivation in utero, which outcome would the health care team be prepared to deal with?
    1. Neonatal jaundice
    2. Preterm delivery with low birth weight
    3. Intrauterine infection
    4. No change in fetal heart rate during contraction

29. The pregnant patient at 37 weeks gestation phones the clinic and reports having some symptoms that are causing discomfort and worry. Which symptom is the **most** serious and warrants immediate evaluation by the HCP ?
    1. Shortness of breath when climbing the stairs
    2. Perineal discomfort and pressure with standing
    3. Muscle aches and difficulty walking
    4. Pain and burning sensation with urination

30. The nurse is discussing sexual activity with the pregnant patient. Which advice would be correct?
    1. Sexual intercourse in the first trimester can increase the risk of miscarriage.
    2. Sexual intercourse should be avoided late in the third trimester.
    3. Sexual intercourse is fine throughout pregnancy if there are no pregnancy complications.
    4. Sexual intercourse increases the risk of spontaneous rupture of membranes.

31. The woman with a low-risk pregnancy tells the nurse that she frequently has to travel for her job. Which questions are **most** relevant? **Select all that apply.**
    1. "Will you have to travel to areas where the water is untreated?"
    2. "Will you be terminated if you refuse to travel?"
    3. "Have you checked the policies of the airline that you usually fly?"
    4. "Are you aware that magnetometers at airports are harmful to the fetus?"
    5. "Are you planning to travel to a foreign country?"
    6. "When you drive, do you use the lap belt and shoulder harness?"

32. The nurse is taking a prenatal history. The patient is currently pregnant. She had one full-term delivery, one baby born at 26 weeks who did not survive, and one abortion. How would the nurse note the patient's obstetric history using the GTPAL system?
    1. G3 P1111
    2. G4 P1111
    3. G4 P2012
    4. G3 P3011

33. The HCP has prescribed an antibiotic to the pregnant woman in the second trimester of pregnancy for a urinary tract infection. The patient calls the nurse and states she read that the antibiotic is Category B in pregnancy and she does not feel it is safe to use. How would the nurse answer the patient?
    1. Category B means that the medication is safe in the second trimester, but not the first.
    2. Category B means that the medication has been shown to cause harm in animal studies but not in human studies.
    3. Category B means that the medication is considered as a second choice medication but the HCP felt it was better for the patient's specific situation.
    4. Category B means that animal studies have not demonstrated fetal risk, but there are no adequate studies of pregnant women.

34. What advice would the nurse give to the pregnant patient in the third trimester who is experiencing pyrosis?
    1. Lay down for a rest period after eating.
    2. Eat three meals a day.
    3. Try a low-sodium chewable antacid tablet after a meal.
    4. Eat foods with a spicier flavor.

CRITICAL THINKING ACTIVITIES

35. The nurse is working at an OB-GYN clinic and is aware that pregnancy is usually a time when women want to improve health habits and that expectant mothers are likely to want and welcome information about how to have a healthy baby.

    a. What counseling should the nurse give patients about self-care according to the trimester checklist?

    _____

    _____

    _____

    b. What factors would the nurse need to consider when the pregnant patient asks about a medication that was prescribed to her?

    _____

    _____

    _____

    c. In addition to selected medications, what other activities or substances should the nurse instruct the woman to avoid during pregnancy?

    _____

    _____

    _____

    _____

    _____

36. The nurse is talking with a woman who is in the first trimester of pregnancy. The patient reports feeling "fat, sluggish, and bloated." She begins to cry and expresses feelings of guilt because she resents the pregnancy for making her feel this way and dreads what is coming because "I'm just going to get bigger; then I'll start waddling like a duck and my skin will get all stretched out." The nurse recognizes that the patient has low self-esteem related to perceived loss of control over lifestyle and a distorted body image related to physiologic changes of pregnancy. What can the nurse do to assist the patient?

_____

_____

_____

_____

_____

_____

37. While it is not the nurse's responsibility to perform genetic counseling, the nurse may be involved in the care of couples who undergo testing for genetic counseling and may have to support families who get bad news or those are conflicted about what to do with the information. Discuss the scenarios with your classmates or instructor.

   a. The nurse is caring for a couple who has just been told that it is likely that their unborn child has Down syndrome. The wife is crying and the husband is very withdrawn. The nurse has a younger brother who has Down syndrome and he is happy and healthy and active in the community. What should the nurse do?

   _____

   _____

   _____

   _____

   _____

   b. The nurse is caring for a couple who have several children with severe congenital and genetic abnormalities. The children are frequently seen in the pediatric clinic and are generally undernourished and not well cared-for. The parents are currently expecting another child but they have no money for genetic testing and they seem unconcerned about the current or any future pregnancies. What is the best way for the nurse to help and support this family?

   _____

   _____

   _____

   _____

   _____

NEXT-GENERATION NCLEX™ (NGN)

38. Matrix

Cognitive Skill: Analyze Cues

Scenario: The nurse is in the prenatal clinic taking calls from pregnant patients with questions about their symptoms. The nurse would need to know what trimester of pregnancy the patient is in to determine if the symptom is normal or abnormal and would need to be reported to the HCP.

Instructions: Use an X to mark the trimester of pregnancy for which the reported symptom would be normal.

Symptom	First Trimester	Second Trimester	Third Trimester
Detects no fetal movement			
Feels pelvic pressure			
Notes tingling of the breasts			
Experiences extreme fatigue			
Perceives occasional contraction			
Identifies first fetal movement			

Labor and Delivery

Answer Key: A complete Answer Key is provided in your Additional Learning Resources on Evolve.

MATCHING

Directions: Match the term/phrase on the left to the correct definition on the right.

Term

____ 1. bloody show
____ 2. effacement
____ 3. primary powers
____ 4. cardinal movements of labor
____ 5. second stage of labor

Definition

a. Begins with complete dilation at 10 cm and ends with the birth of the baby

b. Involuntary uterine contractions that signal the beginning of labor

c. Turns and adjustments that occur as the fetus moves through the maternal pelvis

d. Vaginal drainage and blood-tinged mucus typically increase as term approaches

e. Thinning and shortening or obliteration of the cervix that occurs during late pregnancy, labor, or both

SHORT ANSWER

Directions: Using your own words, answer each question in the space provided.

6. What are the five Ps of the complex process of labor and delivery?

a. _____

b. _____

c. _____

d. _____

e. _____

7. Briefly define the four qualities of uterine contractions that are important to assess.

    a. _____

    b. _____

    c. _____

    d. _____

FIGURE LABELING

8. *Directions:* Label the figure to indicate the fetal position in relation to the quadrant of the maternal pelvis.

Right occipitoposterior (ROP)   Left occipitoposterior (LOP)
Right occipitotransverse (ROT)   Left occipitotransverse (LOT)
Right occipitoanterior (ROA)   Left occipitoanterior (LOA)

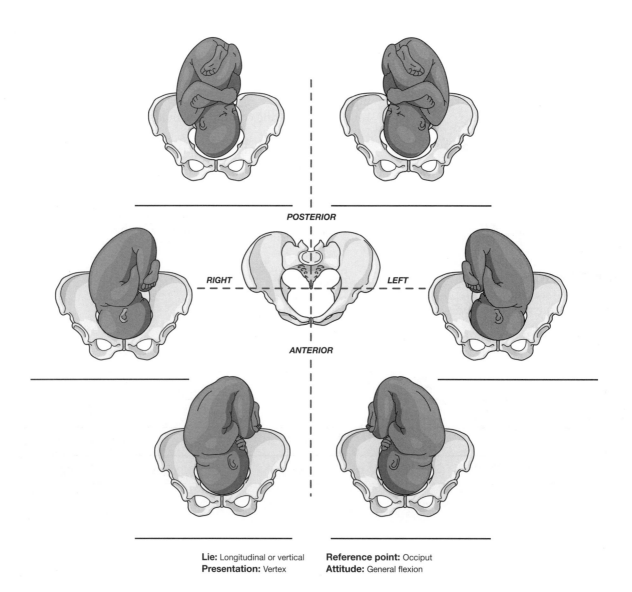

Lie: Longitudinal or vertical   **Reference point:** Occiput
Presentation: Vertex   **Attitude:** General flexion

MULTIPLE CHOICE

Directions: Select the best answer(s) for each of the following questions.

9. Which topics would be included in a discussion about the birth plan? **Select all that apply.**
   1. When to get pregnant
   2. Labor
   3. Delivery
   4. Postpartum period
   5. Fetal development
   6. Genetic counseling

10. Which factor would negate the woman's personal preference to use a birthing center?
    1. Low-risk pregnancy
    2. Unavailability of doula
    3. Need for cesarean section
    4. Limited insurance coverage

11. About 2 weeks before the due date, a nullipara patient reports that the "lightening" that was described in the prenatal classes has occurred. Which physical change is likely to occur because of the lightening?
    1. Urinary frequency
    2. Decreased fetal movement
    3. Shortness of breath
    4. Leakage of amniotic fluid

12. The nurse informs the mother that the results of the nitrazine test are blue-green, pH 6.5. What additional information would the nurse give to the mother?
    1. Advise her that precipitous labor is likely.
    2. Instruct her to go home and resume usual activity.
    3. Inform her that labor will likely start soon.
    4. Tell her that the test is nonreactive and that urine leakage is normal.

13. The patient is 34 weeks gestation and reports an irregular tightening of the uterus and the health care provider (HCP) informs her that these are Braxton Hicks contractions. What additional information would the nurse give the patient?
    1. Anticipate bloody show with Braxton Hicks contractions.
    2. Call the HCP if the tightening sensations become painful and regular.
    3. Anticipate that a headache and backache will accompany these contractions.
    4. Expect leaking amniotic fluid will occur with Braxton Hicks contractions.

14. The provider tells the patient at 39 weeks that it is likely that she is having a vaginal discharge called *bloody show*. What additional information would the nurse provide?
    1. Explain that bloody show can be normal at 39 weeks gestation.
    2. Advise the patient that she must go to the hospital immediately.
    3. Prepare the patient for cesarean section.
    4. Inform the patient that she is now at increased risk for infection.

15. Premature rupture of membranes increases the risk for which complication?
    1. Infection for mother and fetus
    2. Failure to progress
    3. Uterine hemorrhage
    4. Precipitous labor

16. Which behaviors/symptoms would be considered normal and expected a few days before onset of true labor?
    1. Depression and fatigue
    2. Vomiting and loss of appetite
    3. A loss of 5-10 pounds
    4. Renewed energy for cooking and cleaning

17. Which patient is **most** likely to undergo x-ray pelvimetry?
    1. Patient is relatively thin and is in the early part of the first trimester.
    2. Patient is not currently pregnant but has a history of pelvic fracture.
    3. Patient is in the second trimester and multiple fetuses are suspected.
    4. Patient is in the third trimester and placental location is questionable.

18. Which factor increases the risk of transverse lie of the fetus?
    1. A history of seven prior full-term pregnancies
    2. A history of cesarean section.
    3. Placenta implanted in the fundus of the uterus
    4. The pregnant woman is underweight

19. The HCP informs the nurse that the patient has chosen to try for a vaginal birth after cesarean (VBAC). Which practice would be appropriate in the care of this patient during labor?
    1. Restrict position changes.
    2. Use misoprostol for induction of labor.
    3. Avoid use of epidural anesthesia.
    4. Utilize continuous fetal monitoring.

20. What is an acceptable practice in labor and delivery?
    1. Maintenance of a full bladder
    2. Maintenance of supine position
    3. Ambulation before membrane rupture
    4. Administration of enemas in the presence of vaginal bleeding

21. For which patient would the nurse anticipate that the uterine contractions may temporarily become less frequent and intense?
    1. Woman who received an epidural analgesia early in labor
    2. Woman who has been paraplegic for past several years
    3. Adolescent who is nullipara
    4. Older woman who is multipara

22. Which patients would be likely candidates for induction of labor? **Select all that apply.**
    1. Patient had rupture of membranes 6 hours ago and labor has not started.
    2. Patient has high blood pressure with symptoms of headache and dizziness.
    3. Patient has a history of one stillbirth and one fetal demise.
    4. Patient has diabetes mellitus.
    5. Patient has documented placenta previa.
    6. Patient has active herpes simplex infection.

23. Which patients may be candidates for cesarean delivery? **Select all that apply.**
    1. Cephalopelvic disproportion is present.
    2. Mother is a nullipara.
    3. Mother has a cardiac condition.
    4. Prolapse of cord is present.
    5. Presentation is breech.
    6. Fetus has a heart rate of 140 bpm.

24. Put the following steps (1-7) in the mechanism of labor in the order in which they occur for vertex positions.
    _____ a. Extension and restitution
    _____ b. Flexion
    _____ c. Descent
    _____ d. Internal rotation
    _____ e. Expulsion
    _____ f. Engagement
    _____ g. External rotation

25. The HCP informs the nurse that there is a prolapsed umbilical cord. What would the nurse do **first**?
    1. Assist the mother into a high Fowler's position.
    2. Apply a fetal monitoring device and count heart rate.
    3. Prepare the mother for a cesarean birth.
    4. Ensure that the HCP has sterile gloves.

26. The nurse is caring for a patient who has completed the third stage of labor. What is the purpose and goal of massaging the fundus?
    1. Achieve uterine atony
    2. Facilitate separation of the placenta
    3. Regain uterine muscle tone
    4. Determine the number and size of clots

27. The nurse is encouraging the mother to make frequent position changes during labor. Which position facilitates the second stage of labor by increasing the pelvic outlet?
    1. Lateral side-lying
    2. Squatting
    3. Knee-chest
    4. Lithotomy

28. Assessment of the amniotic fluid reveals yellow staining. What is the significance of this finding?
    1. This is associated with hydramnios.
    2. This finding is suggestive of intrauterine infection.
    3. This color is common with abruptio placentae.
    4. This staining is typical with meconium passage in utero.

29. On examination, the patient is found to be 8 cm dilated with contractions every 3 minutes that last for 70 seconds. Which behavior is likely to occur in this transitional phase?
    1. Alert and talkative
    2. Confused and disoriented
    3. Less talkative and focused on breathing
    4. Irritable and deeply focused

30. What is an expected finding for a woman who is in the mid- to active phase of labor?
    1. Cervical dilation of 2 cm
    2. Contractions every 3-5 minutes
    3. A desire to ambulate
    4. Very mild, easily controlled pain

31. When coaching the patient through the early or latent phase of labor, which breathing technique is the nurse **most** likely to encourage?
    1. Shallow panting
    2. Slow, deep chest or abdominal breathing
    3. Acceleration through contractions
    4. Holding the breath for 5 seconds and exhaling

32. All members of the health care team have performed hand hygiene. Which members are appropriately using personal protective equipment while caring for the mother and infant during childbirth? **Select all that apply.**
    1. Unlicensed assistive personnel (UAP) wears clean gloves when cleaning the perineal area after a bowel movement.
    2. HCP wears a sterile waterproof gown and gloves, a mask with shield, cap, and shoe covers when delivering infant.
    3. Nurse wears a gown and gloves when handling the newborn immediately after birth.
    4. Nurse wears clean gloves and gown when inserting an internal scalp electrode.
    5. Nurse wears sterile gloves when inserting a urinary catheter.

33. The patient is receiving intravenous (IV) oxytocin for uterine inertia. The nurse notes that the fetal heart rate (FHR) is dropping below 100 bpm. What would the nurse do?
    1. Stop the infusion.
    2. Slow down the infusion.
    3. Monitor the FHR for 5-10 full cycles of contractions.
    4. Do nothing, as this is an expected response.

34. The baby is assessed after birth and the following are noted: heart rate 124 bpm; respiratory effort good, crying; some flexion of the extremities; grimacing; body pink, extremities bluish. Based on this information, what is the Apgar score?_____

35. What is the **first** intervention that the nurse would perform in the care of an infant who has just been delivered?
    1. Place the infant in contact with the mother's skin.
    2. Assess airway and use a bulb syringe if indicated to clear mucus and fluid from infant's mouth and nose.
    3. Place identification bracelets on both mother and infant.
    4. Immediately dry the infant to help reduce heat loss from evaporation.

36. The neonate has just been delivered. What is an indication that placental separation is occurring?
    1. Uterus is relaxed and flaccid.
    2. Blood can no longer be milked from the umbilical cord.
    3. Contractions are progressively weaker.
    4. The umbilical cord is obviously lengthening.

37. A new nurse is performing fundal massage. When would the supervising nurse intervene?
    1. Explains to patient that rationale is to help placenta to deliver
    2. Supports uterus from below with one hand
    3. Uses upper hand to apply firm downward pressure
    4. Observes perineum for number and size of clots

38. The woman received general anesthesia for a cesarean section. Because the mother has increased risk for uterine relaxation, which action will the nurse perform?
    1. Administer glycopyrrolate as prescribed.
    2. Monitor for increased abdominal pain.
    3. Monitor for postpartum hemorrhage.
    4. Administer magnesium sulfate.

39. Following a precipitous labor and emergency birth, what is likely to be the **greatest** concern?
    1. Grief and loss due to fetal demise
    2. Prolonged contractions and abdominal pain
    3. Severe hypertension and seizures
    4. Postpartum hemorrhage and hypovolemia

40. The patient is experiencing a prolonged but progressive labor in which both she and the fetus are doing well. The father of the baby is irritable and complains repeatedly to the nurse that this is taking too long. What would be the **best** response from the nurse?
    1. "Is there another family member who could take your place here?"
    2. "Labor can take a very long time. You need to think of what your wife is experiencing and how long it must seem to her."
    3. "It is a long labor, but all is going well. If you would like to take a break and get some food, I will stay with your wife until you return."
    4. "Please go home and take a nap and come back when you feel ready to be helpful."

41. Which questions would be **most** important for the admission assessment of a patient in labor? **Select all that apply.**
    1. "When did the contractions begin?"
    2. "How far apart are the contractions?"
    3. "Did you take your prenatal vitamin today?"
    4. "Did your water break?"
    5. "Do you plan to have the baby circumcised if it is a male?"
    6. "Have you noted any vaginal bleeding?"
    7. "How long do you plan to breastfeed your baby?"

42. The woman in labor has chosen to have epidural anesthesia. Which potential side effect would the nurse anticipate?
    1. Postspinal headache
    2. Hypotension
    3. Aspiration
    4. Respiratory depression

CRITICAL THINKING ACTIVITIES

43. a. The admission assessment to the labor area includes: _____

    _____

    _____

    b. Nursing assessment of a patient's status throughout labor includes: _____

    _____

    _____

    c. For the fourth stage of labor, what are the nursing assessments and how often are they done?

    _____

    _____

44. Discuss how the fetus is monitored and circumstances that would warrant notification of the HCP.

    _____

    _____

45. Discuss the use of Standard Precautions during childbirth. _____

    _____

    _____

46. The nurse is caring for a pregnant woman who is in the latent phase of labor. The woman becomes very agitated and panicky during the initial vaginal examination. She begins to cry and apologize after the HCP leaves the room and confides in the nurse that she is a survivor of sexual abuse. She says, "I don't know how I am going to get through this. I feel so vulnerable and exposed."

   a. Discuss how history of sexual abuse may affect patients._____

      _____

      _____

   b. What can the nurse do to help this patient? _____

      _____

      _____

NEXT-GENERATION NCLEX™ (NGN)

47. Matrix

Cognitive Skill: Analyze Cues

Scenario: The nurse has made the following assessments on patients in labor and delivery.

Instructions: Use an X to indicate if the assessment finding is normal or abnormal for a patient in labor and delivery.

Assessment Finding	Normal	Abnormal
Fetal heart rate 145		
Amniotic fluid green		
Minimal variability in FHR		
Contractions every 2 minutes in latent phase of labor		
Blood loss in vaginal delivery 350 mL		
Second stage of labor 2 hours long in nulliparous patient		

Care of the Mother and Newborn

Answer Key: A complete Answer Key is provided in your Additional Learning Resources on Evolve.

TABLE ACTIVITY

1. *Directions:* Complete the table below with the expected values for the newborn.

Assessment of Newborn	Normal Value
Head circumference	
Relationship of head to chest circumference	
Temperature	
Pulse	
Respirations	
Blood pressure	

CLINICAL APPLICATION OF MATH AND CONVERSION

Directions: Calculate or make the necessary conversions for math problems encountered in performing skills for patients.

2. The breastfeeding mother has an intake as indicated in the flow sheet. What would the nurse tell the mother?

24-Hour Fluid Intake	
Time	Amount
7:00	6 oz juice, 8 oz water, 16 oz of low-fat milk
10:00	8 oz juice
12:00	350 mL water
14:00	16 oz of low-fat milk
17:00	250 mL water
20:00	16 oz of low-fat milk

(Continued)

1. Encourage the mother to drink an additional 2-3 servings of liquid each day.
2. Tell the mother that she is drinking more than required, but that's not a problem.
3. Advise the mother that there is a potential for fluid overload; then assess for edema.
4. Reinforce need for fluids and tell her that she is drinking the recommended amount.

3. The healthy neonate weighs 6.8 lbs. How much fluid does the neonate need every day?
_____ mL/day

4. The healthy newborn weighs 3.5 kg. How many kilocalories does the newborn need each day?
_____ kcal/day

MULTIPLE CHOICE

Directions: Select the best answer(s) for each of the following questions.

5. When the let-down reflex occurs, which action would the nurse perform?
   1. Offer the mother oral fluids to prevent dehydration.
   2. Assess the color change and consistency of the lochia.
   3. Assist the mother with breastfeeding as needed.
   4. Observe for frequency of saturation of perineal pads.

6. After an uncomplicated vaginal delivery, the mother reports that her appetite has returned; however, the nurse recognizes that gastric motility may continue to decline. Which action would the nurse perform?
   1. Assess for abdominal discomfort and possible paralytic ileus.
   2. Encourage activity, fluid intake, and increased fiber in the diet.
   3. Obtain an order for antacids as needed and encourage small meals.
   4. Administer a suppository to promote bowel evacuation.

7. The nurse is monitoring the flow of lochia for several postpartum patients. Which condition is cause for the **greatest** concern?
   1. There is a gush of dark lochia as the patient gets out of bed.
   2. Lochia alba changes back to lochia rubra.
   3. Pad with scant lochia serosa has a fleshy smell.
   4. One pad is saturated in 20 minutes with lochia rubra.

8. What instructions would the nurse give to a new mother who has elected to bottle-feed her newborn?
   1. Pump the breasts regularly to prevent engorgement.
   2. Apply warm, moist packs or shower breasts with hot water.
   3. Wear a supportive bra within a few hours of delivery.
   4. Decrease fluid intake to suppress milk production.

9. The nurse hears in report that the woman had a cesarean birth with general anesthesia. The combination of general anesthesia and lost abdominal tone prompts the nurse to be watchful for which potential complication?
   1. Paralytic ileus
   2. Hyperemesis
   3. Loss of sensation in legs
   4. Urinary incontinence

10. The woman is 2 days postpartum following normal spontaneous vaginal delivery. She has no indwelling catheter. The urinary output is noted below. What would the nurse do **first**?

Urine Output	
Time	**Amount**
7:00	50 mL
7:30	75 mL
8:15	30 mL
8:45	60 mL
9:00	30 mL

　　1. Continue to observe output and then record the total at the end of the shift.
　　2. Assess the patient for urgency, dysuria, or bladder distention.
　　3. Obtain an order for urinalysis and culture and sensitivity.
　　4. Obtain an order for straight catheterization to check for residual.

11. The mother has lost a large volume of blood and appears to be in hypovolemic shock following the delivery. Which action would the nurse perform?
　　1. Raise the head of the bed to 80 degrees.
　　2. Discontinue the oxytocic agent in the intravenous infusion.
　　3. Provide skin-to-skin contact with newborn.
　　4. Provide oxygen by face mask at 8-10 L/min.

12. Which action by the mother indicates a need for additional teaching about the care of the infant's umbilicus?
　　1. Gives a tub bath in the first 3 days after delivery
　　2. Uses alcohol on the stump daily
　　3. Folds the diaper down from the umbilicus
　　4. Reports a foul odor or redness from the stump

13. What is included in the care of the circumcision?
　　1. Removing the yellow crusting right away.
　　2. Applying the diaper loosely.
　　3. Assessing for bleeding every hour for 4 hours.
　　4. Using petroleum gauze under the Plastibell.

14. What is an appropriate technique to teach the new mother about the baby's bath?
　　1. Vigorous removal of the vernix caseosa
　　2. Use of plain water on the perineal area
　　3. Washing the baby twice daily
　　4. Having the bathwater at 100° F (37.7° C)

15. The nurse is discussing sexuality with the new mother. What information would the nurse provide?
　　1. Menses usually return in 3-5 months.
　　2. Breastfeeding acts as an effective contraceptive.
　　3. Discomfort and bleeding are expected with sexual activity.
　　4. Intercourse can be resumed when lacerations or episiotomy have healed and bleeding has stopped.

16. In teaching the new mother about breastfeeding, what would the nurse tell her?
　　1. Use one breast for two consecutive feedings.
　　2. Have the baby nurse for 5 minutes at each breast.
　　3. Put as much of the areolar tissue into the baby's mouth as possible.
　　4. Pull the breast straight away from the baby's mouth to break the suction seal.

17. The nurse is teaching the patient about the signs and symptoms that should be reported to the health care provider (HCP). After 5 days from the delivery date, which sign/symptom warrants contacting the HCP?
　　1. Temperature is 99° F.
　　2. Lochia is light pink-brown in color.
　　3. Breast is tender and red.
　　4. Fundus feels like a softball.

18. The patient has opted to bottle-feed her newborn. Which the patient statement indicates that she understood discharge teaching related to breast engorgement?
　　1. "I will most likely not experience breast engorgement if I manually express the milk."
　　2. "If I experience engorgement, I should use a covered ice pack for relief."
　　3. "Engorgement will most likely occur about 10 days from my delivery date."
　　4. "Breast engorgement is unlikely since I am not breastfeeding my baby."

19. The nurse is assessing a newborn infant who was born at 38 weeks gestation. Which findings would be considered normal? **Select all that apply.**
    1. Vernix caseosa
    2. Lanugo
    3. Desquamation
    4. Good skin turgor
    5. Good tissue elasticity

20. The mother reports that the new infant is making a weak, high-pitched crying sound. She has tried feeding, changing, rocking, and ignoring the baby, but the crying continues. What would the nurse do **first**?
    1. Assess the mother-child interaction to see if there are problems with bonding.
    2. Try swaddling or bundling the baby to make him feel secure.
    3. Ask the mother to hold the baby while vital signs are obtained.
    4. Contact the HCP because the crying is excessive.

21. Which are normal variations in the physical characteristics of a newborn? **Select all that apply.**
    1. Acrocyanosis in a 5-day-old infant
    2. The harlequin sign in a 2-day-old infant
    3. Jaundice during the first 24 hours after delivery
    4. Epstein's pearls on the hard palate of a 2-week-old infant
    5. Lacy mottling on pale skin immediately at birth

22. The home health nurse is assessing the mother's peripads 6 days after delivery. What is the expected finding?
    1. Bright-red blood with tissue
    2. Thin pinkish-brown drainage
    3. Slightly yellow to white drainage
    4. Small clots with a fleshy odor

23. After delivery, which patient has the **greatest** risk for life-threatening postpartum hemorrhage?
    1. Has a vaginal hematoma after a forceps-assisted delivery
    2. Has a vulvar hematoma after a normal delivery in a primigravid patient
    3. Has a vaginal hematoma after a repair of a vaginal laceration at delivery
    4. Has a retroperitoneal hematoma after cesarean section.

24. Which treatment related to bowel function would the nurse question for a woman with a fourth-degree laceration of the perineum?
    1. Administer stool softener for constipation as needed.
    2. Assist with ambulation in hall 3 or 4 times / day.
    3. Administer enema for constipation as needed.
    4. Encourage fluid intake of at least 3 L / day.

25. The nurse is explaining to a mother who had an episiotomy how to use a squeeze bottle to clean herself after urination or a bowel movement. Which information is correct?
    1. "First, clean perineal area front to back with toilet tissue."
    2. "Use the whole Peri bottle of water to cleanse the perineum."
    3. "Fill the Peri bottle with sterile water warmed to approximately 98° F (37.7° C)."
    4. "Flush the perineal area twice a day for 20 minutes."

26. The nurse sees that the postpartum patient has a platelet count that is on the high end of the normal range. Based on this observation, which action will the nurse perform?
    1. Observe the patient for fatigue, particularly after exertion.
    2. Monitor temperature and watch for signs of infection.
    3. Encourage the patient to get out of bed and walk around.
    4. Watch for signs and symptoms of hemorrhage.

27. In the postpartum period, the patient has no urge to void, but the nurse notes that the patient's bladder is distended. What complications are **most** associated with bladder distention in postpartum patients?
    1. Uterine hemorrhage and urinary tract infections
    2. Rectocele and uterine prolapse
    3. Kidney dysfunction and painful sexual intercourse
    4. Urinary incontinence and perineal lacerations

28. The postpartum patient complains of a persistent headache. Which action would the nurse perform **first**?
    1. Obtain an order for a mild analgesic, such as acetaminophen.
    2. Reassure that pregnancy-induced headaches will abate.
    3. Check the blood pressure and compare it to baseline measurements.
    4. Check the record for history of epidural or spinal anesthesia.

29. The nurse notes that the patient is profusely diaphoretic during the first night after delivery. Based on the nurse's knowledge of what is expected for the healthy mother in the immediate postpartum period, which action is the nurse **most** likely to take?
    1. Assist the patient to change clothes and explain that diaphoresis is normal.
    2. Monitor the patient's temperature, because diaphoresis suggests a fever.
    3. Check the patient's blood sugar to validate that the patient is not hypoglycemic.
    4. Assist the patient to sit upright to facilitate respiratory effort and oxygenation.

30. The nurse is trying to teach a 15-year-old mother how to swaddle her baby, but the young mother seems more interested in fixing her hair and makeup. She states, "My boyfriend is coming in a little while." How would the nurse respond?
    1. "Let's focus on the swaddling, then you can show him when he gets here."
    2. "You look very pretty. He will be delighted to see you and the baby."
    3. "Don't you want to spend some time holding and snuggling your baby?"
    4. "Well, you finish with your makeup and I'll take the baby back to the nursery."

31. The nurse hears in report that a patient who had a cesarean section should receive liquids for the first day with a gradual reintroduction to a regular diet. How does the nurse know when to offer solid foods?
    1. Follow the protocol or clinical pathway for cesarean section patients.
    2. Give solid food when the dietary kitchen includes it on the meal tray.
    3. Call the HCP to clarify specific parameters.
    4. Assess the abdomen and auscultate for bowel sounds.

32. The woman is interested in returning to her prepregnant weight as soon as possible. She has decided to breastfeed because "it's better for the baby and it will also help me lose weight." What information would the nurse give to the mother about nutrition and diet?
    1. During breastfeeding, consume an additional 300-500 kcal/day.
    2. For gradual weight loss, follow Weight Watchers suggestions and drink 3 L of fluid each day.
    3. Eliminate approximately 300-500 kcal/day for 6-8 weeks for weight loss.
    4. The prepregnant weight will likely be achieved by 6 weeks postpartum.

33. What is the **most** important nursing action to perform before assisting the woman to stand up and ambulate for the first time after the delivery of the baby?
    1. Obtain a wheelchair and place it close to the bedside.
    2. Assist the patient to slowly sit and dangle legs while seated.
    3. Compare the blood pressure in the supine and upright positions.
    4. Assist the patient to apply a pair of slippers with a nonslip sole.

34. The patient received an epidural block. In the early recovery stage, what would be considered a normal finding?
    1. Decreased sensation in both legs
    2. Altered level of consciousness
    3. Elevated blood pressure compared to baseline
    4. Temperature of 102° F (38.9° C)

35. The woman's temperature is slightly elevated 12 hours after delivery of the baby. Which additional assessment would the nurse perform **first**?
    1. Check the appearance and odor of the lochia.
    2. Assess skin turgor and condition of mucous membranes.
    3. Palpate the fundus for height and firmness.
    4. Check a urine specimen for foul odor and cloudiness.

36. The unlicensed assistive personnel (UAP) tells the nurse that there was a gush of brownish vaginal drainage when the patient got out of bed and stood up. What would the nurse do **first**?
    1. Inform the UAP that secretions pool in the supine position and flow is expected.
    2. Ask the UAP to describe the amount and color of the drainage and the patient's response.
    3. Check on the patient and assess for uterine atony, dizziness, or excessive vaginal bleeding.
    4. Tell the patient that there is nothing to worry about and help her clean up.

37. The mother reports to the nurse that the baby doesn't seem to be getting enough breast milk. What would the nurse do **first**?
    1. Suggest that the mother supplement with formula feedings.
    2. Teach the mother how to manually pump the breasts.
    3. Assess the axillary region for engorgement of milk supply.
    4. Assess how the baby is latching onto the breast.

38. The nurse notices that the grandmother seems to be dominating the care of her own daughter and the new infant to the point of excluding the new father. What would the nurse do?
    1. Gently suggest that the grandmother leave so that the new family can bond.
    2. Refer the family to counseling so that parental roles can be clarified.
    3. Assess the father's feelings about his role and his knowledge of child care.
    4. Wait until the grandmother leaves and then teach the father how to hold the baby.

39. The mother reports a mild cramping during the postpartum period. The nurse anticipates that the provider will write an as-needed (PRN) order for which medication?
    1. Morphine
    2. Ibuprofen
    3. Aspirin
    4. Codeine

40. When is infant abduction **most** likely to occur?
    1. During visiting hours
    2. In the middle of the night
    3. During the discharge process
    4. Upon admission to the nursery

41. Which assessment finding in a new infant would be reported to the provider for additional investigation?
    1. Molding
    2. Strabismus
    3. Low-set ears
    4. Nystagmus

42. The nurse notes on assessing the newborn that there is a small tuft of hair at the base of the spine. What is the clinical significance of this finding?
    1. This is the lanugo that frequently covers the newborn's body.
    2. This is part of the vernix caseosa that is usually left in place for 48 hours.
    3. Different skin colorations and hair patterns are related to genetic factors.
    4. Hair tufts indicate possible abnormalities of spinal column development.

43. Which action by the nurse reduces the risk of bleeding in the newborn?
    1. Administer vitamin and mineral supplements as prescribed.
    2. Administer an injection of vitamin K as prescribed.
    3. Administer an injection of $Rh_o(D)$ immune globulin as prescribed.
    4. Administer erythromycin ointment to the eyes.

44. Parents of a newborn have limited funds, but they want to provide something to stimulate their newborn. Which is the **best** response?
    1. "Your baby would like an object that makes happy sounds."
    2. "Your baby prefers to look at your face and eyes."
    3. "Many babies like intricate black and white images."
    4. "Most parents like to get something soft and snuggly."

45. In the first few hours after birth, the neonate who is breastfed has a blood glucose level of 45 mg/dL. The nurse prepares for which intervention?
    1. Oral feeding of sterile glucose water
    2. Oral feeding of prepared formula
    3. Oral feeding of breast milk
    4. Administration of intravenous dextrose

46. Which nursing observation of the newborn's bowel function would be reported to the HCP?
    1. Initial stool is black-green with a sticky consistency.
    2. Stool contains strands of lanugo, mucus, and vernix.
    3. No stool is passed 24 hours after birth.
    4. Newborn appears to be straining when passing stool.

47. Which symptom reported by the patient at 24 hours after vaginal delivery would require further assessment by the nurse?
    1. Fatigue
    2. Mild suprapubic cramping
    3. Vaginal fullness
    4. Breast fullness

48. Which interventions would the nurse recommend to the breastfeeding patient on day 3 with engorged uncomfortable breasts? **Select all that apply.**
    1. Compression of breasts with firm bra
    2. Shower with warm water on the breasts
    3. Manual expression of milk
    4. Ice packs to the breasts
    5. Cabbage leaves to the breasts
    6. Formula-feed until engorgement resolves

49. The breastfeeding newborn in 4 days old and the mother reports that she is worried the baby has diarrhea because he is passing soft yellow stool several times daily, especially after feeding. What would the nurse advise the patient?
    1. This is a normal finding and not diarrhea with a breastfed infant.
    2. The normal stool of a newborn at this time is black and tarry.
    3. That is an unusually large number of stools in 1 day and will be reported to the HCP.
    4. The normal stool of a breastfed infant at this time is brown and formed.

CRITICAL THINKING ACTIVITIES

50. What information would the postpartum nurse expect to get in a transfer report on a new patient who has delivered her baby and is being moved from the recovery area to the postpartum unit?

    _____

    _____

    _____

51. Identify the changes that occur in the mother's body systems after delivery.

    a. Cardiovascular: _____

    _____

    b. Urinary: _____

    _____

    c. Gastrointestinal: _____

    _____

    d. Endocrine: _____

    _____

    e. Integumentary: _____

    _____

NEXT-GENERATION NCLEX™ (NGN)

52. Matrix

Cognitive Skill: Analyze Cues

Scenario: The nurse is assessing a mother and newborn couplet at 8 hours postpartum. The infant was born at full term and is healthy. The mother had a normal spontaneous vaginal delivery with a second-degree perineal laceration and an estimated blood loss of 300 mL. The mother is breastfeeding the baby.

Instructions: Use an X to indicate if the following assessment findings are normal or abnormal.

Assessment Finding	Normal	Abnormal
Mother has small amount of lochia rubra.		
Mother has not voided since delivery.		
Mother with fundus firm at level of umbilicus.		
Mother with slight edema of perineum.		
Newborn has passed two large yellow stools.		
Newborn has not voided since delivery.		
Newborn with molding of skull bones.		
Newborn axillary temperature 97° F (36.1° C).		

Care of the High-Risk Mother, Newborn, and Family With Special Needs

chapter

29

Answer Key: A complete Answer Key is provided in your Additional Learning Resources on Evolve.

CROSSWORD PUZZLE

1. *Directions:* Use the clues on the next page to complete the crossword puzzle.

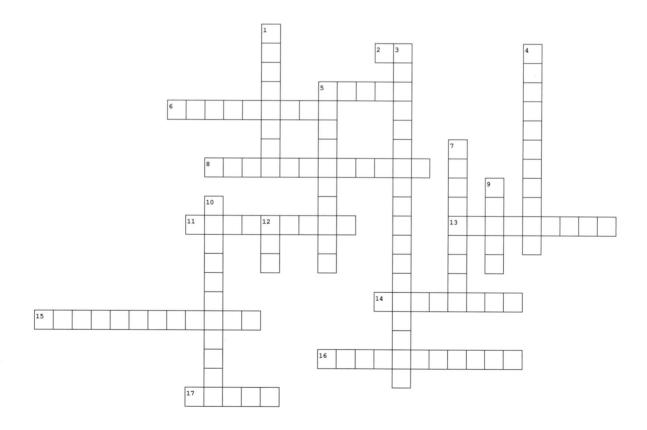

Across
2. Abbreviation for gestational hypertension
5. H, hemolysis; EL, elevated liver enzymes; LP, low platelet count
6. Number of deaths in a given population
8. Increase in blood pressure
11. Fertilization of two separate ova
13. State of having disease
14. Massive, generalized edema
15. Exposing the skin to fluorescent lights
16. Abnormal toxic accumulation of bilirubin in central nervous system tissues
17. Lack of normal tone or strength

Down
1. Uses suture material to constrict the internal os of the cervix
3. Excess of bilirubin in the blood of the newborn
4. Twins begin with one fertilized ovum
5. Excessive amount of amniotic fluid
7. Increased blood pressure after 20 weeks gestation with seizure activity
9. Organisms capable of crossing the placenta: toxoplasmosis, other infections, rubella virus, cytomegalovirus, and herpes simplex viruses
10. Phototherapy at home
12. Abbreviation for gestational diabetes mellitus

SHORT ANSWER

Directions: Using your own words, answer each question in the space provided.

2. Identify examples of high-risk factors in pregnancy for the following areas.

    a. Biophysical:_____

    b. Psychosocial:_____

    c. Sociodemographic: _____

    d. Environmental:_____

3. Identify factors that place the postpartum mother and infant at risk. _____

4. What are the characteristic physical manifestations of a preterm infant? _____

MULTIPLE CHOICE

Directions: Select the best answer(s) for each of the following questions.

5. For a patient with hyperemesis gravidarum, which laboratory value is monitored for the prevention of cardiac arrhythmias?
   1. White blood cell count
   2. Human chorionic gonadotropin level
   3. Potassium level
   4. Clotting factors

6. Which high-risk patient will need support and encouragement for follow-up because of the risk for developing cancer?
   1. Woman has had two multifetal pregnancies.
   2. Woman's first pregnancy was ectopic.
   3. Woman had severe hyperemesis gravidarum.
   4. Woman was diagnosed with hydatidiform mole.

7. A woman comes to the emergency department. She recently had a positive home pregnancy test and is now having severe lower abdominal pain. She is pale, diaphoretic, and reports feeling lightheaded and dizzy. What would the nurse do **first**?
   1. Take vital signs and assess abdominal pain.
   2. Put her on a stretcher and alert the health care provider (HCP).
   3. Obtain an order for a pregnancy test.
   4. Provide privacy and check for vaginal bleeding.

8. What teaching points would be included for a patient who had a spontaneous abortion? **Select all that apply.**
   1. Report any heavy, profuse, or bright-red bleeding to the HCP.
   2. Do not to use tampons until bleeding has stopped.
   3. Avoid sexual intercourse until bleeding has stopped.
   4. Be aware that scant, dark discharge may persist for 1-2 weeks.
   5. Postpone attempts to get pregnant for at least 1 year.

9. The nurse hears in report that the patient needs assessment for 1-2 hours after placement of prophylactic cerclage. What assessments does the nurse plan to make for this patient?
   1. Monitor for dyspnea and abnormal lung sounds.
   2. Assess for headache and hyperreflexia.
   3. Check the fetal heart tones and vital signs.
   4. Observe perineal pad count and signs of pooling.

10. Under which circumstance would the nurse avoid doing a vaginal examination?
    1. Patient has undiagnosed vaginal bleeding in the second trimester of pregnancy.
    2. Patient has sudden onset of chest pain, dyspnea, cyanosis, and frothy blood-tinged sputum.
    3. Patient has a complete abortion and all products of conception are expelled from the uterus.
    4. Patient with no prenatal care and history of substance abuse arrives at hospital in active labor.

11. The nurse hears in report that the patient is at risk for disseminated intravascular coagulation (DIC), but so far the patient has shown no signs/symptoms. What is an assessment finding that alerts the nurse that DIC may be in progress?
    1. Urinary frequency
    2. Elevated blood pressure
    3. Bleeding gums
    4. Low-grade fever

12. What are signs of cold stress in the neonate? **Select all that apply.**
    1. Decreased temperature
    2. Shivering
    3. Pallor
    4. Lethargy
    5. Inconsolable crying

13. The preterm infant's greatest potential problem is respiratory distress syndrome. What is an **early** sign?
    1. Nasal flaring
    2. Substernal retractions
    3. Circumoral cyanosis
    4. Grunting on expiration

14. A patient with which condition may be a candidate for methotrexate therapy?
    1. Unruptured ectopic pregnancy
    2. Incompetent cervix
    3. Gestational hypertension
    4. Vaginal infection

15. The patient is diagnosed with a missed abortion. Which signs and symptoms does the nurse expect to find during assessment of the patient?
    1. Malodorous bleeding, increased temperature, and cramping
    2. Some, but not all, products of conception are expelled
    3. Amenorrhea continues, but no uterine growth is measurable
    4. Bleeding increases and membranes rupture

16. What is the target outcome for a woman experiencing hyperemesis gravidarum?
    1. Relief of painful uterine contractions
    2. Absence of fetal withdrawal symptoms
    3. Normalization of partial thromboplastin time
    4. Adequate caloric intake for maternal and fetal health

17. In the care of a patient who has just been admitted for hyperemesis gravidarum, which tasks can be delegated to the unlicensed assistive personnel (UAP)? **Select all that apply.**
    1. Provide education and support to patient's family.
    2. Measure and report frequency and amount of emesis.
    3. Assess for and report signs of dehydration.
    4. Assist with oral hygiene after episodes of vomiting.
    5. Administer antiemetic as ordered.
    6. Weigh the patient every day.

18. A patient is diagnosed with placenta previa. The HCP indicates to the patient that she is stable enough to manage the condition at home. Which instructions will the nurse give?
    1. Take small amounts of clear fluid until vomiting subsides.
    2. Maintain bedrest, but getting up to the bathroom is allowed.
    3. Painless, bright-red bleeding is expected to continue.
    4. The prescribed tocolytic drug is used to relax the uterus.

19. The nurse's assignment on the postpartum unit includes patients with the following assessment data. Which patient would the nurse see **first**?
    1. The patient has saturated one peripad within the last 2 hours.
    2. The patient has a blood glucose of 160 mg/dL.
    3. The patient had a spontaneous abortion and is experiencing moderate dark bleeding.
    4. The patient has had a continuous headache, upset stomach, and blurred vision.

20. The patient has a fasting blood glucose of 130 mg/dL. What sign/symptom would the nurse expect to find in conjunction with this laboratory result?
    1. Cool, pale skin
    2. Increased appetite
    3. Frequent urination
    4. Irritability and tremors

21. The nurse is assisting an inexperienced HCP in training to examine a patient with unexplained vaginal bleeding in the third trimester of pregnancy. When would the nurse intervene?
    1. The HCP measures the fetal heart rate with a Doppler device.
    2. The HCP sets up for a vaginal examination.
    3. The HCP places the patient in a side-lying position.
    4. The HCP orders an ultrasound scan.

22. Which patient is **most** likely to need vital signs every 15 minutes until stable and then every hour as indicated?
    1. Has probable hydatidiform mole
    2. Had placement of prophylactic cerclage
    3. Has low-implantation placenta previa
    4. Has abruptio placentae requiring cesarean section

23. The nurse recognizes that the chance of hemolytic disease in the newborn is very low if which findings are present?
    1. Mother blood type O, infant blood type A
    2. Mother Rh negative, father Rh negative
    3. Mother Rh negative, father Rh positive
    4. Mother blood type O, infant blood type B

24. What are significant signs of gestational hypertension that would be immediately reported?
    1. Weight gain with edema
    2. Vomiting and low potassium
    3. Tachycardia and fever
    4. Hyperglycemia and polyuria

25. Which medication does the nurse anticipate for the patient who is experiencing severe gestational preeclampsia?
    1. Meperidine
    2. Heparin
    3. Oxytocin
    4. Magnesium sulfate

26. The nurse is working with an adolescent mother who has just delivered her first child. Which is the **most** likely problem for this patient?
    1. Insufficient knowledge
    2. Inadequate fluid volume
    3. Poor health maintenance
    4. Insufficient cardiac output

27. The nurse is teaching the pregnant woman about prevention of infection. Which is the **most** important teaching point related to toxoplasmosis?
    1. Hand hygiene after using the bathroom
    2. Vaccination with an attenuated virus
    3. Delay of sexual relations
    4. Avoidance of cat litter

28. The nurse suspects that a postpartum patient being seen for her 6-week postdelivery checkup is experiencing postpartum depression (PPD). Which patient behavior is evidence of PPD?
    1. Demonstrates little interest in her baby
    2. Talks extensively about her labor experience
    3. Reports fatigue due to infant's feeding schedule
    4. Admits to having some problems with breastfeeding

29. A woman who had an incomplete abortion several days ago reports sudden onset of chest pain and dyspnea. The nurse notes bleeding gums, petechiae, and ecchymoses. To support suspicion of DIC, which laboratory results will be immediately investigated and reported to the HCP?
    1. Cardiac enzymes
    2. Electrolyte levels
    3. Clotting factor studies
    4. Type, screen, and crossmatch

30. In the early postpartum period, the nurse notes a boggy uterus and the flow of lochia is heavy. What would the nurse do **first**?
    1. Report suspected hemorrhage.
    2. Start intravenous oxytocin.
    3. Perform fundal massage.
    4. Continue routine assessments.

31. In the early postpartum period, the mother complains of severe, deep rectal pain. She has an increased pulse and respiratory rate and her skin is pale and cool. There are no obvious signs of hemorrhage that the nurse can see. What assessment would the nurse make to detect a possible hematoma?
    1. Take the patient's blood pressure and compare it to baseline.
    2. Examine the perineum for a bulging mass or skin discoloration.
    3. Palpate the suprapubic area and listen for bowel sounds.
    4. Save all pads, linen savers, and linen to estimate blood loss.

32. The patient is diagnosed with gestational hypertension that is severe enough to warrant a prescribed antihypertensive medication. The morning blood pressure is 150/95 mm Hg. What would the nurse do **first**?
    1. Administer the medication as ordered.
    2. Call the HCP and clarify parameters for holding the medication.
    3. Compare blood pressure to baseline; then administer medication.
    4. Call the pharmacy and ask for contraindications.

33. The pregnant patient with HELLP (*H*, hemolysis; *EL*, elevated liver enzymes; *LP*, low platelet count) syndrome reports right upper quadrant and lower right chest pain, with nausea and vomiting. Which assessment technique would **not** be performed on this patient?
    1. Auscultation of lung sounds
    2. Abdominal palpation
    3. Inspecting for hemorrhage
    4. Monitoring fetal status

34. To prevent mastitis, which teaching point would the nurse emphasize?
    1. Take prophylactic antibiotics as ordered.
    2. Increase fluid intake to flush organisms from breasts.
    3. Empty both breasts regularly by feeding or pumping.
    4. Apply cold packs between feedings to reduce edema.

35. Which outcome statement **best** indicates that the plan of care for the patient with gestational diabetes is successful?
    1. Patient continues in euglycemic state.
    2. Patient reports dietary compliance.
    3. Patient shows weight gain as expected.
    4. Patient is able to self-administer insulin.

36. The nurse is caring for a postpartum mother who was diagnosed and managed for peripartum cardiomyopathy. During labor, the mother required oxygen and demonstrated some transient arrhythmias, but otherwise had a normal delivery. What will the nurse plan to do in the care of this patient?
    1. Routine care and assessment, because labor was the critical time for cardiac problems to occur.
    2. Obtain an order for oxygen as needed and continuous telemetry monitoring.
    3. Increase frequency of assessment for cardiac decompensation during the 48 hours after birth.
    4. Consult the HCP to see if transfer to the coronary care unit is warranted.

37. In caring for the postpartum patient during the hospital stay, which intervention would the nurse use to prevent thromboembolic disease?
    1. Assist to elevate both legs.
    2. Gently massage the legs.
    3. Administer oral anticoagulant.
    4. Encourage early ambulation.

38. The nurse is reviewing the laboratory results for a woman who comes to the clinic for routine prenatal visits. The nurse sees that the mother is Rh negative. Which question is the **most** important to ask the mother?
    1. "How many children do you have?"
    2. "Do you know the blood type of the father?"
    3. "Have you ever received Rh_o(D) immune globulin?"
    4. "Do you plan on having an amniocentesis?"

39. For a pregnant patient who is having an eclamptic seizure, what would the nurse do? **Select all that apply.**
    1. Provide oxygen by mask at 8-10 L/min.
    2. Notify the HCP.
    3. Protect the airway, inserting an oral airway if needed after the convulsion.
    4. Remain with the patient and press the emergency call light for assistance.
    5. Observe fetal monitor patterns for bradycardia, tachycardia, or decreased variability.
    6. Place the patient in supine position.
    7. Prepare for emergency cesarean section.

40. The patient has been diagnosed with a molar pregnancy asks the nurse for further explanation of the condition. What would the nurse tell the patient? **Select all that apply.**
    1. In a molar pregnancy, the fetus has died but been retained in the uterus.
    2. A molar pregnancy usually implants in the fallopian tube rather than the uterus.
    3. In a molar pregnancy, the sperm has fertilized an egg whose nucleus is lost or inactivated.
    4. The patient can be advised to wait 2 months to try to get pregnant again.
    5. A molar pregnancy carries a risk for choriocarcinoma.
    6. A patient with a molar pregnancy may experience excessive nausea and vomiting.

41. What would the nurse teach the pregnant patient with a history of genital herpes?
    1. A cesarean section will be necessary to prevent transmission of herpes to the newborn.
    2. If the bag of waters breaks, the patient may stay home for a few hours until contractions start.
    3. The patient should not breastfeed if genital herpes is present.
    4. The decision about whether to have a vaginal delivery will be made upon admission in labor.

42. The patient had gestational diabetes that was not well controlled. What complication would be most likely in her newborn?
    1. Hypoglycemia
    2. Poor feeding
    3. Hyperbilirubinemia
    4. Positive Coombs test

CRITICAL THINKING ACTIVITIES

43. During a routine prenatal appointment, the patient's blood pressure is 140/90 mm Hg. The nurse sees that this is an elevated reading compared to the past several appointments. The patient is currently at 22 weeks gestation.

    a. Describe the additional assessments that the nurse will make that will assist the HCP in determining if the patient is developing gestational hypertension.

    _____

    _____

    _____

    _____

    _____

    _____

    b. What is the treatment for mild preeclampsia? _____

    _____

    _____

44. The nurse is interviewing a woman who comes into the clinic for prenatal care. She reports feeling thirstier than before with frequent urination and excessive hunger. When the nurse performs urine testing, the results indicate the presence of glucose. The provider recommends testing for gestational diabetes.

    a. Which diagnostic tests may be performed for gestational diabetes?_____

    _____

    _____

    b. What complications for mother and infant are related to gestational diabetes? _____

    _____

    _____

    _____

    _____

NEXT-GENERATION NCLEX™ (NGN)

45. Extended Multiple Response

Cognitive Skills: Analyze Cues, Take Action

Scenario: The nurse is admitting a patient to the postpartum unit after normal vaginal delivery 2 hours ago. The following assessment findings are noted.

Vitals:
99.2° F (37.3° C)
BP 58/40
P 120
R 16

Physical assessment:
Fundus is soft, 3 centimeters above umbilicus, and nontender
Vaginal bleeding: Lochia rubra filling pad with clots present

Based on these assessment findings, which actions would the nurse take?

Instructions: Use an X to indicate the correct actions.

_____	1.	Stop IV infusion with oxytocin (Pitocin).
_____	2.	Massage fundus firmly.
_____	3.	Check if patient has voided since delivery.
_____	4.	Notify HCP.
_____	5.	Anticipate need for magnesium sulfate administration.
_____	6.	Place patient in left lateral position.
_____	7.	Administer acetaminophen.

Health Promotion for the Infant, Child, and Adolescent

Answer Key: A complete Answer Key is provided in your Additional Learning Resources on Evolve.

SHORT ANSWER

Directions: Using your own words, answer each question in the space provided.

1. Identify strategies to promote dental health for the following age groups.

    a. Infant: _____

    _____

    b. Preschooler: _____

    _____

    c. Adolescent: _____

    _____

2. Identify at least one nutritional consideration for the following age groups.

    a. Infant: _____

    b. Preschooler: _____

    c. Adolescent: _____

3. Identify three barriers to immunization for children.

    a. _____

    b. _____

    c. _____

MULTIPLE CHOICE

Directions: Select the best answer(s) for each of the following questions.

4. Which lunch tray includes the top three caloric sources for children ages 2-17 years?
   1. Fruit juice, granola bar, and ham sandwich
   2. Pizza, garlic bread, and a chocolate chip cookie
   3. Hamburger with French fries and a soda
   4. Chicken nuggets, potato chips, and ice cream

5. Which lunch tray for a school-age child **best** reflects the Dietary Guidelines for Americans (USDA)?
   1. Low-fat milk, vegetable soup, and orange slices
   2. Orange juice, whole-wheat crackers and jelly
   3. Chocolate milk, plain pasta, and a cookie
   4. Skim milk, nachos with queso and sour cream

6. A group of adolescents decides to experiment with a hookah. Which adolescent is **most** likely to experience an immediate adverse effect?
   1. Has a significant family history for throat and stomach cancer
   2. Has a significant family history for stroke and heart problems
   3. Has recently started taking antidepressant medication
   4. Had a recent episode of bronchitis with underlying asthma

7. The nurse is talking to an adolescent about responsible sexual behavior. Which question **best** demonstrates use of the principle of anticipatory guidance?
   1. "What kind of precautions do you plan to use for protection during sexual intercourse?"
   2. "Are you sexually active now or thinking about having sex in the near future?"
   3. "Would you like to have information about sexually transmitted infections?"
   4. "Abstinence is 100% effective; is this consistent with your beliefs and behavior?"

8. What would be the **best** way for the nurse to contribute to the overall achievement of the *Healthy People 2030* goals?
   1. Administer immunizations to infants during routine well-baby visits.
   2. Teach health promotion classes for parents/children at a community center.
   3. Pass out healthy snack samples in the waiting room at a local children's hospital.
   4. Give burn prevention brochures to parents when children are treated for minor burns.

9. A young couple is seeking advice about how to help their toddler develop good lifelong health habits. What would the nurse recommend as the **best** method?
   1. Schedule the child for regular medical and dental check-ups.
   2. Encourage the parents to obtain the recommended immunizations.
   3. Enroll the child in a daycare program that includes exercise.
   4. Role-model a lifestyle that includes exercise and healthy foods.

10. Which male child has the **greatest** risk for developing obesity?
    1. A 3-year-old who drinks whole milk
    2. A 9-year-old who eats at a fast-food restaurant every day
    3. A 13-year-old who spends 2-4 hours/day at the computer
    4. A 17-year-old who eats five meals a day with large portions

11. When an infant begins to transition from breastfeeding or formula to solid foods, which is recommended as the introductory food?
    1. Strained applesauce
    2. Farina with whole milk
    3. Thinned rice cereal
    4. Strained bananas

12. The nurse is assisting a toddler to eat a healthy diet tray. Based on the child's developmental age, what would the nurse say?
    1. "Drink your milk, then you can continue to play."
    2. "Let's have a race to see who can eat the most."
    3. "Would you like cheese or peanut butter on your bread?"
    4. "If you eat your vegetables, you will be strong like Daddy."

13. The nurse has a 14-year-old daughter who is refusing to wear sunscreen because "I want a tan just like my best friend." Using knowledge of growth and development for adolescents, what is the nurse's **best** response?
    1. Tell the daughter that she can't go out unless she wears sunscreen.
    2. Review the dangers of skin cancer that are linked to sun exposure.
    3. Suggest that the best friend has heredity for naturally darker skin.
    4. Point out that red, peeling skin takes away from summer fashions.

14. Which age group is **most** at risk for foreign-body aspiration?
    1. 1-5 months
    2. 6-12 months
    3. 1-2 years
    4. 2-4 years

15. The nurse is developing a nutrition plan with the parents of an overweight 12-year-old child. Which statement(s) by the parents demonstrate(s) an understanding of the plan? **Select all that apply.**
    1. "Our child's calories from saturated fats should be no more than 7% daily."
    2. "We should not allow our child to drink milk that is less than 2% milk fat."
    3. "Our child should participate in physical activity for at least 60 minutes a day."
    4. "We should give our child foods from all the food groups except for grains."
    5. "Children outgrow obesity and complications when they reach adolescence."

16. Which statement by a 7-year-old child indicates an understanding of safety principles to reduce injury caused by motor vehicle accidents?
    1. "I won't play outside anymore unless somebody goes with me."
    2. "I will wear my helmet if I am going a long ways on my bike."
    3. "I will 'stop, look, and listen' if I have to run to get my ball."
    4. "I won't play behind parked cars or at the curbside of the street."

17. Which child has the **highest** risk for accidental ingestion of a poisonous substance?
    1. Infant who is just learning to crawl
    2. A toddler who is visiting grandma
    3. A school-age child who is cleaning paintbrushes
    4. An adolescent who is studying chemistry

18. The health care team seeks to reduce or eliminate substance abuse among all persons; however, which child represents the group that is currently of particular concern?
    1. 15-year-old girl who admits to smoking cigarettes to impress older boys
    2. 17-year-old reports his parents allow him to drink beer whenever they do
    3. 12-year-old reports he and his friends experiment with any drugs they can get
    4. 9-year-old admits to watching her older brother smoke marijuana in the park

19. A nursing student is interested in a career in pediatrics and asks several pediatric nurses about common pediatric disorders and conditions. Which response **best** matches the health concerns for the current pediatric population in the United States?
    1. "Childhood obesity is a problem and we are now treating kids for hypertension and heart problems."
    2. "We see a lot of physically abused or neglected children who are usually from low-income single-parent homes."
    3. "We see children with chronic illnesses or physical limitations and they are usually bullied at school."
    4. "Mental health issues that we see in pediatrics include depression, suicide, eating disorders, and substance abuse."

20. The father of an 11-year-old boy is hesitant to let his son get the recommended human papillomavirus (HPV) vaccine because he sees it as permission for the boy to have sex. What information would the nurse provide to him about this vaccine?
    1. "The purpose of the vaccine is to give your son protection against certain types of cancers."
    2. "The vaccine prevents several sexually transmitted infections and since he will eventually be sexually active, it is good to get the vaccines now."
    3. "The vaccine is required for school so it would be better to get it now."
    4. "The vaccine can be delayed until the boy is sexually active."

21. What instructions would the nurse give the parents of a 1-year-old child who weighs 20 pounds about car seat use?
    1. Transition the child from the rear-facing car seat to front-facing car seat in the back seat at this time.
    2. Allow the child to try a booster seat in the back seat of the car.
    3. Keep the child in a rear-facing car seat in the back seat.
    4. Read the weight limits on the car seat, and transition the child to afront-facing seat if he exceeds the weight limits.

22. The nurse is teaching the mother of a 10-month-old infant about the dangers of aspiration. As well as securing the home to prevent access to coins and toys with small parts, what foods would the nurse teach the mother to avoid or to use with extreme caution? **Select all that apply.**
    1. Grapes
    2. Cottage cheese
    3. Popcorn
    4. Nuts
    5. Hot dogs
    6. Chopped carrots
    7. Puréed beans

CRITICAL THINKING ACTIVITIES

23. Discuss benefits of physical activity and suggest ways that the nurse can promote physical activity for children.

_____

_____

_____

_____

_____

_____

_____

24. The nurse is preparing a discussion for a community group about how to prevent accidental poisoning. What strategies will the nurse share that will help participants prevent accidental poisoning?

_____

_____

_____

_____

_____

_____

_____

25. Explain the factors that contribute to tobacco use among adolescents and suggest interventions that the nurse can use to help teens stop or never start using tobacco.

_____

_____

_____

_____

_____

_____

_____

_____

NEXT-GENERATION NCLEX™ (NGN)

26. Cloze

Cognitive Skills: Recognize Cues, Take Action, Evaluate Outcome

Scenario: The nurse is providing education to a 14-year-old and her family regarding safety issues.

Instructions: Choose the most likely option for the information missing from the statements below by selecting from the lists of options provided.

The nurse knows that an adolescent is in the ___1___ stage of psychosocial development and that usually the peer group influence is of great importance. The greatest risk of death during this stage of life is ___2___. Due to this, the nurse will engage the teen in conversation and ask her if ___3___. The nurse will know that the teaching had impact if the teen ___4___.

Options for 1	Options for 2	Options for 3	Options for 4
initiative versus guilt	cancer	she or her friends are interested in taking driver education	takes a brochure on seatbelts
autonomy versus shame	suicide	she has known anyone who committed suicide	discloses that her friend went driving with an older teen who had been drinking
industry versus inferiority	accidents	she and her friends use sunscreen	decides she will not take driver education
identity versus role confusion	homicide	there are household medications in childproof bottles	tells her mother she has smoked marijuana
trust versus mistrust	heart disease	she know the importance of seatbelts	denies that she has feelings of depression

Basic Pediatric Nursing Care

Answer Key: A complete Answer Key is provided in your Additional Learning Resources on Evolve.

FIGURE LABELING

1. *Directions:* Look at the Wong-Baker FACES Pain Rating Scale below and label each face with the appropriate description, then write an explanation that the nurse would give to a child about the scale so he or she could assess the child's pain.

TABLE ACTIVITY

2. *Directions:* Complete the table below with the average vital signs for each age.

Vital Signs (Averages)

Age	Heart Rate/Min	Respirations/Min	Blood Pressure
Newborn			
1-11 months			
2 years			
4 years			
6 years			
10 years			
12 years			
16 years			

CLINICAL APPLICATION OF MATH AND EQUIVALENTS

Directions: Calculate or make the necessary conversions for math problems encountered in pediatrics.

3. The mother reports that her 4-year-old has grown 3 inches (1 inch = 2.54 cm) in the last year. How many centimeters has he grown? _____ cm   Is this growth within the normal range? _____

4. A 12-year-old is voiding 35 mL/hr. Over a period of 8 hours, how many mL of urine will he void? _____ mL

5. The mother tells the nurse that she gave the child 4 cc (cubic centimeters) of liquid acetaminophen according to the instructions on the package. How many mL did the mother administer? _____ mL

6. The nurse is measuring the urine output for an infant. The wet diaper weighs 20 g more than the dry diaper. How many mL does the nurse record as urine output? _____ mL

7. A 6-year-old proudly hands the nurse an 8-ounce plastic cup full of urine, because he knows that "nurses like you to pee in a cup." Convert this to mL, so that the total can be added to the intake and output for the day. _____ mL

8. A 16-year-old male weighs 161 lbs. He tells the nurse that he intentionally eats around 1500 kcal/day to lose weight to secure his position on the wrestling team. What is the deficit of kcal/day according to daily caloric needs for his age and weight? _____ kcal/day. What should the nurse do?

_____

9. A 15-year-old girl tells the nurse that obesity runs in her family and she would like to avoid gaining weight. She currently weighs 105 lbs. How many kilocalories per day does she need? _____ kcal/day

10. A child has a temperature of 98.3° F. The nurse needs to record the temperature in Fahrenheit and Centigrade. Convert Fahrenheit to Centigrade. _____ ° C

11. Determine the expected systolic blood pressure of a 5-year-old using the quick formula to calculate normal systolic blood pressure. What is the calculated systolic blood pressure? _____ mm Hg

12. Determine the expected diastolic blood pressure of a 6-year-old using the quick formula to calculate normal diastolic blood pressure. What is the calculated diastolic blood pressure? _____ mm Hg

MULTIPLE CHOICE

Directions: Select the best answer(s) for each of the following questions.

13. A teenager is brought to the clinic by a male "guardian" for treatment for a sexually transmitted disease. The girl is withdrawn, submissive, and the guardian answers all of the questions. Based on suspicion of possible abuse, what would the nurse do **first**?
    1. Call Child Protective Services (CPS).
    2. Escort the teen to a private exam room.
    3. Call the police for possible sex trafficking.
    4. Notify the RN and health care provider (HCP) about suspicion of abuse.

14. Which parents are using the **best** approach to guide an adolescent child?
    1. Mother advises daughter that she will look better and weigh less if she skips dessert.
    2. Parents tell son to pay attention to sex education at school and stop looking at the Internet.
    3. Parents discuss with daughter the pros and cons of delaying college for travel to Europe.
    4. Father asks the coach to excuse son for skipping practice so he does not get cut from the team.

15. Which nursing actions will help gain the parents' trust when the child is admitted to the hospital? **Select all that apply.**
    1. When obtaining a nursing history, select a quiet place on the unit to listen to parents' responses.
    2. Emphasize that the HCP considers hospitalization as a routine event.
    3. On admission, give parents specific information on routines, hospital policies, and limitations.
    4. Explain the tests and treatments thoroughly and repeat information as needed.
    5. Ask for parents' assistance in establishing goals or revising a care plan.
    6. Tell parents they are responsible for procedures such as tube feeding and suctioning.

16. Which family is **most** likely to be eligible for and benefit from a referral to the Women, Infants, and Children (WIC) program?
    1. 22-year-old mother who needs emotional support to cope with a child who sustained a serious head injury
    2. 53-year-old mother of a 13-year-old child who is developmentally disabled and needs a new wheelchair
    3. 35-year-old single working mother of a toddler and preschooler, who is currently expecting her third child
    4. 15- and 16-year-old sisters who need counseling for prevention of pregnancy and sexually transmitted infections

17. Which nurse is **best** demonstrating the family-centered concept of enabling?
    1. Nurse A tells the parents that the adolescent needs privacy and independence.
    2. Nurse B encourages the mother to show her partner how to burp the infant.
    3. Nurse C gives the child a small reward after a painful procedure is completed.
    4. Nurse D is truthful with the child and the family and follows up on promises.

18. The nurse reads in the HCP's notes that the toddler is having physiologic anorexia. Which intervention is the nurse **most** likely to use?
    1. Suggest three meals per day with planned snacks so the child eats every 2-3 hours.
    2. Obtain an order from the HCP for a referral to a registered dietitian.
    3. Teach the parents how to do calorie counts and measure intake and output.
    4. Tell the mother that this is normal and that the child will eat when he gets hungry.

19. The nurse is working at a health fair performing growth measurements on children. Which children need follow-up for further investigation? **Select all that apply.**
    1. 9-year-old male with height in the 10th percentile and weight in the 90th percentile
    2. 10-year-old male who had a sudden increase in height putting him in the 90th percentile
    3. 17-year-old male who has had no increase in height or weight since age 13
    4. 11-year-old male who continues in the 50th percentile for weight and height
    5. 13-year-old male with height in the 90th percentile and weight in the 10th percentile

20. A student nurse is performing routine measurements on an 18-month-old child. When would the supervising nurse intervene?
    1. Student positions the child recumbent and extends the child's legs to measure length.
    2. Student uses a paper measuring tape to measure arm circumference
    3. Student asks the nurse if the child's clothes should be removed prior to weighing.
    4. Student puts the tape under the chin and over the top of the head for head circumference.

21. Which child is **most** likely to benefit from the en face position?
    1. Toddler falls down and looks up at mother to gage her response.
    2. School-age child wants parent to look at a completed school project.
    3. Newborn infant shows quiet alertness after breastfeeding.
    4. Adolescent wants privacy while talking to friends on the phone.

22. A 4-year-old child has a sore throat and cough. She is holding a doll and peering from behind the mother's leg. A history, vital signs, and focused assessment on the throat and upper airway are necessary. Which action would the nurse perform **first**?
    1. Say hello to the child and ask what her doll's name is.
    2. Stand at eye level of the child and welcome her.
    3. Talk to the doll and show the stethoscope to the doll.
    4. Ask the mother to sit and hold the child on her lap.

23. The mother tells the nurse that her 9-year-old daughter has pain on urination with frequency, and some brown spotting in her underpants. The mother also says the child seems more anxious than usual. What would the nurse do **first**?
    1. Ask the mother to elaborate on symptoms and behavior.
    2. Ask the child about the discomfort and the brown spots.
    3. Alert the HCP about possibility of sexual abuse.
    4. Help the child obtain a midstream urine specimen.

24. There is a cry for help; a child is having a grand mal seizure and the mother is cradling his head and sobbing. The child recovers quickly, but the mother repeatedly sobs, "I didn't know what to do." What can the nurse do to empower the mother?
    1. Stay with the family and observe for complications.
    2. Reinforce the fact that the child is going to be fine.
    3. Tell her that managing the head was the correct action.
    4. Ask her if this was the first time she witnessed a seizure.

25. Which nursing action **best** exemplifies partnering with the parent of a toddler who has been admitted for an exacerbation of asthma?
    1. Suggests that the mother take the toddler to the play area
    2. Instructs the mother on how to hold the nebulizer
    3. Asks the mother for advice about the child's preferred rituals
    4. Maintains a cheerful and warm attitude toward the toddler

26. Which factors does the nurse consider when selecting a method to measure a temperature on a pediatric patient? **Select all that apply.**
    1. Child's ability to cooperate
    2. Parent's preference for route
    3. Child's developmental age
    4. Parent's familiarity with route
    5. Child's need for precise temperature
    6. Child's psychological response to method

27. Which set of vital signs is closest to the average findings for a 2-year-old child?
    1. P 110, R 25, BP 94/66
    2. P 100, R 20, BP 110/80
    3. P 90, R 22, BP 108/70
    4. P 70, R 24, BP 120/76

28. Which vocalization exemplifies the vocabulary of a typical 1-year-old child?
    1. "Mama, me; dada, me"
    2. "Burrr, ahhh, eeeehhhh"
    3. "Give me cookie cup."
    4. "When is daddy coming?"

29. Which set of vital signs for a 12-year-old child requires a follow-up intervention?
    1. P 124, R 32, BP 126/66
    2. P 90, R 20, BP 100/80
    3. P 88, R 20, BP 110/70
    4. P 74, R 22, BP 110/76

30. The nurse is reviewing infant development. What is an expected finding?
    1. Having a visual acuity of 20/100 at birth
    2. Enjoying "peek-a-boo" games throughout infancy
    3. Controlling bladder elimination by 18 months
    4. Tripling of birth weight by 6 months

31. The nurse is preparing to administer an immunization to a 4-year-old child in the pediatric clinic. What is the **best** way to communicate this event to the child?
    1. "This may feel like a pinch."
    2. "Don't move when I give you this."
    3. "Do you want to take this medicine now?"
    4. "I will be coming back to give you a shot."

32. The nurse has to administer a liquid medicine that has a bitter taste to a 5-year-old. Which strategy would be the **best** to use?
    1. Use a syringe to squirt the liquid along the side of the mouth.
    2. Give the child an ice pop to suck on beforehand to numb the tongue.
    3. Give the child a glass of sweetened juice immediately after the medicine.
    4. Hand the child the medication cup and allow independent sipping.

33. The nurse is evaluating the bath given to the infant by the adult caregiver. Identify which actions indicate a need for additional teaching. **Select all that apply.**
    1. Using soap around the eyes
    2. Using a cotton-tipped swab to clean the ear canal
    3. Supporting the head while bathing the infant in a tub
    4. Washing the extremities after washing the face
    5. Washing the perineum in an anterior to posterior direction
    6. Retracting the foreskin of the male infant

34. An older school-age child will be having surgery with anesthesia. What would the nurse do to reduce anxiety?
    1. Show the child the mask that will be used for the anesthesia.
    2. Introduce the child to a peer so they can talk about the experience.
    3. Reassure the child that the procedure is safe and necessary for health.
    4. Explain the special type of sleep that will occur with the anesthetic.

35. The mother of a toddler asks the nurse how to get him to eat right. Which advice would the nurse give?
    1. "Food should be left out, so the child can eat when he feels like it."
    2. "The child should be restrained in the high chair for meals."
    3. "The child should sit at the table for scheduled meals."
    4. "Meals should be arranged about every 5 hours for the child."

36. Which statements by the mother of a 3-month-old indicate that health promotion teaching has been successful? **Select all that apply.**
    1. "My baby's birth weight should be doubled at the age of 6 months."
    2. "My baby should be actively exploring his environment."
    3. "My baby should enjoy parallel play by the age of 8 months."
    4. "My baby should enjoy toys that bang, shake, or can be pulled."
    5. "My baby should start eating rice cereals just before bedtime."

37. The nurse prepares to give an injection to an infant in the vastus lateralis muscle. Why does the nurse select this site?
    1. This is the easiest area to expose on the baby.
    2. No blood vessels or nerves are near this site.
    3. This site is the least painful site for injections.
    4. The leg muscle is the least developed in an infant.

38. Which child is exhibiting behavior that warrants additional assessment?
    1. 6-month-old infant coos and babbles to himself
    2. 2-year-old refuses to eat as much as he used to
    3. 10-year-old exhibits apprehension when another child cries
    4. 17-year-old is resistant to any parental suggestions

39. Which question **best** demonstrates the nurse's use of anticipatory guidance in helping the parents of an 8-month-old child?
    1. "Has your child been eating and drinking like he should?"
    2. "Have you looked at floor space from his perspective?"
    3. "Would you like to have a brochure on infant growth?"
    4. "Have you talked to the HCP about immunizations?"

40. The nurse is trying to auscultate the bowel sounds of a 4-year-old child, but the child is resisting the placement of the stethoscope. What would the nurse do **first**?
    1. Document the attempt as "deferred by patient."
    2. Let the child handle the stethoscope.
    3. Obtain the assistance of a helper.
    4. Ask the parent if the child has been eating.

41. Which vital sign would be performed **first** on an infant?
    1. Temperature
    2. Pulse
    3. Respirations
    4. Blood pressure

42. Which assessment findings would be reported to the HCP for follow-up? **Select all that apply.**
    1. Two palmar flexion creases in a newborn
    2. Tufts of hair along the spine of a newborn
    3. Preference for en face position in newborn
    4. Bumping into obstacles by 1-year-old
    5. Lack of babbling by a 9-month-old
    6. Tongue protrusion by a toddler

43. The mother who is breastfeeding her infant tells the nurse that the infant's bowel movements "look terrible." What would the nurse say to the mother?
    1. "Infant stool is supposed to look different from ours because of immaturity."
    2. "The stool of breastfed babies is a light mustard color with seedlike particles."
    3. "The stool should be soft and formed with a pale greenish-yellow color."
    4. "As long as the baby does not have runny diarrhea, you should not worry."

44. What is the **best** rationale for advising the parent to withhold whole cow's milk until the child passes the 12-month mark?
    1. Breast milk is cheaper and a better source of high-quality protein.
    2. The child is more likely to develop allergies to milk later in life.
    3. The protein and minerals in whole milk place stress on immature kidneys.
    4. Whole milk is more likely to cause vomiting, diarrhea, and flatus.

45. The aunt of an 11-month-old infant is making homemade baby food using materials that she has on hand. When would the mother intervene?
    1. Aunt adds white sugar.
    2. Aunt uses a blender.
    3. Aunt mixes in honey.
    4. Aunt uses frozen peaches.

46. What is the **best** indicator of readiness to wean in a 9-month-old breastfed infant?
    1. The HCP says that most children wean around 9 or 10 months.
    2. The infant reaches for his siblings' or parents' cup or drinking glass.
    3. The father remembers that the sibling was weaned at 8 months.
    4. The mother has to return to work, so breastfeeding is increasingly difficult.

47. Which child needs cholesterol testing somewhere between the age of 2 and 10 years?
    1. Mother has a total cholesterol level of 200 mg/dL.
    2. Father has a total cholesterol level of 300 mg/dL.
    3. Grandfather died of a heart attack at age 65.
    4. Grandmother had a coronary bypass at age 70.

48. While examining a child, the nurse finds human bite marks, linear ecchymosis patterns, and round red sores. According to the parent, "he frequently gets into fights at school." What would the nurse do **first**?
    1. Assist the HCP to examine for occult injuries.
    2. Contact Child Protective Services and report suspected abuse.
    3. Ask the child to give details about how he sustained specific injuries.
    4. Assess the parent for signs of hostility toward the child.

49. How does the nurse use knowledge of body position and space to engage the preschooler and begin the nurse-patient relationship?
    1. Stands in the doorway and greets the child by making a funny face.
    2. Directs the child to sit on mother's lap; then nurse holds child's hand.
    3. Puts chairs in a small circle and invites everyone to sit down.
    4. Allows the child to get comfortable; then nurse gets to child's eye level.

50. The nurse is placing electrodes on the chest of a 4-year-old child. What would the nurse say to the child?
    1. "Feel this; like little round band-aids with a bit of cold jelly."
    2. "These snaps will hook you to the machine, so we can watch you."
    3. "The electrodes allow us to watch your heart beat all the time."
    4. "This won't hurt. It's just a way for us to see your heart."

51. Which action is included when performing gavage feeding for a small infant?
    1. Administer warm formula, 10 mL/min, and allow gravity flow into the stomach.
    2. Keep the infant positioned on the right side for at least 1 hour after feeding.
    3. Obtain an order for an x-ray to confirm tube placement before every feeding.
    4. Check placement by injecting 10 mL of air into the tube and auscultating for a gurgle.

52. Which patient is the **most** likely candidate for an elbow safety reminder device (SRD)?
    1. Active toddler needs to safely sit in a highchair.
    2. Infant needs a lumbar puncture procedure.
    3. Infant has a newly repaired cleft palate.
    4. Toddler needs nasogastric tube insertion.

CRITICAL THINKING ACTIVITIES

53. A 9-year-old child is being admitted to the hospital for surgical repair of a hernia. The nurse knows that the procedure should have an uncomplicated outcome, but the parents appear very nervous. The child is carefully watching his parents' reactions and the nurse sees that he is also fearful and distrustful of this new experience.

    a. What should the nurse do to reduce anxiety for the child and the parents? _____

    b. What strategies can the nurse use when communicating with the child? _____

54. a. Identify the guidelines for performing a physical assessment on a child. _____

b. Describe methods that can be used to have the child assist while you auscultate his/her lungs.

_____

_____

_____

_____

55. Identify characteristics in yourself that would make you a good pediatric nurse._____

_____

_____

_____

_____

_____

_____

_____

NEXT-GENERATION NCLEX™ (NGN)

56. Extended Multiple Response

Cognitive Skill: Take Action

Scenario: An experienced nurse who usually works on the adult medical-surgical unit is asked to temporarily float to the pediatrics unit. The nurse asks the charge nurse for some reminder tips about how to manage pain in pediatric patients.

Which management tips would the charge nurse share with the float nurse?

Instructions: Place a check mark next to interventions and pain management tips for pediatric patients. **Check all that apply.**

_____ 1. Encourage parents to participate and use soothing talk when giving care.

_____ 2. For infants, nonpharmacologic interventions include pacifiers, swaddling, rocking, or being held.

_____ 3. In smaller children, opioids have a greater risk for respiratory depression compared to adults.

_____ 4. Observe children for reluctance to report or express pain; they may fear medication injection.

_____ 5. Observe vocalization, facial expressions, and body movements for infants and children who are unable to verbalize or indicate the location of pain

_____ 6. When a child is playing or reading, it is likely that he or she feels comfortable and pain-free.

_____ 7. Reduce noise and disturbing sensations to create a calm environment for the child in pain.

Care of the Child With a Physical and Mental or Cognitive Disorder

Answer Key: A complete Answer Key is provided in your Additional Learning Resources on Evolve.

MATCHING

Directions: Match the disorder with the clinical manifestations. Indicate your answer in the space provided.

Physical Disorder

_____ 1. hypertrophic pyloric stenosis

_____ 2. nephrotic syndrome

_____ 3. pneumonia

_____ 4. septic arthritis

_____ 5. cerebral palsy

_____ 6. hyperthyroidism

_____ 7. severe diarrhea

_____ 8. otitis media

_____ 9. hypothyroidism

_____ 10. Duchenne's muscular dystrophy

Clinical Manifestations

a. Cough, wheeze or crackles, respiratory distress, chest pain, fever, malaise, myalgia, nasal discharge

b. Cool, pale skin; sunken eyes and fontanelles; poor skin turgor; lethargy; rapid pulse and respirations; weight loss

c. Projectile vomiting, hungry, weight loss, peristaltic waves from left to right, palpable olive-shaped mass

d. Delayed growth, dry skin, constipation, lethargy, mental slowness, cold intolerance

e. Nervous, irritable, hyperactivity, tremors, excessive appetite, exophthalmos, palpable thyroid gland, tachycardia

f. Involuntary movement, hypertonic movements, arching of back, delayed gross motor development, drooling

g. Increased body weight, decreased urine output, ascites, periorbital edema, vomiting, anorexia, diarrhea, irritability

h. Clumsy, frequent falls, a waddling gait, difficulty running or climbing, Gowers' sign

i. Limited range-of-motion (ROM) to affected joint with erythema, edema, warmth, and exquisite pain; fever; limps or refuses to walk

j. Pulling, tugging, or rubbing the affected ear; fever; rhinitis; fussiness; irritability; decreased appetite

TABLE ACTIVITY

11. *Directions:* Complete the table below by filling in the signs and symptoms for each assessment that indicates the clinical manifestations of dehydration.

Clinical Manifestations of Dehydration

Assessment	Signs and Symptoms
Skin	
Mucous membranes	
Eyes	
Fontanelles	
Behavior	
Pulse	
Blood pressure	
Respirations	

FIGURE LABELING

12. *Directions:* On the figure below, identify the assessment findings for the infant.

CLINICAL APPLICATION OF MATH AND CONVERSIONS

Directions: Calculate or make the necessary conversions for math problems encountered in pediatrics.

13. The nurse is performing a physical examination on a 6-month-old infant. At birth, the infant weighed 7 lbs. The current weight is 14 lbs. How much weight has the child gained in kilograms? _____ kg

14. Toddlers require 7 mg/day of iron. The mother has purchased a bottle of liquid iron and the label indicates that there are 40 mg/15 mL. The mother is unable to determine how much to give. How many mL does the nurse tell her to give the child to achieve the correct dose? _____ mL

15. The nurse must calculate an infant's urine output by weighing the wet diaper. The wet diaper weighs 35 g more than the dry diaper. What does the nurse record for urine output? _____ mL

MULTIPLE CHOICE

Directions: Select the best answer(s) for each of the following questions.

16. A child who has leukemia shows the symptoms of fatigue, fever, and bruising. Which relevant laboratory results would the nurse seek out and report to the health care provider (HCP)?
    1. Complete blood count (CBC) and platelet count
    2. CD4+ lymphocyte count and viral load
    3. CBC, serum ferritin, and serum iron concentration
    4. Erythrocyte sedimentation rate and C-reactive protein

17. An infant is rubbing and pulling at the right ear and demonstrates fever, rhinitis, fussiness, and decreased appetite. In addition to antibiotics, which comfort measure would make the infant feel better?
    1. Place infant in a supine position during bottle-feeding.
    2. Give clear fluids to thin secretions, withhold formula and breast milk.
    3. Apply a clean, warm, moist washcloth over the affected ear.
    4. To decrease pain during sleep, position the infant on the unaffected side.

18. Which child is **most** likely to benefit from the use of adaptive eating devices?
    1. Child has spina bifida
    2. Child has cerebral palsy
    3. Child with talipes equinovarus
    4. Child with idiopathic scoliosis

19. The mother of a 7-year-old child reports seeing head lice and nits in the child's hair. Which instructions would the nurse give? **Select all that apply.**
    1. Wash hair once or twice a day with a mild shampoo.
    2. Remove dead lice and remaining nits with a fine-toothed comb.
    3. Wash clothing, towels, and bed linens in hot water; run dryer at the highest setting for 20 minutes.
    4. Vacuum carpets, car seats, rugs, mattresses, and upholstered furniture.
    5. Seal nonwashable items in plastic bags for 14 days.
    6. Soak combs, brushes, and hair accessories in boiling water for 10 minutes.
    7. Isolate child from others until lice and nits are no longer observed.

20. A 9-month-old infant appears uncomfortable, fussy, irritable, and restless. There is a red rash on the skin underneath the diaper. The HCP directs the nurse to review the standard interventions to control diaper rash with the mother. **Select all that apply.**
    1. Keep skin dry.
    2. Use cloth diapers covered by rubber pants.
    3. Change diapers as soon as they are soiled and once during the night, whenever possible.
    4. Expose healthy or slightly irritated skin to air and dry completely.
    5. Apply generous amounts of talcum powder between skin folds.
    6. Apply zinc oxide or petrolatum jelly if skin is red or has moist, open areas.

21. Which assessment is the HCP **most** likely to ask the nurse to perform to assist in the diagnosis of possible coarctation of the aorta?
    1. Take the blood pressure (BP) in the arms and the legs.
    2. Take manual BP in both arms, rather than using the automatic cuff.
    3. Take orthostatic BP in lying to sitting to standing positions.
    4. Take BP every 15 minutes for 1 hour, then every 30 minutes for 2 hours.

22. Which lunch tray provides the **best** food sources to help a toddler get the required 7 mg/day of iron?
    1. Milk, chicken fingers, and biscuit
    2. Fruit punch, cheese and crackers
    3. Orange juice, and beef and bean burrito
    4. Low-fat milk and egg salad sandwich

23. An 11-month-old infant presents with fever, vomiting, and irritability. He has a bulging fontanelle, a high-pitched cry, and generalized petechiae over the trunk area. What is the **best** rationale for immediately notifying the HCP about the infant's symptoms?
    1. Infant shows signs/symptoms of meningococcal meningitis.
    2. It is likely that infant has something contagious and requires isolation.
    3. Infants have an increased risk for sepsis and septic shock.
    4. Signs/symptoms suggest an illness that requires immediate attention.

24. For a child in sickle cell crisis, what are the **priority** interventions? **Select all that apply.**
    1. Analgesics
    2. Comfort measures
    3. Sickle-turbidity test
    4. Oxygenation
    5. Hydration

25. Which child and family are **most** likely to need emotional support for anticipatory grief and loss immediately after being told about the medical diagnosis of their child?
    1. 3-year-old boy is diagnosed with acute bronchitis
    2. 4-year-old boy is diagnosed with Legg-Calvé-Perthes disease
    3. 2-year-old girl is diagnosed with Duchenne's muscular dystrophy
    4. 3-year-old girl is diagnosed with idiopathic thrombocytopenia purpura

26. The nurse is reviewing the child's medication list and sees that etanercept is prescribed. Based on the nurse's knowledge of pharmacologic therapy for juvenile rheumatoid arthritis, which intervention is the nurse likely to use **first**?
    1. Encourage normal routines, such as homework and playing with friends.
    2. Plan a time for physical therapy to review ROM exercises.
    3. Discuss how to use heat and cold to reduce swelling.
    4. Ask the parent and child about strategies they use to reduce pain.

27. Which nurse is **most** likely to encounter a child who needs care for respiratory distress syndrome?
    1. Nurse A works in an after-school drop-in center.
    2. Nurse B works in a newborn intensive care unit.
    3. Nurse C works in a general pediatric hospital unit.
    4. Nurse D works in an allergy and asthma clinic.

28. The nurse is sitting at the front desk of a walk-in clinic. Simultaneously, several children come in with their parents. Which child would the nurse attend to **first**?
    1. 12-year-old has no symptoms, but parents report that a sibling was recently diagnosed with tuberculosis
    2. 5-year-old has low-grade fever, malaise, anorexia, pharyngeal erythema, and sore throat
    3. 2-year-old demonstrates hoarseness, nasal flaring, intercostal retractions, and a barking cough
    4. 3-year-old is anxious with a high fever, muffled voice, drooling, and progressive respiratory distress

29. Which child is **most** likely to gain therapeutic benefit from blowing bubbles or pinwheels?
    1. 4-year-old diagnosed with cystic fibrosis
    2. 6-year-old with acute epiglottitis
    3. 3-year-old with cough and sore throat
    4. 5-year-old who just had a tonsillectomy

30. The nurse sees that the child takes fluticasone. Which assessment is the nurse **most** likely to perform to evaluate the efficacy of the medication?
    1. Auscultate for bowel sounds.
    2. Auscultate for breath sounds.
    3. Assess for relief of pain.
    4. Assess for relief of itching.

31. A nursing student is participating in the care of a child who is undergoing diagnostic testing for possible Wilms' tumor. When would the supervising nurse intervene?
    1. Student assists the child to obtain a mid-stream urine specimen.
    2. Student takes the child's weight and compares it to baseline.
    3. Student engages the child in quiet play to conserve energy.
    4. Student palpates the abdominal mass to assess for pain.

32. Which infant is **most** likely to benefit from a pacifier?
    1. Infant who recently had a cleft palate repair
    2. Infant who is being treated for a thrush infection
    3. Infant whose mother abused drugs during pregnancy
    4. Infant who has difficulty latching to the nipple for breastfeeding

33. In reviewing diabetic dietary management with a child and the family, which point is the **most** important to emphasize?
    1. Avoid candy, desserts, and sodas with sugar.
    2. Maintain a consistent intake and timing of food.
    3. Learn to monitor blood sugar and adjust food accordingly.
    4. Eat the same food at the same time as the rest of the family.

34. The nurse hears in report that the child has nephrotic syndrome. Which assessments is the nurse **most** likely to perform? **Select all that apply.**
    1. Assess for worsening abdominal pain.
    2. Monitor intake and output.
    3. Check abdominal girth.
    4. Monitor platelet count.
    5. Monitor body weight.

35. The child has a hemoglobin (Hgb) value of 8 g/dL. Which symptom would the nurse expect to see at this Hgb level?
    1. Fatigue
    2. Pallor
    3. Glossitis
    4. "Spoon" fingernails

36. What sign/symptom would be common to both patent ductus arteriosus and septal defects?
    1. Murmurs
    2. Chest pain
    3. Hypotension
    4. Headache

37. What is the **most** commonly recommended treatment for the majority of congenital heart defects?
    1. Diet therapy
    2. Exercise
    3. Surgery
    4. Medication

38. The walk-in clinic is conducting screenings on children for blood disorders. Which blood disorder is the **most** likely to be detected during general screenings?
    1. Hemophilia
    2. Sickle cell anemia
    3. Iron deficiency anemia
    4. Idiopathic thrombocytopenic purpura

39. The nurse is instructing the parents of a child with iron deficiency anemia. Which action enhances iron absorption?
    1. Giving the supplement with milk.
    2. Giving the supplement with citrus juice or fruits.
    3. Offering a chewable form once each day.
    4. Giving the tablet 30 minutes before eating.

40. Which children are **most** likely to need an iron supplement? **Select all that apply.**
    1. A 5-month-old infant who is exclusively breastfed
    2. A healthy toddler with age-appropriate eating habits
    3. A 16-year-old girl who is trying to lose weight
    4. A preterm infant with low birth weight
    5. A 10-month-old infant who eats commercial infant cereal

41. A high school senior with sickle cell disease wants to take a vacation with friends. Which trip would be the **best** choice to avoid the precipitating factors of a sickle cell crisis?
    1. Cross-country ski trip
    2. Hiking in the mountains
    3. Road trip to the beach
    4. Flying to Europe

42. The nurse is talking to the mother of a 10-year-old boy who has hemophilia. Which toy would be the **best** to recommend for this child?
    1. Skateboard
    2. Football
    3. Swim fins
    4. Hockey skates

43. Which blood disorder places a child at **greatest** risk for intracranial bleeding if a head injury occurs?
    1. Sickle cell anemia
    2. Sickle cell trait
    3. Iron deficiency anemia
    4. Idiopathic thrombocytopenia purpura

44. The child with leukemia has been placed on neutropenic precautions. Which persons would be allowed to enter the room? **Select all that apply.**
    1. A 5-month-old sibling who was born prematurely
    2. A 3-year-old sibling who is coughing and sneezing
    3. A nursing student who is 5 months pregnant
    4. A parent who works at a waste management plant
    5. An aunt who completed antibiotics for chlamydia infection
    6. A sibling who is showing the symptoms of conjunctivitis

45. For human immunodeficiency virus (HIV) testing on a child who is younger than 18 months, what is the physiologic explanation that discourages the use of standardized testing procedures (Western blot test and enzyme-linked immunosorbent assay [ELISA])?
    1. Infant's immune system is too immature to produce antibodies.
    2. It is unclear whether antibodies are the mother's or the infant's.
    3. The polymerase chain reaction test is safer for infants.
    4. Standardized tests yield too many false negatives for infants.

46. The nurse is talking to a 17-year-old who recently found out that he is HIV positive. He says, "I guess I really messed up. I'm in serious trouble." What is the **most** therapeutic response?
    1. "Yes, you made a serious mistake, but you can take the medications."
    2. "You are very young and you shouldn't blame yourself for making a mistake."
    3. "You are thinking about your future and how to live with being HIV positive."
    4. "You sound really scared. Well, don't worry. With treatments, you'll be okay."

47. The child has recently been diagnosed with juvenile idiopathic arthritis. The nurse will prepare an educational brochure for which type of drugs?
    1. Tumor necrosis factor blockers
    2. Disease-modifying antirheumatic drugs
    3. Slower-acting antirheumatic drugs
    4. Nonsteroidal antiinflammatory drugs

48. In caring for a neonate who was intubated for respiratory distress syndrome, when does the nurse perform endotracheal tube suctioning?
    1. Routinely every 2 hours or according to facility policy
    2. According to the HCP's written orders
    3. After auscultation of lungs and noting moisture in the tube
    4. When the neonate begins to secrete and cough up mucus

49. In the acute phase of respiratory distress syndrome, which route of feeding is **most** likely to be used for the neonate?
    1. Bottle-feeding
    2. Breastfeeding
    3. Parenteral nutrition
    4. Gavage feeding

50. The nurse is reinforcing the instructions to treat the child's viral pharyngitis with lozenges, gargles, and acetaminophen. The mother tells the nurse that she wants a prescription for antibiotics. What is the **best** response?
    1. "The HCP didn't order any antibiotics."
    2. "Viral pharyngitis is always treated conservatively."
    3. "Let me call the HCP so that you can talk to him."
    4. "The throat culture showed no evidence of bacterial infection."

51. Which two conditions can develop if streptococcal infections are inadequately treated?
    1. Hydrocephalus and nephrotic syndrome
    2. Rheumatic fever and acute glomerulonephritis
    3. Iron deficiency anemia and gastroenteritis
    4. Bronchopulmonary dysplasia and pneumonia

52. The nurse is caring for a child who had a tonsillectomy. Which report from the unlicensed assistive personnel (UAP) is the **greatest** concern?
    1. "I put the bed flat, because he wanted to go to sleep."
    2. "His pulse is 140 bpm, and earlier in the shift it was 90 bpm."
    3. "I gave him a cup of red soda, because that's what he wanted."
    4. "He got out of bed and has been running up and down the hall."

53. The nurse is assisting an inexperienced HCP to examine a child who appears acutely ill with high fever, muffled voice, drooling, and progressive respiratory distress. The nurse would intervene if the HCP started to perform which action?
    1. Suggests that the mother hold the child on her lap
    2. Calls the operating room to alert them about the child
    3. Examines the back of the throat using a tongue blade
    4. Takes a history of preceding upper respiratory infection

54. The child presents with a nonproductive, hacking cough that worsens at night. The HCP makes the diagnosis of bronchitis. Which instruction will the nurse give to the parent?
    1. "Complete all antibiotics as prescribed."
    2. "Cough suppressants will cause drowsiness."
    3. "Use a cool-mist humidifier to relieve cough."
    4. "Withhold fluids at night to decrease secretions."

55. The nurse is working on the pediatric unit and five patients have bronchiolitis caused by respiratory syncytial virus. What infection-control measure would be considered in making care assignments?
    1. Health care personnel with minor infections should not be assigned to these patients.
    2. Each patient is placed in a negative pressure room and care is more time-consuming.
    3. All of these patients should be placed in the same room with one nurse to give care.
    4. Nurses who care for these patients should not be assigned to other high-risk patients.

56. For patients with cystic fibrosis, which body system is targeted to prevent the **most** likely complications?
    1. Cardiac
    2. Renal
    3. Gastrointestinal
    4. Respiratory

57. Immediately following cleft palate surgery, the infant is to receive nothing by mouth. After the nurse determines that the effects of the anesthesia have disappeared, which fluid would be fed to the infant **first**?
    1. Breast milk
    2. Regular formula
    3. Dextrose water
    4. Normal saline

58. For the child experiencing gastroenteritis with diarrhea, which treatment does the nurse anticipate?
    1. Nothing by mouth
    2. Oral rehydration
    3. No solid foods for 48 hours
    4. Traditional BRAT diet

59. There are several different types of hernias that children may experience. Which type of hernia usually has spontaneous closure by the time the child is 2 years old?
    1. Hiatal
    2. Inguinal
    3. Umbilical
    4. Diaphragmatic

60. Within hours of delivery, the neonate is diagnosed with the most severe type of hernia that requires immediate surgical repair. What signs/symptoms is the nurse **most** likely to observe with this condition?
    1. Regurgitation after eating
    2. No bowel movements
    3. Outpouching around umbilicus
    4. Difficulty breathing

61. Which pharmacologic treatment does the nurse anticipate for a child who has gastroesophageal reflux?
    1. Prochlorperazine
    2. Calcium chloride
    3. Cimetidine
    4. Fosphenytoin

62. The nurse is caring for an 8-year-old child who has severe diarrhea. IV fluid with potassium is prescribed by the HCP and prepared by the pharmacy. Before the nurse hangs the IV solution, which function must be verified?
    1. Auscultate the lungs for the presence of crackles or wheezes.
    2. Check the urine output to ensure that output is at least 30 mL/hour.
    3. Auscultate for bowel sounds to determine presence of peristalsis.
    4. Check blood sugar for evidence of hypoglycemia.

63. A mother brings the 6-year-old child to the clinic for constipation. The mother reports that the child eats what the family eats, takes no medication, has no known health problems, and is active. Which questions will the nurse ask the child? **Select all that apply.**
    1. "What does it feel like when you try to go to the bathroom?"
    2. "When you feel like you have to go, do you go right away or wait?"
    3. "Do you take time to use the bathroom when you are at school?"
    4. "What do you think is making you so constipated?"
    5. "Would you like to eat more fruit, or would you rather take medicine?"

64. The nurse is caring for a child who had hydrostatic reduction for intussusception. Which outcome statement indicates that the goal of the therapy was met?
    1. "Barium enema procedure was well-tolerated."
    2. "Parents understand the criteria for surgery if needed."
    3. "Bowel sounds are present; passing stool with barium."
    4. "Nasogastric tube is patent and suction is maintained."

65. Which treatment does the nurse anticipate for the child with nephrotic syndrome?
    1. Frequent ambulation
    2. Increased sodium
    3. Decreased protein
    4. Adrenocortical steroids

66. An infant is diagnosed with hypothyroidism. Which teaching point would be reinforced?
    1. Prompt treatment is needed to avoid permanent cognitive impairment.
    2. A delay in treatment could result in damage to the heart and great vessels.
    3. Noncompliance with therapy will result in unusually short stature.
    4. Hypothyroidism will contribute to psychological disorders if untreated.

67. The nurse recognizes that hyperthyroidism is **most** common in which age group?
    1. Neonates
    2. Toddlers
    3. Preschoolers
    4. Adolescents

68. For a child with talipes equinovarus, which care is the nurse **most** likely to provide?
    1. Frequent assessment of breath sounds
    2. Assess for pain and administer medication
    3. Ensure that traction is maintained
    4. Teach parents about cast care

69. A 1-year-old child has a spiral fracture of the right forearm. The x-ray shows an old, healed spiral fracture in the same arm. Using knowledge of musculoskeletal development and fracture pathology, which situation is the nurse prepared to deal with?
    1. Parents will be devastated by possible diagnosis of bone cancer.
    2. Parents must be questioned about possible physical abuse.
    3. Parents must be counseled about possible genetic bone disorder.
    4. Parents need teaching about safety issues related to the child's age.

70. Which intervention is **most** important for the nurse to implement in the care of a child with varicella?
    1. Initiate airborne and contact precautions.
    2. Use cool-mist humidifier for cough.
    3. Monitor cardiac and respiratory status.
    4. Initiate bleeding precautions.

71. Which clinical manifestations would the nurse observe in a school-age child with scoliosis? **Select all that apply.**
    1. Unequal hip and shoulder height
    2. Scapular and rib prominence
    3. Protrusion of the spine in the lumbar region
    4. Posterior rib hump that is visible when bending forward
    5. Taller than expected for age group

72. For a child with strabismus, which condition can develop if the strabismus is not treated?
    1. Myopia
    2. Hyperopia
    3. Presbyopia
    4. Amblyopia

73. After hearing in report that the child has a history of unpredictable sudden-onset status epilepticus, the nurse is **most** likely to check the availability of which medication and obtain a standing as-needed (PRN) prescription?
    1. Valproic acid
    2. Phenytoin
    3. Lorazepam
    4. Carbamazepine

74. Which interventions would the nurse use during a child's seizure? **Select all that apply.**
    1. Ask charge nurse to immediately call the HCP.
    2. Move the child to the bed when the seizure begins.
    3. Loosen restrictive clothing.
    4. Turn the child's head to the side.
    5. Push a tongue blade between the teeth.
    6. Stay with the child throughout the seizure.

75. Which assessment is the **most** important for the early detection of hydrocephalus?
    1. Weigh the infant at every visit and compare to the previous weights.
    2. Routinely measure head circumference and compare for rapid changes.
    3. Check the infant's pupillary response and accommodation.
    4. Ask parents about subtle changes in mental status or behavior.

76. The mother is quite frustrated because the child has attention-deficit/hyperactivity disorder, and it is taking several hours each night to help the child finish his homework. What is the **best** recommendation to give to the mother?
    1. Use a large variety of brightly colored shapes to hold the child's attention.
    2. Create an interactive approach that stimulates all of the senses.
    3. Have the child run and do very active play to tire him out before studying.
    4. Create a calm and quiet space with limited objects and fewer distractions.

77. Which medication is **most** likely to be prescribed for a child who has depression?
    1. Fluoxetine
    2. Methylphenidate
    3. Diphenhydramine
    4. Dextroamphetamine

78. The nurse hears in report that the child with Down syndrome has atlantoaxial instability. Which assessment finding would the nurse watch for and immediately report to the HCP?
    1. Persistent neck pain
    2. Persistent constipation
    3. Protruding tongue
    4. Drooling saliva

79. How can the nurse assist and support the parents if the child is experiencing school avoidance?
    1. Reassure parents that the behavior is normal and related to stress.
    2. Tell the parents to allow the child to stay home if he is too stressed.
    3. Tell the child that no one will pressure him if he doesn't want to go.
    4. Suggest getting the homework assignments when he misses school.

80. What are appropriate interventions for a child with autism? **Select all that apply.**
    1. Bring favorite possessions during hospitalization.
    2. Give written material about treatment options for cure.
    3. Vary routine and schedule from day to day.
    4. Provide brief, concrete communication with the child.
    5. Promote increased auditory and visual stimulation.
    6. Use gentle touch to get the child's attention.

CRITICAL THINKING ACTIVITIES

81. For bronchial asthma, identify the following.

    a. Signs and symptoms: _____

    _____

    b. Diagnostic tests: _____

    _____

    c. Medical treatment:_____

    _____

    d. Nursing interventions: _____

    _____

82. For lead poisoning, identify the following.

    a. Sources of lead:_____

    _____

    b. Prevention: _____

    _____

    c. Parent guidelines to reduce lead levels: _____

    _____

83. The school nurse is talking to a 15-year-old girl. The girl tells the nurse that one of the teachers accused her of using drugs because she thought "I was acting weird." The nurse asks her to describe the "weird behavior" and the girl talks about being withdrawn, with less interest in schoolwork, school activities, or socializing with her friends. Further assessment reveals that the girl often feels sad, down, and empty and has fantasized about committing suicide.

    a. Which questions would the nurse ask? _____

    _____

    _____

b. How would the nurse determine whether to contact others, such as parents, HCP, or school administrators?

_____

_____

_____

NEXT-GENERATION NCLEX™ (NGN)

84. Matrix

Cognitive Skill: Analyze Cues

Scenario: A 19-year-old Native American woman brings her 3-month-old son to the clinic for a check-up. The infant was premature, had low birth weight, and experienced respiratory dysfunction at birth. For financial reasons, the mother did not have adequate prenatal care. The health care team identifies that the infant has several risk factors for sudden infant death syndrome (SIDS). The RN and LPN/LVN collaborate to teach the mother actions that would help prevent SIDS.

Instructions: Use an X to indicate which actions are essential, nonessential, or contraindicated. All should be used and can be used only once.

Action	Essential	Nonessential	Contraindicated
Remove stuffed animals, towels, and quilts from the crib.			
Place the infant on his abdomen at night and turn his head to the side.			
Monitor the infant when he is awake for irregular respirations.			
Continue breastfeeding the infant.			
Firmly attach soft bedding material to pad the side rails of the crib.			
Dress infant in lightweight clothing; maintain comfortable room temperature.			
Ensure adequate space if the infant shares a bed with parents or siblings.			
Advise smoking cessation for parents and others who live in the infant's household.			

Health Promotion and Care of the Older Adult

Answer Key: A complete Answer Key is provided in your Additional Learning Resources on Evolve.

TABLE ACTIVITY

1. *Directions:* Fill in the blank boxes to complete the table for comparison of characteristics associated with delirium, dementia, and depression.

	Delirium	**Dementia**	**Depression**
Onset	Sudden		
Cognitive impairment		Minimal cognitive impairment initially; progresses to impaired abstract thinking, judgment, memory, thought patterns, calculations, agnosia	
Activity	Increased or decreased; may fluctuate		
Speech and language		Disordered, rambling, or incoherent; struggles to find words	
Reversibility			Can be treated

CLINICAL APPLICATION OF MATH AND CONVERSIONS

Directions: Calculate or make the necessary conversions for math problems encountered in caring for older adults.

2. The nurse is performing a physical examination on an 83-year-old resident. On admission to the long-term care unit, the resident weighed 106 lbs. The current weight is 110 lbs. How much weight has the resident gained in kilograms? _____ kg

3. The patient, age 80 years, weighs 130 lbs (59 kg). To maintain this weight, the patient needs to take in approximately 30 calories per kilogram of body weight per day. How many calories per day should the patient consume? _____ calories

4. An older woman weighed 120 lbs (54 kg) in January. In June, the patient weighs 108 lbs (49 kg). The patient denies any intentional efforts to lose weight. What percent of the total body weight was lost in 6 months? _____ %

   What should the nurse do? _____

5. The patient's fluid intake is shown below. What is the total fluid intake in mL? _____ mL

   What should the nurse do? _____

Time	Amount
700	6 oz of low-fat milk, 6 oz of coffee
1000	8 oz of water
1200	250 mL of water
1400	4 oz of water
1700	250 mL of iced tea
1900	3 oz of juice

6. The nurse is monitoring the patient's urinary output because the patient is on several medications that can be affected by changes in renal excretion. If the patient voids 500 mL over a period of 8 hours, how many mL is the patient producing per hour? _____ mL

MULTIPLE CHOICE

Directions: Select the best answer(s) for each of the following questions.

7. Which assessment finding of the integumentary system is the **most** important to report to the health care provider (HCP) or dermatologist?
   1. Tan or brown macule spots
   2. Thick, brittle, yellowed nails
   3. Thin skin with purple patches
   4. Irregular, raised, crusted lesion

8. The nurse determines that a resident is fatigued today, so a partial bath would be acceptable in place of a full bath. Regarding the partial bath, which instructions will the nurse give to the unlicensed assistive personnel (UAP)?
   1. "Assist the patient to wash the perineal area and then the hands."
   2. "Help the resident wash his face, hands, armpits, and perineal area."
   3. "Before breakfast, help the resident wash his hands and face."
   4. "Perform a partial bath on the patient, just for today."

9. The nurse sees that patient is taking a diuretic medication. Which laboratory result is the nurse **most** likely to monitor?
   1. Serum potassium
   2. Urinalysis results
   3. Blood glucose
   4. Serum calcium

10. The nurse is **most** likely to question the prescription for an enteral feeding tube for which patient?
    1. 68-year-old patient who was in an auto accident
    2. 73-year-old patient who has advanced dementia
    3. 65-year-old patient who sustained severe burns
    4. 70-year-old patient who had surgery for lip cancer

11. The UAP tells the nurse that for the past 3 days, a thin brown liquid has been oozing from the resident's rectal area, but there is no formed stool. What would the nurse do **first**?
    1. Tell the UAP to assist the resident to the bathroom every 2 hours.
    2. Instruct the UAP to continue to change the incontinence pants as needed.
    3. Check the resident for a fecal impaction and assess the surrounding skin.
    4. Obtain an order for a stool hemoccult and culture and sensitivity.

12. The patient retired years ago. He was very involved with community, family, and friends, but now appears content to spend more time alone and others support his privacy. Which theory of aging **most** directly explains his behavior?
    1. Disengagement theory
    2. Exchange theory
    3. Continuity theory
    4. Activity theory

13. Which nurse is **most** likely to need an extensive knowledge and understanding of the Patient Self-Determination Act?
    1. Nurse A helps patients and families understand Medicare benefits.
    2. Nurse B cares for patients and families during end of life.
    3. Nurse C works at an outpatient surgical and diagnostic center.
    4. Nurse D counsels older people at a community senior citizen center.

14. The patient has a history of peripheral vascular disease. Which symptom is the cause for **greatest** concern?
    1. Gradual and progressive edema going up both legs
    2. Excessive warmth of the leg on the dominant side
    3. Sudden onset of a cold foot on the non-dominant side
    4. Cramping of the calf muscles after exertion

15. The patient is recovering from a stroke, but some residual symptoms continue. Which statement by a nursing student demonstrates an understanding that precautions need to be taken during meals?
    1. "The aphasia improves as the condition improves."
    2. "Dysphagia creates a risk for developing pneumonia."
    3. "Presbyopia will improve with corrective devices."
    4. "Appropriate exercises will counteract akinesia."

16. The patient reports that nocturia usually occurs once each night, but recently the urge has increased to 4-5 times. What would the nurse suggest as the **first** measure?
    1. Observe for fall hazards in the environment.
    2. Take diuretic medication in the morning.
    3. Contact the HCP for medical evaluation.
    4. Limit fluids and semisolid foods at bedtime.

17. The UAP is assigned to assist an older adult who is experiencing pruritus with bathing and hygiene. The nurse would intervene if the UAP performs which action?
    1. Uses tepid water for washing and rinsing the body.
    2. Uses an antibacterial soap to reduce potential for infection.
    3. Gives a partial bath of face, hands, axillary, and perineal areas.
    4. Applies a water-based lotion with gentle, even strokes.

18. For the older adult patient with dysphagia, which intervention is appropriate to use during mealtimes?
    1. Add thickeners to liquids.
    2. Feed the patient quickly to reduce fatigue.
    3. Place the patient in low-Fowler's position.
    4. Provide opportunities for socialization while eating.

19. The patient is taking alendronate. Based on knowledge of this medication, which intervention will the nurse use when caring for the patient?
    1. Handle gently when assisting to move or change position.
    2. Encourage pursed-lip breathing to control breathlessness.
    3. Frequently note the rate, regularity, and strength of the pulse.
    4. Teach the patient how to perform Kegel exercises.

20. For a patient who has kyphosis, which symptom is cause for the **greatest** concern?
    1. Heartburn sensation after eating large meal
    2. Weak stream when urinating
    3. Swelling of ankles with prolonged sitting
    4. Difficulty coughing up secretions

21. The nurse is giving a health promotion presentation to a community group of older people. What would be included as primary prevention strategies? **Select all that apply.**
    1. Quit smoking to reduce the risk of heart disease.
    2. Eat a well-balanced diet without excess sugar, fat, or alcohol.
    3. Receive the recommended vaccinations.
    4. Take prescribed medications according to instructions.
    5. Do 20-30 minutes of moderate exercise three to five times a week.

22. Which statement by a senior citizen **best** indicates an understanding of the "donut hole" in the Medicaid prescription plan?
    1. "My dental bills are covered if my dentist prescribes any medication."
    2. "I don't have any money to pay for extra nongeneric medications."
    3. "A percentage of the cost of medications is paid to a certain amount."
    4. "The Affordable Care Act is going to take care of all my medical expenses."

23. The nurse is talking to the daughter of a patient who has dementia. Which comment by the daughter **most** strongly indicates problems related to the caregiver role?
    1. "Would you think I was a horrible person if I asked about respite care?"
    2. "Dealing with Dad is pretty exhausting, but I try to focus on happier times."
    3. "Well, I had to decrease my hours at work, but they do let me telecommute."
    4. "My sister says that I am too impatient with Dad, but she doesn't offer to help."

24. The patient reports feelings of grief related to multiple losses and recent death of her spouse. She appears sad and withdrawn. What is the **best** intervention to help this patient deal with grief and loss?
    1. Role-model cheerful and optimistic behavior.
    2. Encourage alone time and introspection.
    3. Help to set realistic short-term goals.
    4. Suggest temporarily moving in with an adult child.

25. The nurse is caring for a very thin patient who is bedridden. Which intervention is the **best** method to prevent damage to the skin at pressure points?
    1. Gently massage fragile skin with water-based lotion.
    2. Reposition the patient at least every 2 hours.
    3. Use a mechanical lifting device to prevent shearing forces.
    4. Place pressure-reducing pads and aids over bony prominences.

26. The nursing student is caring for a patient with fragile skin. The nurse would intervene if the student performed which actions? **Select all that apply.**
    1. Asks the patient to grab side rail and slide across the bed to change wet linens
    2. Secures the patient's IV with several pieces of tape to prevent dislodgement
    3. Washes dried fecal material from rectal area and rubs to dry moisture
    4. Asks for lifting help when trying to move patient from bed to stretcher
    5. Firmly grasps the patient on the forearm when moving from bed to chair

27. The nurse hears during handover report that the patient has a diminished gag reflex. Which morning assessment would be particularly important?
    1. Checking other reflexes
    2. Auscultating lung fields
    3. Assessing for pain in the neck area
    4. Assessing nutritional status

28. The nurse is encouraging the older adult to reduce calories and consume quality foods. Which breakfast choice is the **best** to supply vitamins, minerals, and fiber?
    1. Biscuits and gravy with coffee and artificial sweetener
    2. Orange juice and a low-fat banana-nut muffin
    3. Bacon with white toast and skim milk
    4. Oatmeal with fresh berries and hot tea

29. The patient reports controlling incontinence by limiting fluid intake. To encourage the patient to meet the minimum daily intake of 1500 mL of fluid, which intervention would be the **most** helpful?
    1. Suggest the use of an adapted cup with a double handle.
    2. Propose voiding every 2 hours during the day and every 4 hours at night.
    3. Divide the 1500 mL of fluid into portions to be taken during waking hours.
    4. Emphasize the importance of adequate fluid for body function.

30. The patient reports sensation of abdominal distention and early satiety. Based on knowledge of how aging affects gastric motility, which intervention would the nurse suggest?
    1. Walking for short distances several times a day
    2. Cooking food with a variety of different seasonings
    3. Preparing homemade frozen dinners with extra portions
    4. Performing oral hygiene to remove offensive tastes and odors

31. Which patient statement is **most** relevant to the medical diagnosis of gastric reflux?
    1. "I have never really liked the taste of milk."
    2. "I have gained a lot of weight within the last year."
    3. "Lately, my stool seems to be a very dark brown color."
    4. "Recently, I noticed a sore in mouth that won't heal."

32. The patient requests a laxative because "I feel constipated." What would the nurse do **first**?
    1. Find out when the last laxative was administered.
    2. Assist the patient to the bathroom and observe afterward.
    3. Ask the patient to describe the typical bowel pattern.
    4. Offer a high-fiber snack of prune juice and bran muffin.

33. The nurse is teaching the patient about self-care measures for modifiable cardiac risk factors. Which teaching points would be included? **Select all that apply.**
    1. Take blood pressure medications as prescribed.
    2. Decrease intake of complex carbohydrates and vegetable proteins.
    3. Perform moderate exercise 30 min/day at least twice a week.
    4. Aim for body mass index of 18.5-24.9 kg/m².
    5. Get adequate sleep and rest.
    6. Avoid exposure to secondhand smoke.

34. The patient with chronic obstructive pulmonary disease (COPD) states, "I can't cough up this phlegm in the back of my throat." Which intervention is the **best** to address this problem?
    1. Teach purse-lipped breathing.
    2. Promote moderate exercise 3-5 days/week.
    3. Use oxygen therapy as prescribed.
    4. Encourage plenty of fluids to liquefy secretions.

35. A normally cheerful and alert resident in a long-term facility demonstrates lethargy, disorientation, and her skin is very warm. Which action would the nurse take **first**?
    1. Allow the patient to rest for several hours and then reassess mental status.
    2. Increase lighting, give sips of fluid, and control ambient room temperature.
    3. Check vital signs, blood glucose, and pulse oximeter reading.
    4. Use reality orientation and give simple, brief commands.

36. The nurse walks into a room and finds the patient on the floor. The patient reports severe pain in the hip area and the affected leg appears shorter than the other side. What would the nurse do **first**?
    1. Assist the patient back into bed.
    2. Assess for other injuries.
    3. Immobilize the affected side.
    4. Report the findings to the HCP.

37. The nurse is interviewing a 56-year-old woman who reports that over the past year she has had frequent minor infections, minor wounds that seem slow to heal, blurred vision, and weight gain. Which laboratory finding is **most** likely to be observed?
    1. Elevated thyroid-stimulating hormone level
    2. Elevated blood glucose level
    3. Elevated estrogen level
    4. Elevated serum cholesterol level

38. The nurse notes that the patient's total cholesterol level is elevated. Which dietary information is the **most** relevant to this laboratory finding?
    1. Elevation of cholesterol is not related to current diet.
    2. Consumption of fluid and fiber should be increased.
    3. Amount of saturated fat in diet should be decreased.
    4. Reduce caloric intake to achieve a body mass index of 18.5-24.9 kg/m².

39. Patient reports "running out of my levothyroxine several weeks ago." Which sign/symptom would the nurse expect because the patient has not been taking the medication?
    1. Apathy
    2. Heat intolerance
    3. Diarrhea
    4. Weight loss

40. A newly graduated nurse, age 22, is starting an interview with a 68-year-old patient who presents himself as very proper and conservative. The nurse feels that she will have trouble asking questions related to sexuality. What is the **best** strategy for this situation?
    1. Get another nurse to complete the interview.
    2. Have the patient wait and quickly assess own discomfort.
    3. Ask the patient for permission to initiate the discussion about sex.
    4. Defer the questions until after rapport is established.

41. The nurse is making a home visit and notices that the patient is squinting while reading the newspaper. There is no eye chart available to test the patient's vision. What would the nurse do **first**?
    1. Ask the patient to read the newspaper out loud.
    2. Suggest an appointment with an eye doctor.
    3. Assess the eyes for yellowing of the lens.
    4. Use a small flashlight to check pupil reaction.

42. Which symptom is an **early** sign of primary open-angle glaucoma?
    1. Severe eye pain
    2. Rainbow halo surrounding lights
    3. Pupil dilation
    4. Deteriorating peripheral vision

43. The patient watches the speaker's lips and tilts head towards the person who is speaking. Which position would the nurse assume when interviewing the patient?
    1. Stand near the window, so that there is bright light behind the nurse.
    2. Sit at the patient's eye level and directly face the patient.
    3. Sit beside the patient with mouth at the level of best ear.
    4. Stand over the patient, but lean into eye level when speaking.

44. The nurse works in a long-term care facility and is concerned about the quality of care. Which concern would be supported by the Omnibus Budget Reconciliation Act of 1987?
    1. A resident cannot file a complaint because there is no assigned ombudsman.
    2. A resident's chronic health condition was never assessed or documented.
    3. A resident is treated disrespectfully and there are no consequences for the offender.
    4. A resident dies and the room is immediately assigned to a new resident.

45. A patient has Parkinson's disease. Which long-term outcome is considered the **most** important?
    1. Adapting to long-term memory loss through reminiscence
    2. Maintaining mobility through exercise and activity
    3. Decreasing confusion by using reality orientation
    4. Managing pain with pharmacologic and nonpharmacologic intervention

46. The patient is slowly recovering from a cerebrovascular accident, but hemianopia has not resolved. Which reminder will the nurse give during mealtimes?
    1. Sit upright before attempting to eat and swallow.
    2. Ask for help if having trouble with utensils or opening wrapped items.
    3. Move head to the right and left when looking at the food tray.
    4. Minimize distractions and focus on chewing and swallowing.

47. Which factors contribute to polypharmacy where the risk for the patient outweighs the benefits? **Select all that apply.**
    1. Takes five or more prescription medications
    2. Sometimes borrows medication
    3. Uses a pill box with pockets for each day of the week
    4. Uses over-the-counter medications including vitamins and herbal preparations
    5. Sees primary HCP on a regular basis
    6. Fills prescriptions at local pharmacies and through the mail

48. The nurse is discharging an older woman to return home where her daughter is the primary caregiver. Which patient response is **most** likely to prompt the nurse to gather more information about possible elder abuse?
    1. "My daughter leaves me alone when she goes to work."
    2. "You are nice. Would you come and visit me sometime?"
    3. "Could I have a lunch tray before I go home?"
    4. "When you are old, family can do whatever they want with you."

49. The patient had minor surgery 8 hours ago. He refuses to walk to the bathroom. "I'm old and I just had surgery. You should bring me the urinal. That's what you get paid for." What is the **best** response?
    1. "I'll bring you the urinal, but you have to promise to get up soon."
    2. "Actually, I get paid to make sure that you recover from your surgery."
    3. "Getting up helps prevent constipation, pneumonia, and blood clots."
    4. "Sir, your HCP has ordered that you get up and walk around."

50. Which nursing action helps meet goals for older adults according to *Healthy People 2030*?
    1. Checks the patient's blood pressure every 4 hours while in the hospital
    2. Reminds patients that testing stool for occult blood should be done monthly
    3. Teaches fall prevention tips to community-dwelling older adults
    4. Reports onset of new symptoms promptly to the HCP

51. The resident in a long-term care facility has lost 2 pounds within a month and shows a lack of interest in eating. Which interventions would the nurse use? **Select all that apply.**
    1. Assess reasons for loss of interest
    2. Monitor daily intake
    3. Determine food preferences
    4. Instruct UAP to feed patient
    5. Give liquid protein shakes
    6. Ask UAP to assist with oral hygiene before meals

52. A patient reports blood in the stool and expresses fears about having colon cancer. Which question will the nurse ask **first**?
    1. "Can you give me a stool sample for testing?"
    2. "What makes you think you have cancer?"
    3. "Did anyone in your family ever have bowel cancer?"
    4. "What other changes or symptoms have you noticed?"

53. Which patient is **most** likely to benefit from practicing Kegel exercises every day?
    1. A bedridden patient is incontinent of small amounts of liquid stool
    2. An older woman passes small amounts of urine with coughing or sneezing
    3. A patient with severe arthritis passes urine before he can unfasten his pants.
    4. A woman who is postmenstrual reports has pain during intercourse.

54. The patient says he is fine now, but he reports an episode that lasted about 20 minutes with blurred vision, headache, disorientation, impaired coordination and he fell but did not lose consciousness. The patient should have follow-up care because he has risk for which complication?
    1. Stroke within 5 years
    2. Accidental fall within 1 year
    3. Early onset Alzheimer's disease
    4. Insidious onset of Parkinson's disease

55. Which older patient's comment reflects expected changes in memory that occur with aging?
    1. "I know that aide who helped me bathe, but I don't recognize you."
    2. "I can't remember what my eldest daughter looks like."
    3. "Have you seen my reading glasses? I am always misplacing them."
    4. "The weather is so cold today, what month is this? "

56. For a patient who has a sudden change in mental status, which laboratory values would the nurse check and report to the HCP? **Select all that apply.**
    1. Cholesterol levels
    2. Electrolyte levels
    3. Liver function tests
    4. Thyroid function tests
    5. Hemoglobin A1C (HbA1c)

CRITICAL THINKING ACTIVITIES

57. For the following systems, describe the nursing assessment of the older adult.

    a. Integumentary: _____

    _____

    b. Cardiovascular: _____

    _____

    c. Respiratory: _____

    _____

    d. Gastrointestinal: _____

    _____

    e. Urinary: _____

    _____

f. Musculoskeletal: _____

_____

g. Neurologic: _____

_____

h. Vision and hearing: _____

_____

58. The nurse is caring for a 78-year-old woman who comes to the clinic with reports of "problems with my stomach and bowels."

a. What questions would the nurse use to obtain data about the patient's concerns? _____

_____

_____

_____

_____

b. The HCP examines the patient and informs the nurse that the patient is likely having gastric reflux and constipation. What nursing interventions may be implemented for the older adult who is experiencing gastric reflux and constipation?

_____

_____

_____

_____

59. At the beginning of her new job, the nurse is open to any suggestions from others and tries to get along with everyone. As time goes by, she feels comfortable and likes working with a group of younger nurses. There are several older staff members who are nice, but working with them is less stimulating and interesting. In fact, she finds the older staff members to be rigid in their outlook and slow to complete assigned tasks. When the nurse is assigned to precept an older nursing student, she hesitates, because her impression of older people is that they don't make the best nurses.

a. Do you think that this nurse is guilty of ageism? Why or why not? _____

_____

_____

b. How could the nurse create a better situation for herself and others? _____

_____

_____

_____

60. The nurse is making a home visit to a 75-year-old woman who lives with her 80-year-old husband. Both the wife and husband are alert and oriented. Both are taking medication to treat hypertension. The wife has recently returned from a rehabilitation center following a hip fracture that she sustained in a fall. The nurse notes that the home is overfilled with a collection of items. Many of the rooms in the house tend to be poorly lighted. The house has an upstairs and downstairs bathroom. Identify the factors that are fall risks and make suggestions about how this older couple can prevent future falls.

_____

_____

_____

_____

_____

_____

_____

NEXT-GENERATION NCLEX™ (NGN)

61. Cloze

Cognitive Skill: Analyze Cues

Scenario: The home health nurse is doing a follow-up visit with an older patient who is being treated for a urinary tract infection (UTI). The patient also takes several medications for chronic health conditions. One of the goals for the visit is to review teaching points related to the medications.

Instructions: Choose the most likely options to complete the statement below.

For the UTI and the antibiotic medication, the nurse would remind the patient the importance of ___1___. The patient takes an oral hypoglycemic agent for type 2 diabetes. For this type of medication, the most important side effects that the patient must watch for are ___2___. Because the patient takes an oral anticoagulant medication, the nurse cautions the patient to watch for and report ___3___.

Options for 1	Options for 2	Options for 3
avoiding alcohol	bradycardia, angina, hypotension	yeast infection
taking the medication 1 hour after meals	weakness, headache, malaise	depression
increasing fiber to reduce constipation	nausea, vomiting, gastrointestinal (GI) bleeding	hearing loss
drinking plenty of fluids	depression, vertigo, lethargy	diarrhea
reporting tremor or spasms	hallucinations, agitation, disorientation	bleeding

Concepts of Mental Health

chapter

34

Answer Key: A complete Answer Key is provided in your Additional Learning Resources on Evolve.

MULTIPLE CHOICE

Directions: Select the best answer(s) for each of the following questions.

1. Which person is acting according to an ascribed role?
   1. Nurse arrives at work 15 minutes before the start of the shift.
   2. Patient with cancer listens as oncologist describes treatment options.
   3. Police officer brings a confused person to the hospital for evaluation.
   4. Child chooses to take dance lessons rather than doing team sports.

2. Which physical signs/symptoms are associated with higher levels of anxiety? **Select all that apply.**
   1. Rapid speech and vocal changes
   2. Increased pulse and respiration
   3. Decreased level of consciousness
   4. Tremors and restlessness
   5. Nausea and occasional vomiting
   6. Diarrhea and frequent urination

3. The nursing student feels overwhelmed by study, working part-time, and neglecting relationships. What is the **best** intervention that the nursing instructor could use to decrease the level of the student's anxiety?
   1. Allow him to skip a clinical experience.
   2. Ask about his work-study schedule.
   3. Talk about importance of his relationships.
   4. Help him prioritize responsibilities.

4. Which patient is demonstrating the **strongest** motivation to participate in the plan of care?
   1. Patient asks the nurse to show his wife how to change and manage his colostomy bag.
   2. Patient does leg exercises because he wants to dance at his 50th wedding anniversary.
   3. Patient does a return demonstration of finger exercises for the occupational therapist.
   4. Patient tells the nurse he must leave the hospital because his dog is alone at the house.

5. Which person is demonstrating the **most** maladaptive behavior?
   1. Nursing student who does poorly on tests places emphasis on skills performance.
   2. Woman is a poor driver and explains that other drivers are too impatient.
   3. Man says his drinking, followed by the occasional sick day, are no big deal.
   4. College student admires her roommate and starts dressing and acting like her.

6. The nurse is assessing a patient's use of defense mechanisms. He reports having a bad day at work and going home and shouting at the children. Which defense mechanism is he displaying?
   1. Projection
   2. Displacement
   3. Identification
   4. Reaction formation

7. Which person is demonstrating regressive behavior?
   1. Victim of sexual abuse laughs while talking about the incident.
   2. Aggressive adolescent participates in numerous competitive sports.
   3. An 80-year-old acts as if an incident of incontinence did not occur.
   4. An 8-year-old sucks his thumb when hospitalized for the first time.

8. An adolescent female patient tells the nurse that she often feels very "uneasy," but can't identify any specific reasons for this feeling. What is this patient experiencing?
   1. Stress
   2. Anxiety
   3. Crisis
   4. Mental illness

9. Based on factors that possibly affect mental health, which adolescent is **most** likely to have the **best** mental health later in life?
   1. Participates in several school activities and has reasonably good grades
   2. Competitive in sports and displays ongoing rivalry with older brother
   3. Has a successful father, but mother died shortly after adolescent was born
   4. Has exceptional academic record and parents expect superior performance in all areas

10. A nurse is talking to people who are in a substance abuse support group. Which statement is evidence of the **best** level of mental health?
    1. "I don't have any problems with drinking anymore."
    2. "I just try to avoid drinking, one day at a time."
    3. "As long as my wife doesn't drink, then I won't drink either."
    4. "I have had a really hard time in life and I don't like being judged."

11. What is the **best** rationale for all nurses to study and be familiar with the concepts of basic mental health?
    1. Every nurse must study mental health concepts that are tested for licensure.
    2. Nurses need excellent mental health to help their patients.
    3. Nurses have daily contact with patients who are at risk for mental health problems.
    4. Younger nurses may lack personal experience in dealing with loss or mental illness.

12. Based on Freud's theory of personality development, the superego would cause the nurse to perform which action?
    1. Focus on own duties and ignore extraneous requests to perform additional tasks.
    2. Disagree with patient's decision to refuse treatment, but show respect and support.
    3. Minimize the importance of a medication error to facilitate patient care.
    4. Obtain the continuing education units required to maintain licensure.

13. The nurse suffered a terrible traumatic event during childhood, but now appears happy and satisfied with her life and career. According to Freud's theory on preconsciousness, which behavior is the nurse **most** likely to manifest?
    1. Is unable to recall any memory of the traumatic event.
    2. Frequently thinks about the event and experiences growth in reflection.
    3. Remembers the event, but generally represses the unpleasant aspects.
    4. Attempts to experience pleasure and avoids pain at all costs.

14. There is a fire in the facility and the nurse is attempting to instruct patients to go to a safe area. Which patient is **least** likely to be able to understand and appropriately respond to a simple command?
    1. Using a wheelchair to assist bedbound roommate to safe area
    2. Frantically searching through belongings to find her wedding ring
    3. Standing in the corner, crying, and clinging to the bedrail
    4. Walking towards safe area, but arguing about the need to leave

15. Which nursing student is **most** likely to experience stress during the final examination for a course?
    1. Has done well throughout the semester, but did not get much sleep the night before the exam
    2. Knows that the test is important, but believes that testing is just another hurdle to get over
    3. Is a smart student, has two children, works full-time, and spouse has chronic illness
    4. Has studied hard for final examination, but graduating is contingent on test results

16. A newly admitted patient appears upset. She says, "I'm going to wear my own clothes. I'm not going to answer any more questions and I'm not giving anyone any blood or pee or anything else!" How would the nurse respond?
    1. "You can wear your own nightgown if you would prefer."
    2. "Let me call your health care provider (HCP) so you can talk to her."
    3. "Coming into the hospital is really difficult. What can I do to help?"
    4. "Looks like you are having a bad time. I'll come back later."

17. An older home health patient is socially isolated but he is resistant to all suggestions related to social activities. Based on knowledge of how aging affects mental health, what would the home health nurse do **first**?
    1. Conclude that the resistance to socialization is an exaggeration of younger behavior.
    2. Assess for physical, financial, or relationship limitations that exist for the patient.
    3. Assist the patient to reminisce about happier times with friends and family.
    4. Locate and contact family members and suggest that they visit the patient.

18. An 8-year-old child complains of feeling sick on school days, although there is no fever, pain, change in behavior, or any other physical symptoms. Which question would the nurse ask to determine if the child is using the sick role as a coping strategy related to a problem at school?
    1. "Don't you like your school and your teachers anymore?"
    2. "Did something happen at school that made you feel uncomfortable?"
    3. "What will happen if you keep missing school all the time?"
    4. "What do you and your friends like to do during recess and lunch break?"

19. Which development related to the care and treatment of mental health patients was the **most** influential in the movement of deinstitutionalization in the United States?
    1. Provision of community-based services
    2. Availability of psychotherapeutic drugs
    3. Use of electroconvulsive therapy (ECT)
    4. Establishment of the National Institute of Mental Health

20. An older woman who lives in a long-term care facility seems to get sick whenever her son tries to take vacation time with his wife. He feels frustrated, but also guilty, so he never leaves. What would the nurse do **first**?
    1. Validate the son's feelings of frustration and guilt and offer emotional support.
    2. Reassure the mother that she will be well cared for while her son is gone.
    3. Suggest that the son take an overnight trip as a trial run for everyone.
    4. Tell the son that the mother is manifesting a secondary gain by being sick.

21. The HCP has just informed a woman that her husband, who is in a coma, is likely to die during the night. The woman is sitting at the husband's bedside and silently weeping. Which action would be the **most** therapeutic?
    1. Silently step outside and call other family members to come and support the wife.
    2. Ask the HCP for a prescription for an anti-anxiety medication for the wife.
    3. Make the patient as comfortable as possible and reassure the wife that he is pain-free.
    4. Quietly stand nearby and watch for the wife's receptiveness to touching or hugging.

22. A 70-year-old woman has chronic health problems. Her husband confides to the home health nurse that "Martha just doesn't seem to be herself; she seems so lackluster." Which data are included in the assessment of the wife's emotional state? **Select all that apply.**
    1. Appears disheveled; clothes are clean but mismatched
    2. Ambulates independently to the bathroom
    3. Answers questions correctly in monotone voice
    4. Sits slumped, gazes out the window during interview
    5. Maintains a quiet and subdued affect during interview
    6. Correctly relates recent and distant past events

CRITICAL THINKING ACTIVITIES

23. Based on the characteristics of a mentally healthy individual, select characteristics that currently apply to yourself and give an example of an action, behavior, or event that illustrates your good mental health.

    _____

    _____

    _____

    _____

24. Think about times in the past where you have witnessed (or personally experienced) various levels of anxiety. Briefly describe the behaviors that you observed (or feelings that you personally experienced) in each case.

    a. Mild anxiety:_____

    _____

    _____

    b. Moderate anxiety: _____

    _____

    _____

    c. Severe anxiety: _____

    _____

    _____

    d. Panic: _____

    _____

    _____

NEXT-GENERATION NCLEX™ (NGN)

25. Extended Drag and Drop

Cognitive Skill: Analyze Cues

Scenario: Everyone uses defense mechanisms to deal with problems and stressors of everyday life. Nurses must recognize when patients are overusing certain defense mechanisms or when they undermine acquisition of healthy behaviors. Nurses can also teach patients to recognize triggers that prompt the use of a defense mechanism.

Instructions: In the left column are some common defense mechanisms. Examples are listed in the right column. In the space provided, write in the letter of the defense mechanism that is represented. Each defense mechanism will be used only once.

Defense Mechanism	**Example**
a. Compensation	_____ 1. A teenager starts talking and dressing like the "popular girls" in her high school.
b. Conversion	_____ 2. A man has an argument with his daughter so he destroys the birthday card she sent to him.
c. Denial	_____ 3. A student who fails a test blames her study partner for goofing around and failing to contribute to achieving educational goals.
d. Displacement	_____ 4. A man frequently criticizes and berates his son, and his wife starts having seizures whenever the arguments begin.
e. Identification	_____ 5. An employee takes extra office supplies for personal use, saying, "Everybody takes supplies because we are so underpaid."
f. Projection	_____ 6. A nursing student who typically gets low scores on multiple choice tests focuses on creating comprehensive care plans.
g. Rationalization	_____ 7. A patient who is diagnosed with liver failure continues to overuse alcohol, he says, "because it's just a few drinks."

Care of the Patient With a Psychiatric Disorder

Answer Key: A complete Answer Key is provided in your Additional Learning Resources on Evolve.

MATCHING

Directions: Match the therapy to the correct description. Indicate your answers in the spaces provided.

Therapy

_____ 1. electroconvulsive therapy

_____ 2. behavior therapy

_____ 3. cognitive therapy

_____ 4. group therapy

_____ 5. play therapy

_____ 6. hypnosis

_____ 7. psychoanalysis

_____ 8. adjunctive therapies

Description of Therapy

a. Breaking negative thought patterns and developing positive feelings about memories

b. Using toys, such as a puppet, to be a "spokesperson" for feelings

c. Helps recover deeply repressed emotions

d. A small amount of electrical current is used to trigger a tonic-clonic seizure

e. Group of patients with similar problems gain insight through discussion

f. Includes occupational, recreational, music, magnetic, and art therapy, and hydrotherapy

g. Intense therapy that brings unconscious thoughts to the surface

h. Conditioning and retraining of behavioral responses by repetition

MULTIPLE CHOICE

Directions: Select the best answer(s) for each of the following questions.

9. The nursing students are preparing to enter a clinical rotation on an acute care psychiatric unit. Which types of disorders are the students **most** likely to observe during this clinical experience? **Select all that apply.**
   1. Major depression
   2. Schizophrenia
   3. Somatic illness
   4. Dementia
   5. Bipolar disorder
   6. Panic attack disorder

10. A Good Samaritan brings an unidentified, confused older woman who was found wandering. The woman is dressed in clean clothes, but is disoriented to self, place, and time. She cannot give appropriate answers to simple questions. Which assessments can the nurse perform to help the health care provider (HCP) differentiate dementia from delirium? **Select all that apply.**
    1. Use pulse oximeter and count respirations.
    2. Give simple directions and assess for response.
    3. Check blood pressure and assess peripheral pulses.
    4. Use glucometer to check blood glucose.
    5. Check temperature and assess for dehydration.

11. In a care plan for a patient with paranoid schizophrenia, a nursing student correctly includes "observe for signs of agitation and ensure safety." During the clinical day, when would the nursing instructor intervene?
    1. Student reports that patient tilts his head adopts a listening pose when there is no one around.
    2. Student observes that patient is pacing and muttering and helps other patients to move away.
    3. Student suggests to the patient that they go to his room and spend quiet time talking together.
    4. Student assists the medication nurse to administer medication and watches for pouching.

12. The nurse has a family member who is diagnosed with cyclothymic disorder. What is the **primary** reason that the nurse would encourage follow-up visits with the psychiatrist?
    1. Many patients with cyclothymic disorder progress to bipolar disorder.
    2. Cheerfulness will progress to poor judgment and provocative behavior.
    3. If untreated, delirium may lead to death from exhaustion.
    4. Cyclothymic disorder is prodromal to major depressive disorder.

13. Which educational brochure is the nurse **most** likely to prepare for a patient who has seasonal affective disorder?
    1. "SSRIs: A New Class of Antidepressant Medications"
    2. "How Phototherapy Helps Relieve Your Symptoms"
    3. "The Benefits and Risks of Hydrotherapy"
    4. "How to Make Selections for Your Music Therapy"

14. Which psychiatric disorder is **most** likely to manifest signs/symptoms similar to those of a myocardial infarction?
    1. Somatoform disorder
    2. Anorexia nervosa
    3. Schizophrenia
    4. Panic attack

15. In disaster planning and management, which intervention is recommended to prevent post-traumatic stress disorder?
    1. Initiating group therapy for survivors of trauma
    2. Reviewing pre-event instructions with participants
    3. Debriefing immediately after a traumatic event
    4. Identifying people at risk for anxiety disorders

16. The nurse is assessing a patient and notices tooth erosion and callused knuckles. Which behavior would the nurse watch for around mealtimes?
    1. Hiding the food or throwing it away
    2. Pushing the food around the plate
    3. Eating an extraordinarily large amount
    4. Self-induced vomiting

17. Which patient has a sexual concern that could be treated with surgery?
    1. Patient A has premature ejaculation.
    2. Patient B has transvestic fetishism.
    3. Patient C has transsexualism.
    4. Patient D has hypoactive sexual desire.

18. The patient has been taking olanzapine for several years. Which patient response indicates that the medication therapy is successful?
    1. Says that nightmares and flashbacks have decreased
    2. Reports that his compulsive behavior is under control
    3. Says he still misses his dead wife, but doesn't ruminate
    4. Smiles as he tells the nurse about his new job

19. The nurse has just finished taking shift report. Which patient would the nurse check on **first**?
    1. Patient has a serum lithium level of 1.5 mEq/L (1.5 mmol/L) with slurred speech.
    2. Patient has bizarre movements of the face with torticollis and oculogyric crisis.
    3. Patient has hyperthermia, muscle rigidity, and labile blood pressure.
    4. Patient has rigidity, resting tremors, and a shuffling gait.

20. The nurse is caring for an older resident in a long-term care facility who develops confusion, delirium, agitation, and mutism. The nurse sees that the patient takes sertraline. Which additional assessment findings would accompany serotonin syndrome?
    1. Blood pressure fluctuation and ataxia
    2. Headaches and anxiety
    3. Vomiting and muscle pain
    4. Crying spells and irritability

21. The patient is in the manic phase of bipolar affective disorder. What is the **primary** aim of the nurse's therapeutic communication?
    1. Reinforce assertive behaviors.
    2. Provide focus and consistency.
    3. Orient to surroundings and time.
    4. Encourage expression of feelings.

22. Which medication is **most** likely to be prescribed for a patient with an obsessive-compulsive disorder?
    1. Lithium carbonate
    2. Haloperidol
    3. Chlorpromazine
    4. Clomipramine

23. For a patient who is receiving lithium therapy, which electrolyte level is **most** important to monitor?
    1. Calcium
    2. Sodium
    3. Magnesium
    4. Potassium

24. A patient tells you that he is hearing voices right now that are telling him not to eat. What is the **best** response?
    1. "What specifically did the voices tell you not to eat?"
    2. "Did the voices say why they didn't want you to eat?"
    3. "Just ignore the voices. Lunch is served at 1:00 PM."
    4. "I don't hear any voices. What you are experiencing now?"

25. Based on the information provided in the change-of-shift report, which patient will the nurse see **first**?
    1. Patient had electroconvulsive therapy 30 minutes ago.
    2. Patient has refused to take the morning medication.
    3. Patient has said, "I am going to meet my [dead] wife."
    4. Patient identified "voices" with a message from God.

26. The patient was admitted to the acute care facility for drug-induced psychosis. He tells the nurse that he has smelled his own flesh rotting for the past 2 days. Which positive symptoms is the patient is experiencing?
    1. Delusion
    2. Avolition
    3. Akathisia
    4. Hallucination

27. In caring for a patient who has schizophrenia, which behaviors does the nurse interpret as negative signs and symptoms? **Select all that apply.**
    1. Makes no attempts to maintain hygiene or appearance.
    2. Says, "I am the Queen of the Nile, bow down before me."
    3. Does not smile or react when his mother brings a birthday cake.
    4. Assumes a listening pose and then talks loudly to an empty corner of his room.
    5. Repeatedly washes his hands even though they are red and raw.
    6. Prefers to be alone and refuses to join group activities.

28. Which patient statement would indicate a compulsion?
    1. "I can't stop thinking about my hand towels being out of place on the towel rack."
    2. "I had to drive back home eight times this morning to be sure I locked my front door."
    3. "Those voices in my head are driving me crazy. Can you make them stop?"
    4. "It terrifies me to think about going fishing; I know there may be spiders in the boat."

29. A woman has bipolar disorder and is currently displaying an outgoing personality, productivity in her work, and great optimism. Which phase of bipolar disorder is she experiencing?
    1. Manic
    2. Depressive
    3. Cyclothymic
    4. Hypomanic

30. A wife complains that her husband must be neurotic. Which signs and symptoms would the nurse expect the husband to display? **Select all that apply.**
    1. Nervousness
    2. Low self-esteem
    3. Out of touch with reality
    4. Phobias
    5. Impaired judgment

31. The patient asks the nurse not to tell anyone that he wants to end his life. What would the nurse tell the patient?
    1. "Information must be shared with the rest of the health care team."
    2. "All disclosures from patient to nurse are always confidential."
    3. "Consider talking to a spiritual advisor before acting impulsively."
    4. "Information is documented in writing, but not verbally discussed."

32. The unlicensed assistive personnel (UAP) reports that an older patient said, "You have been kind and I want you to remember me," and then she gave the UAP her grandmother's necklace. What would the nurse do **first**?
    1. Investigate the relationship between the patient and the UAP.
    2. Instruct the UAP to return the necklace to the patient.
    3. Talk to the patient about the gesture of gift-giving to employees.
    4. Praise the UAP for having trust and rapport with the patient.

33. Which patient is **most** likely to be experiencing a panic attack?
    1. Patient A reports fear of being followed and demonstrates hypervigilance.
    2. Patient B reports an excruciating headache with blurred vision and nausea.
    3. Patient C reports an aura followed by tonic-clonic seizure activity.
    4. Patient D reports chest pain, fear of going crazy, sweating, and trembling.

34. It's lunchtime and a staff member walks into the dayroom of an acute psychiatric unit and announces, "It's chow time folks! Hop on down." Which patient is **most** likely to start physically hopping?
    1. Has major depression with apathy and flat affect
    2. Has panic disorder with agoraphobia and anxiety
    3. Has dysthymic disorder with suicidal ideations
    4. Has disorganized schizophrenia with concreteness

35. A parent reports that her adolescent child displays poor hygiene and odd, excessive religious beliefs. What could the nurse do to assist the HCP to differentiate between the prodromal phase schizophrenia and normal adolescent behavior?
    1. Help the parent to compare current behavior to childhood behaviors.
    2. Talk directly to the adolescent and ask about beliefs and interests.
    3. Assess and compare the parent's religious beliefs to the adolescent's.
    4. Ask the parent if there is a family history of mental illness.

36. The patient reports recurrent nausea, vomiting, diarrhea, stomach pain, and headaches. She reports stress related to her marital relationship. If physical causes are ruled out, these symptoms are consistent with which mental health disorder?
    1. Somatoform disorder
    2. Posttraumatic stress disorder
    3. Generalized anxiety disorder
    4. Bulimia nervosa

37. The nurse is trying to assess a patient who is newly diagnosed with schizophrenia. The patient refuses to speak, but whispers, "They are listening to my conversations through the intercom." What would the nurse do?
    1. Conduct the interview in whispers or by writing.
    2. Walk over to the intercom and turn it off.
    3. Suggest that they move to the garden area.
    4. Acknowledge his feelings of fear and anxiety.

38. The patient says, "The man on the television is telling me to buy that motorcycle." What is the **most** therapeutic response?
    1. "It's just a television program; he wasn't really talking to you."
    2. "You can't buy a motorcycle right now; you are in the hospital."
    3. "Have you been thinking about buying a motorcycle?"
    4. "Television advertisements try to persuade us to buy products."

39. The nurse is caring for a patient who is scheduled to have surgery in the morning, but she also happens to have an anxiety disorder. What would the nurse do **first** to decrease stimuli for this anxious patient?
    1. Close the door and give the patient some privacy.
    2. Ask if sounds, light, or movement are disturbing.
    3. Turn off the lights so that the patient can sleep.
    4. Limit the number of visitors to decrease noise.

40. Which information is appropriate when preparing a patient for electroconvulsive therapy? **Select all that apply.**
    1. "Pain will be experienced, but it only lasts a few seconds."
    2. "Confusion may last for a few hours."
    3. "A grand mal seizure occurs, but it is brief and controlled."
    4. "Temporary memory loss is experienced after treatment."
    5. "Most patients are kept in the hospital for 2-3 days afterward."
    6. "Medication is given through an IV catheter during the procedure."

41. A woman reports that her teenage daughter is counting calories, practicing unusual food rituals, making excuses to avoid eating, and losing weight. Which vital sign abnormality is **most** likely to accompany the pattern of behavior that the mother is describing?
    1. Shallow breathing
    2. Irregular pulse
    3. High blood pressure
    4. High fever

42. Which medications are typically used to treat depression? **Select all that apply.**
    1. Fluoxetine
    2. Lorazepam
    3. Sertraline
    4. Venlafaxine
    5. Citalopram
    6. Paroxetine

43. For a patient taking haloperidol, which nursing interventions are used for the anticholinergic side effects? **Select all that apply.**
    1. Suggest sugarless candy or gum.
    2. Suggest high-fiber foods in the diet.
    3. Perform periodic blood tests to assess haloperidol level.
    4. Explain need to rise slowly from sitting to standing.
    5. Administer prn diphenhydramine.
    6. Assess for urinary retention.

44. In caring for a patient with borderline personality disorder, which behavior would the nurse expect?
    1. Patient would be suspicious of the nurse and distrustful of the care.
    2. Patient would be dependent on the praise and attention of the nurse.
    3. Patient would be focused on self and view the nurse as insignificant.
    4. Patient would be manipulative and erratic towards the nurse.

CRITICAL THINKING ACTIVITIES

45. The nurse is working in a long-term care facility. There are two residents who have been living there for several years. Both are showing signs of new-onset mental health change. A resident with quadriplegia was recently admitted to the hospital for treatment of pressure injuries. He returned to the long-term care facility several weeks ago, but now he seems sullen and withdrawn and frequently talks about death. The other resident is an older man with no family. He has a history of chronic depression. He is ambulatory and able to independently perform most activities of daily living. He has been talking about the loss of friends and family and his desire to join them. He mentions feeling "lonely, old, and useless." He asked the nurse if she would "give him a few extra pills."

    a. What are the warning signs of suicide? _____

    _____

    _____

    _____

    b. Compare and contrast precautions that should be taken for these two residents who are suicidal.

    _____

    _____

    _____

    _____

    _____

    _____

46. The nurse is caring for a patient with chronic pain who displays sadness, loss of interest in activities, and pessimistic thoughts. The nurse reports these findings. A consulting psychiatrist makes the medical diagnosis of depression. What specific treatments for depression should the nurse anticipate?

_____

_____

_____

_____

NEXT-GENERATION NCLEX™ (NGN)

47. Matrix

Cognitive Skill: Take Action

Scenario: The patient was recently diagnosed with bipolar disorder and admitted to the acute care psychiatric unit. The HCP has prescribed lithium carbonate to stabilize the patient's behavior. It may take 7-10 days to reach a therapeutic level and lithium toxicity is a potential danger. Which interventions are used to safely manage the use of lithium to treat the patient's condition?

Instructions: Use an X to indicate which nursing interventions are essential, nonessential, or contraindicated. All should be used and can be used only once.

Nursing Intervention	Essential	Nonessential	Contraindicated
Maintain stable salt use.			
Ensure periodic blood tests to assess drug level.			
Reassure patient that serum level >1.5 mEq/L (1.5 mmol/L) is within the therapeutic range.			
Observe for nausea, vomiting, diarrhea, drowsiness, muscle weakness, and ataxia.			
Encourage smoking cessation.			
Give medication with food to prevent indigestion.			
Restrict fluid intake in the evening.			

Care of the Patient With an Addictive Personality

Answer Key: A complete Answer Key is provided in your Additional Learning Resources on Evolve.

TABLE ACTIVITY

1. *Directions:* In the table below, indicate at least one or two disorders that are associated with chronic alcohol use for each body system.

Disorders Associated With Alcoholism

System	Disorders
Gastrointestinal	
Hepatic	
Cardiovascular and hematologic	
Respiratory	
Urologic and reproductive	
Musculoskeletal	
Neurologic	

SHORT ANSWER

Directions: Using your own words, answer the question in the space provided.

2.   CAGE is an assessment tool that is used to identify problems with alcohol abuse. Two or more affirmations to the four questions indicate probable alcoholism. What are the four questions?

a.   _____

b.   _____

c.   _____

d.   _____

MULTIPLE CHOICE

Directions: Select the best answer(s) for each of the following questions.

3.   Which person is displaying the four elements that indicate an addiction?
   1.   Teenager gets drunk at weekend parties to reinforce peer relationships.
   2.   Nurse frequently takes patients' opioids and falsifies the documentation.
   3.   Construction worker goes to a bar every day after work to drink with friends.
   4.   Older couple has wine every day with dinner and a cocktail before bed.

4.   A patient comes into the walk-in clinic for a prescription refill. She admits to recently taking a hit of "Molly." What assessment findings would the nurse expect?
   1.   Pinpoint pupils and memory loss
   2.   Increased pulse and blood pressure
   3.   Slurred speech and listlessness
   4.   Confabulation and lack of coordination

5.   Which person is displaying the five personality traits that are associated with an addictive personality?
   1.   Stay-at-home mom feels dependent, insecure, and easily upset. She is frequently depressed and sees herself as having no marketable skills.
   2.   Manager feels overwhelmed by work. She overcompensates, is aggressive and competitive, and frequently displays false bravado around others.
   3.   College student is quiet, shy, and unsure of herself around others. She studies and stays at home to avoid social situations.
   4.   Woman feels angry about her husband's infidelity. She becomes flirtatious and has a series of one-night stands to express her hostility toward men.

6.   Which person has the **most** risk factors for alcohol dependency?
   1.   A 50-year-old French female who drinks after death of a spouse
   2.   A 30-year-old Irish female who does recreational drinking and cocaine
   3.   A 14-year-old Native American male who drinks and father is an alcoholic
   4.   A 42-year-old Jewish male with depression related to liver cancer

7. In the United States, there has been a decrease in alcohol use over the years. According to experts, there are factors that account for this decrease. Which nursing action is consistent with these identified factors?
   1. Nursing assessment includes standardized tools to identify alcohol abuse.
   2. Nursing programs include substance and alcohol abuse in the curriculum.
   3. There are increased roles for nurses at residential treatment centers.
   4. Patient teaching includes short- and long-term health effects of alcohol abuse.

8. Which behaviors are seen in the **early** stage of substance dependency? **Select all that apply.**
   1. Stops using to prove control over substance use
   2. Makes light of concerns expressed by family or friends
   3. Socializes more with other users and less with family
   4. Takes the substance to just feel "normal"
   5. Demonstrates mood swings, guilt, and resentment

9. Infective endocarditis is **more** likely to occur with which route of substance abuse?
   1. Smoking a bong
   2. Snorting opioids
   3. Huffing inhalants
   4. Injecting drugs

10. When a person is drinking an alcoholic beverage, which function of the central nervous system will be affected **first**?
    1. Frontal cortex is affected and person experiences memory loss and loss of judgment.
    2. The limbic system is affected and disrupts regulation of hunger, thirst, and sexual desire.
    3. Higher centers of the brain are affected and person starts to lose self-control.
    4. Basal ganglia of the brain are affected, and this leads to obsessive-compulsive behavior.

11. The nurse is talking to a group of people who are likely to be in denial about alcohol abuse, but each is describing a typical drinking pattern for a Saturday night. Which person has the **highest** amount of reported alcohol intake for a single day?
    1. Drinks a six-pack of beer (12 ounces per can)
    2. Drinks three glasses of red wine (4 ounces per glass)
    3. Drinks one beer (12-ounces) and two glasses of wine (4 ounces per glass)
    4. Drinks three mixed drinks (1 1/2 ounces hard liquor per drink)

12. For the patient who has Wernicke encephalopathy, which assessment finding indicates that the prescribed thiamine is effective?
    1. Hallucinations cease and delirium is resolved.
    2. Memory and muscle coordination show improvement.
    3. Tremors are decreased and there is no seizure activity.
    4. Vomiting, cramps, and diarrhea have resolved.

13. A patient has a blood alcohol level of >500 mg/dL (108.55 mmol/L) (>0.50%). Which action is the nurse likely to use **first**?
    1. Assess for changes in mental status.
    2. Assist with ambulation because of clumsiness.
    3. Set limits for loosening of inhibitions.
    4. Assist health care provider (HCP) with intubation.

14. A coworker states that he consumes too much caffeine and wants to eliminate it from his diet. Which question would the nurse ask **first**?
    1. "Are you aware that you will have withdrawal symptoms?"
    2. "Do you take any supplements or over-the-counter medications?"
    3. "Have you ever tried to give up or cut down on your consumption?"
    4. "What would you typically eat and drink during a 24-hour period?"

15. A patient who had smoked for years suddenly stopped smoking cigarettes after he was admitted to the hospital. Which symptom is associated with withdrawal from nicotine?
    1. Lethargy
    2. Improved concentration
    3. Decreased heart rate
    4. Decreased appetite

16. The nurse is working at a facility that assists workers who have substance abuse problems. Which worker is **least** likely to need assistance to get through withdrawal?
    1. Person A has been smoking cannabis for several years.
    2. Person B admits to a steady increase in amphetamine use.
    3. Person C reports using heroin whenever it is available.
    4. Person D frequently uses hallucinogens on the weekends.

17. A college student has used marijuana since early high school. Which nursing assessment will assist the HCP to substantiate the diagnosis of amotivational cannabis syndrome?
    1. Ask the student about vaping as a vehicle for marijuana use.
    2. Obtain data about the frequency and content of hallucinations.
    3. Assess for bruises, cuts, or other signs of physical aggression.
    4. Ask the student about his studies and goals after graduation.

18. A patient was prescribed an opioid analgesic for a fractured femur. He states that he has noticed that he doesn't seem to get the relief that he used to, despite the fact that his leg is healing. What would the nurse tell the patient?
    1. "Tolerance to opioids develops rapidly, but abstinence reverses tolerance."
    2. "You should switch to nonsteroidal antiinflammatory drugs (NSAIDs)."
    3. "Addiction to opioid medications is common for those who have chronic pain."
    4. "This is an expected effect; I will contact the HCP to increase your dosage."

19. The nurse's friend believes that her boyfriend may have an alcohol problem. Which question will elicit indicators of the **early** stage of alcoholism?
    1. "What form of alcohol does he drink?"
    2. "Is the drinking controlling him?"
    3. "What makes you think there's a problem?"
    4. "Have you talked to him about this?"

20. The nurse is caring for a teenager who crashed his parents' car while he was intoxicated. The mother, wracked with guilt, confides that she knew he had a drinking problem, but didn't do anything about it. What is the **most** therapeutic response?
    1. "You can't watch your kids all of the time, especially when they are teenagers."
    2. "The accident may be a blessing; now you can get help for his drinking."
    3. "You feel like you are to blame, but it was his choice to drink and drive."
    4. "It's hard for parents to really believe that their child has a drinking problem."

21. The nurse is a assessing a patient who has been in the middle stage of substance abuse for years. Which factor is **most** likely to hasten the progression from the middle stage to the late stage?
    1. Poor family relationships
    2. Multiple substances of abuse
    3. Gastrointestinal problems
    4. Substance abuse on the job

22. From a cultural standpoint, which patient is the **least** likely to develop alcoholism?
    1. Asian
    2. Irishman
    3. Mormon
    4. Inuit

23. Which patient represents the leading national health problems in the United States?
    1. An infant who has birth defects and fetal alcohol syndrome (FAS)
    2. An adolescent with cancer who smokes medicinal cannabis
    3. An executive who uses cocaine to counteract his depression
    4. An older patient who is an alcoholic with heart disease

24. What is the physiologic reason for the vitamin B_1, folic acid, and vitamin B_{12} deficiencies that occur in alcoholism?
    1. Alcohol affects the intestinal mucosa and results in decreased absorption.
    2. One ounce of alcohol provides 200 kcal but has no other nutritional value.
    3. Alcohol has a diuretic effect, so most nutrients are excreted in the urine.
    4. The liver metabolizes most of the alcohol; thus the liver is damaged.

25. The nurse is caring for a postoperative patient who has a history of alcoholism. The patient demonstrates restlessness, tachycardia, and mild diaphoresis. How could the nurse differentiate between suspected alcohol withdrawal and postoperative complications, such as bleeding or infection?
    1. Call the HCP and obtain an order for blood alcohol level.
    2. Monitor vital signs and assess for pain related to the surgery.
    3. Explain concerns and then ask the patient about alcohol use.
    4. This differentiation is beyond the nurse's scope of practice.

26. Which substance has the **most** dangerous consequences during withdrawal?
    1. Alcohol
    2. Heroin
    3. Amphetamine
    4. Nicotine

27. The nurse is interviewing a patient who has an alcohol problem and his wife has decided to file for divorce. Which patient statement typifies the **most** common defense mechanism used by substance abusers?
    1. "My wife is the one who has a drinking problem. I am glad she is gone."
    2. "I don't have a drinking problem. My wife just used that as an excuse."
    3. "Have you ever been married? I wouldn't recommend it to anyone."
    4. "My wife got on my nerves, so sometimes I would have a few drinks."

28. Which laboratory findings are likely to be seen for a patient who has chronic alcoholism? **Select all that apply.**
    1. Elevated liver enzymes
    2. Decreased hemoglobin
    3. High cholesterol
    4. Abnormal blood proteins
    5. Hyperglycemia
    6. Abnormal clotting times

29. A person is brought to the hospital for an acute opioid overdose, which is probably a suicide attempt. The patient is difficult to arouse, and the family is hysterical. What is the **priority** action?
    1. Assess for time of ingestion.
    2. Check airway and respirations.
    3. Calm the family to obtain a history.
    4. Administer IV naloxone.

30. Which complications are associated with FAS? **Select all that apply.**
    1. Stillbirth
    2. Cardiac arrest
    3. Wide-set eyes
    4. Cognitive delays
    5. Spontaneous abortion
    6. Alcohol withdrawal symptoms

31. During physical assessment, the nurse observes that the patient with a substance abuse problem has excessive gum and tooth erosion and extreme vasoconstriction. Which abnormal vital sign change is **most** likely to accompany these objective findings?
    1. Elevated temperature
    2. Low blood pressure
    3. Increased pulse rate
    4. Decreased respiratory rate

32. The nurse finds her teenage son and his friends laughing and drinking alcohol. One of the boys is on the floor. He is breathing steadily, but drifting in and out of consciousness. What would the nurse do **first**?
    1. Find out what they drank, how much, and when they started.
    2. Establish the boy's airway and put him in a side-lying position.
    3. Call 911, monitor the boy for decompensation, and watch the others.
    4. Call the parents, report the event, and ask them to come to the house.

33. The nurse monitors patients who are being treated for substance abuse problems. Which question is the nurse **most** likely to ask related to evaluate the effectiveness of bupropion?
    1. "How many servings of alcohol are you having per week?"
    2. "Has the medication lessened your desire for heroin?"
    3. "Have you discontinued contact with your supplier?"
    4. "How many cigarettes are you smoking each day?"

CRITICAL THINKING ACTIVITIES

34. A daughter of a home health patient very hesitantly approaches the nurse and asks for information about alcohol abuse. At first, the daughter is very vague and claims to be asking out of general interest. As rapport develops, the daughter discloses that her mother (home health patient) and her stepfather seem to be drinking more alcohol. The daughter is not sure if they are true "alcoholics," but is worried about how their drinking is affecting the rest of the family.

    a. The nurse decides to collect data to determine if the family members have risk factors that could contribute to alcoholism. What are some contributing factors?

    _____

    _____

    _____

    b. What can the nurse tell the daughter about the possible effects of alcoholism on relationships between family members who abuse alcohol and family members who do not?

    _____

    _____

    _____

    _____

35. The nurse suspects that something unusual is happening during the night shift. The patients frequently complain that the pain medication that they receive at night seems ineffective. These complaints seem to occur when the same two nurses are working together; however, the nurse hesitates to report these complaints because he recognizes that subjective reports of pain could be influenced by a number of factors.

    a. What should the nurse do? _____

    _____

    _____

    _____

    _____

b. What are the specific role-related signs or behaviors that may be seen if nurses are chemically impaired?

_____

_____

_____

_____

36. How would you feel about reporting a friend/coworker for stealing opioid medication?

_____

_____

_____

_____

NEXT-GENERATION NCLEX™ (NGN)

37. Extended Drag and Drop

Cognitive Skill: Recognize Cues

Scenario: A nurse has recently started a new job at a clinic that specializes in outpatient treatment of various substance abuse problems. The supervisor tells the nurse that while many of the drugs will be familiar, reviewing the purpose and application of these drugs for substance abuse problems will be helpful in the new job.

Instructions: Indicate which medications listed in the right column would be used for the substance abuse treatment listed in the left column. Each medication will used only once.

Substance Abuse Treatment

_____ 1. Facilitate smoking cessation

_____ 2. Suppress withdrawal symptoms from morphine or heroin addiction

_____ 3. Treat seizures associated with delirium tremens

_____ 4. Reduce craving for cocaine

_____ 5. Reverse respiratory depression associated with opioid overdose

_____ 6. Reverse or prevent Wernicke encephalopathy

_____ 7. Treat cardiac dysrhythmias caused by cocaine

_____ 8. Reduce tremors associated with delirium tremens

_____ 9. Encourage alcohol abstinence

Medications

a. disulfiram
b. thiamine
c. lorazepam
d. phenytoin
e. naloxone
f. bromocriptine
g. methadone
h. nicotine gum
i. propranolol

Home Health Nursing

Answer Key: A complete Answer Key is provided in your Additional Learning Resources on Evolve.

MULTIPLE CHOICE

Directions: Select the best answer(s) for each of the following questions.

1. Which patient is **most** likely to be eligible for Medicare coverage for home health services?
   1. 71-year-old who needs help with bathing, grooming, and toileting
   2. 67-year-old who is discharged from the hospital after hip surgery
   3. 83-year-old who has dementia and needs around-the-clock supervision
   4. 45-year-old who needs prefilling of insulin syringes and diabetes education

2. Which nursing action indicates that the nurse understands how diagnosis-related groups impact nursing practice?
   1. Collaborates with RN to ensure that nursing problems align with the medical diagnosis
   2. Reviews the pathophysiology and chronic effects of medical diagnosis for all assigned patients
   3. Does focused assessments related to medical diagnosis and reports findings to prevent complications
   4. Reinforces information about the medical diagnosis and teaches self-care measures to prevent relapse

3. Which patient situation is an example of the major impact that diagnosis-related groups have on hospitalized patients?
   1. Patient A has to change health care provider (HCP) for insurance purposes.
   2. Patient B has a medical diagnosis that is not covered by Medicare.
   3. Patient C has more out-of-pocket costs because of medical diagnosis.
   4. Patient D is discharged, but still needs ongoing home care.

4. For families and patients who receive Medicare home services, what is the significance of the 60-day period?
   1. The family or patient must pay for the first 60 days of home services, then Medicare coverage starts.
   2. The patient must need skilled nursing or therapy for at least 60 days to be eligible for home care coverage.
   3. Recertification by physician and primary disciplines must be completed for each subsequent 60-day period.
   4. Persons who are eligible for Medicare get a maximum coverage of 60 days of home care each year.

5. The nurse is making a home visit with an older woman who has an indwelling urinary catheter because of urinary retention. The nurse notes that the urine has a strong, foul odor and the woman seems lethargic and listless. What would the nurse do **first**?
   1. Call the supervising RN and ask for a second opinion about possible urosepsis.
   2. Take vital signs, and do a head-to-toe assessment to identify sources of infection.
   3. Clamp the catheter and then obtain a fresh urine specimen using sterile technique.
   4. Remove the indwelling catheter and save the tip of the catheter for culture.

6. Which evaluative statement indicates that the "improvement" goal of service is being met for a patient who has type 2 diabetes mellitus and was recently discharged after a toe amputation related to a diabetic foot ulcer?
   1. Patient loses 5 lbs after adherence to exercise routine and healthy eating.
   2. Wound edges are well approximated; tissue is pink with no evidence of infection.
   3. Patient gives return demonstration of inspection, cleaning, and care of feet.
   4. Patient resumes routine blood glucose testing and self-administration of insulin.

7. Which assessments will the nurse perform on a patient who uses a mask for delivery of home oxygen therapy? **Select all that apply.**
   1. Checks the patient's skin underneath the straps.
   2. Observes the tops of ears for skin breakdown.
   3. Assesses oral and mucous membranes.
   4. Observes the amount and quality of secretions.
   5. Checks and replaces the oxygen equipment as needed.

8. After a stroke, a patient exhibits difficult swallowing and is at high risk for aspiration. Which member of the health care team could **best** assist the patient?
   1. Speech-language therapist
   2. Ear, nose, and throat specialist
   3. Occupational therapist
   4. Primary HCP

9. The documentation shows that it has been a month since the RN made a home visit or interacted directly with the home health aide. Which action would the LPN/LVN take?
   1. Contact the director of the agency to review the documentation.
   2. Assess the patient, supervise the aide, and update the documentation.
   3. Remind the RN that the onsite visit and supervision of the aide are overdue.
   4. Continue to provide care and documentation under the existing plan.

10. Which nurse is demonstrating the **best** collaboration with the patient, family, and Spanish interpreter to improve communication?
    1. Nurse A speaks a little Spanish but defers to the interpreter.
    2. Nurse B asks the interpreter to use very simple language.
    3. Nurse C gives all information directly to the interpreter.
    4. Nurse D speaks directly to the patient and family.

11. The nurse observes that the home health patient has trouble with tasks that require fine motor skills such as writing or manipulating eating utensils. Which member of the health care team is **best** able to assist the patient with these problems?
    1. Physician
    2. Physical therapist
    3. Home health aide
    4. Occupational therapist

12. The home health nurse is reviewing use of home oxygen with the patient and family. Which information would be included?
    1. Use petrolatum-based lubricant on the lips.
    2. Place "No Smoking" signs where they are clearly visible.
    3. Change disposable equipment once a month.
    4. Use wool blankets to provide warmth and static control.

13. Which home health patient would be the **best** candidate for a telehealth program?
    1. Lacks fine motor control to perform ostomy care
    2. Needs infusion of total parenteral nutrition every morning
    3. Recently prescribed insulin and blood glucose monitoring
    4. Requires assessment of home environment for safety

14. What do Medicare and Medicaid require for the patient to be entered into the formalized system?
    1. An evidence-based clinical pathway that relates to the primary medical diagnosis
    2. A standardized nursing care plan that is linked to the hospital discharge diagnosis
    3. An individualized nursing care plan that is developed by the RN and LPN/LVN
    4. An interdisciplinary treatment plan that is reviewed and signed by the HCP

15. Which evaluative statement indicates that the "restorative" goal of service is being met?
    1. Patient who had a stroke 4 weeks ago is now able to feed self without signs of choking.
    2. Patient who had smoking cessation classes reports no smoking for the past 2 months.
    3. Patient who had bariatric surgery reports exercising routinely with no weight gain.
    4. Patient who has hypertension reports compliance with low-cholesterol, low-sodium diet.

16. A patient was treated in the hospital for an exacerbation of emphysema. The home health team is providing follow-up care and includes an RN, LPN/LVN, home health aide, and a respiratory therapist. Which tasks can be delegated to the home health aide? **Select all that apply.**
    1. Take and report vital signs.
    2. Assist with hygiene and bathing.
    3. Accompany for short walks in the garden.
    4. Assess for fatigue after exertion.
    5. Report shortness of breath.
    6. Set up and replace oxygen equipment.

17. An older patient with severe arthritis requires physical therapy and assistance with activities of daily living (ADLs). The family is enquiring about the eligibility for Medicare home health coverage. Which set of activities is **most** likely to require out-of-pocket payment?
    1. Bathing and oral hygiene
    2. Walking and transfers
    3. Shopping and cooking
    4. Eating and toileting

18. A home health aide is assigned to assist a patient with a bath several times a week. Which instruction would the nurse to give to the aide?
    1. "Try to do everything for the patient, so he feels nurtured."
    2. "Ask the patient if he prefers a shower, tub bath, or a partial bath."
    3. "If you or the patient has any problems, just let me know."
    4. "Watch for redness of the skin, particularly on the buttocks and back."

19. A nurse is spending 3 or more hours with each patient for home visits. The supervisor sees this as a problem. What would the supervisor do **first**?
    1. Explain that clinical efficiency is critical within the industry.
    2. Describe how the current Medicare prospective payment system works.
    3. Ask the nurse to describe what happens on a typical home visit.
    4. Review the nurse's documentation for evidence of how the time is spent.

20. What are the purposes of documentation in home health care? **Select all that apply.**
    1. Provides an accurate picture of the type and quality of care
    2. Replaces verbal nursing reports that are used in facilities
    3. Allows the health care team to make internal evaluations as needed
    4. Provides evidence required for reimbursement and payments
    5. Serves as a legal document that is subject to close scrutiny
    6. Allows family to have access to all patient information

21. A 63-year-old woman is referred to home health care because she is having trouble with colostomy management. She takes antihypertensive medication and an oral hypoglycemic. Which interventions can be assigned to LPN/LVN? **Select all that apply.**
    1. Setting up medications
    2. Ostomy care and teaching
    3. Admission physical assessment
    4. Fingersticks for blood glucose readings
    5. Emotional support related to change of body image
    6. Teaching about dietary restrictions to prevent blockage

CRITICAL THINKING ACTIVITIES

22. Today, the home health patient with heart failure seems short of breath, has 4+ pitting edema in the lower extremities, and a weight gain of 5 lbs within a week. The pulse oximeter reading is 89% on oxygen at 4 L/min per nasal cannula. The nurse calls the HCP and receives an order to have the patient transported by ambulance to the hospital for an exacerbation of heart failure. The nurse informs the patient about the HCP's plan. The patient says, "I don't want to go to the hospital. Can you stay with me and give me an IV diuretic? That's all they will do at the hospital."

    a. What should the nurse do first? _____

    _____

    _____

    _____

    b. If the patient continues to refuse to go to the hospital despite the nurse's best efforts to convince him, should the nurse stay? If so, for how long and under what conditions should the nurse continue to stay with the patient?

    _____

    _____

    _____

23. Identify qualities/attributes in yourself that would indicate that a career in home health would either be suitable (or not) for you.

    _____

    _____

    _____

    _____

    _____

NEXT-GENERATION NCLEX™ (NGN)

24. Extended Multiple Response

Cognitive Skill: Take Action

Scenario: The RN completed the home health intake assessment of an older patient who is 3 weeks postoperative for amputation of the 4th and 5th digits on the right foot. The patient has poorly controlled diabetes and hypertension. The LPN/LVN is assigned to do weekly home visits and the physical therapist is consulting because of gait and balance problems related to the amputation.

Which interventions would be assigned to the LPN/LVN?

Instructions: Place a check mark next to interventions that would be assigned to the LPN/LVN. **Check all that apply.**

_____	1.	Assess and clean the wound site.
_____	2.	Assess gait and balance.
_____	3.	Assist with showering and hygiene.
_____	4.	Monitor blood pressure and weight.
_____	5.	Perform fingersticks for blood glucose readings.
_____	6.	Prefill insulin syringes.
_____	7.	Teach tips for medication compliance.
_____	8.	Reinforce therapeutic diabetic diet information.
_____	9.	Evaluate treatment outcomes at the end of the 60-day period.

Long-Term Care

chapter

38

Answer Key: A complete Answer Key is provided in your Additional Learning Resources on Evolve.

MULTIPLE CHOICE

Directions: Select the best answer(s) for each of the following questions.

1. An older couple who are in good health express the desire to "age in place." Which action would the nurse take **first**?
   1. Arrange for regular home health visits.
   2. Consult with the RN to make a comprehensive plan.
   3. Gather data about the resources that they may need.
   4. Suggest that they talk to the family about their wishes.

2. For which patient circumstance is the nurse **most** likely to suggest respite care?
   1. Older patient who occasionally wanders needs supervision when wife goes to work
   2. Older couple needs assistance with shopping and going to medical appointments
   3. Older couple is in relatively good health and needs some assistance for ADLs
   4. Older patient has advanced dementia, daughter performs around-the-clock care

3. Which person is **most** likely to qualify for Program of All Inclusive Care for the Elderly (PACE)?
   1. 73-year-old woman with moderate Alzheimer's disease who lives with 77-year-old spouse
   2. 60-year-old woman with mild dementia who needs adult daycare when her daughter is at work
   3. 80-year-old man who needs tube feedings and respiratory treatments every 6 hours
   4. 55-year-old man who lives in a rural area and needs transportation to the veteran's hospital

4. The LPN/LVN staffing coordinator receives an incomplete report about an older person (Mr. X) who is requesting home care. Which question is the **most** important to ensure appropriate scheduling and assignment?
   1. "Has Mr. X ever had home health before? If so, would he like the same caregiver?"
   2. "What is Mr. X's medical diagnosis and what is the name of his primary health care provider?
   3. "Does Mr. X need assistance with activities of daily living or skilled nursing care?"
   4. "How many days of the week and hours per day does Mr. X need care and assistance?"

5. Which outcome statement indicates that the **primary** goal of hospice care has been met?
   1. Family is notified to attend patient because death is near.
   2. Family is aware of and agrees to plan of care.
   3. Patient signals readiness to let go and then dies.
   4. Patient is clean, dry, comfortable, and pain-free.

6. Which patient is **most** likely to benefit from palliative care?
   1. Patient who sustained a hip fracture needs additional time for rehabilitation.
   2. Patient with a feeding tube and oxygen therapy shows slow but steady deterioration.
   3. Patient with dementia frequently cries, but no organic cause of pain is identified.
   4. Patient with rheumatoid arthritis has chronic pain and long-term disabilities.

7. Which action would the nurse suggest to avoid a "precipitating event" that could lead to sudden need for long-term care placement for a family member who has early stage Alzheimer's disease?
   1. Check home for safety hazards.
   2. Ask family/friends to visit frequently.
   3. Reminisce and decorate with nostalgic items.
   4. Establish a simple daily routine.

8. The LPN/LVN is caring for 60 residents at a long-term care facility with a team of four certified nursing assistants (CNAs) and two certified medication aides (CMAs). What role/responsibilities related to medication administration is the LPN/LVN **most** likely to assume?
   1. CMAs will administer all medications and LPN/LVN will supervise all CNA and CMA actions.
   2. LPN/LVN will administer opioids, nonopioids, enteral tube, and as-needed (PRN) medications.
   3. LPN/LVN and CMAs can give medications, so each caregiver administers to 20 residents.
   4. LPN/LVN can delegate medication administration to CMAs or CNAs if they have experience.

9. Which person requires assistance with instrumental activities of daily living (ADLs)?
   1. Able to stand, but can't independently ambulate to the bathroom
   2. Can brush own teeth if someone applies the toothpaste
   3. Can pay bills by check, but doesn't understand online payments
   4. Owns a car, but vision and psychomotor coordination are poor

10. Before a clinical rotation at a long-term care center, the nursing instructor advises a group of first-year nursing students to do some reading about health problems that are likely to be found among the older adult residents. Which list represents the **most** common disorders that the students will see?
    1. Chronic obstructive pulmonary disease, paraplegia, and hip or long bone fractures
    2. Cardiovascular disease, hypertension, depression, dementia, and type 2 diabetes
    3. Amyotrophic lateral sclerosis, stroke, urinary incontinence, and end-stage renal failure
    4. Hypothyroidism, schizophrenia, traumatic injury, and peripheral vascular disease

11. The nurse is training a new CNA at a long-term care facility. Which topics would the nurse include in the CNA's training regarding ADLs? **Select all that apply.**
    1. Equipment needed for bathing or showering
    2. Ways to maintain independence in brushing teeth
    3. Communication techniques for social activities
    4. Safety measures to use during ambulation
    5. Money management during shopping
    6. Ways to maintain privacy during toileting

12. A patient requires extensive wound care and intravenous antibiotics due to an infection of a surgical wound. Which type of care will **best** meet this patient's needs?
    1. Long-term care facility
    2. Subacute unit
    3. Residential care facility
    4. Hospice unit

13. Which nursing action reflects the positive influence of the Omnibus Budget Reconciliation Act (OBRA) on long-term care?
    1. Instructs CNA to safely apply safety reminder devices
    2. Reviews and updates the residents' advance directives
    3. Reviews the qualifications of a CNA who applied for a job
    4. Ensures that each resident qualifies for Medicaid or Medicare

14. An older couple needs some assistance with bathing, dressing, and taking their medication. Both are always alert and oriented. They are mobile but constrained by arthritis. Which setting would be the **most** beneficial for this couple?
    1. Skilled nursing facility
    2. Subacute unit
    3. Adult daycare facility
    4. Assisted-living community

15. The interdisciplinary team at a long-term care facility is meeting to discuss the care plan of one of the residents. Who should attend this meeting? **Select all that apply.**
    1. Physical therapist
    2. Activities director
    3. CNA
    4. Nursing unit manager
    5. Other interested residents
    6. Resident

16. What is the **priority** concept that the supervising nurse will emphasize during the nursing student's orientation to the nursing home facility?
    1. Respectful communication
    2. Complete documentation
    3. Residents' safety and security
    4. Assistance with ADLs

17. What is the purpose of a resident assessment instrument?
    1. Identifies the problems that residents will have in communicating needs
    2. Allows residents to self-assess and report on what they can do for themselves
    3. Used by surveyors during unannounced visits to assess residents' quality of life
    4. Facilitates assessment of functional, medical, mental, and psychosocial status

18. How does documentation in a long-term care facility differ from that in a hospital setting?
    1. Documentation occurs at the beginning and end of each 24-hour period.
    2. The assistants do most of the physical care, so they do most of the documentation.
    3. Summaries of resident status are usually recorded on a monthly basis.
    4. Documentation occurs only if there is a sudden change in a resident's status.

19. An older person who is alert, ambulatory, and independent with ADLs has started to wander and the police have brought him home twice. Which question would the nurse use **first** to help the family determine if long-term care is needed?
    1. "Who has the power of attorney for health care?"
    2. "What are the current living arrangements for family members?"
    3. "What kinds of options have you considered for your father?"
    4. "Is there any way to plan 24-hour care among the family?"

20. An interdisciplinary team meeting is planned to discuss the needs of a resident who is hostile about being in the long-term care facility. The CNA who has the best relationship with the resident is not invited to attend. What would the nurse do?
    1. Ask the resident to invite the CNA.
    2. Advocate for the CNA to attend.
    3. Ask the CNA to do a written statement.
    4. Inform the CNA of the outcomes.

21. Which nursing action complies with the Emergency Support for Nursing Homes and Elder Justice Reform Act of 2020 for the management of the COVID-19 pandemic in long-term care facilities?
    1. Ensures that high-risk residents are isolated
    2. Files a daily report about the staffing levels
    3. Tracks vaccination/health status of all employees
    4. Takes visitors' temperatures before allowing entry

CRITICAL THINKING ACTIVITIES

22. You are considering a job in a long-term care facility. Your clinical experiences in nursing school included acute care and long-term care facilities. You recognize that part of selecting a job is to match your interests and experiences with the setting, patients, other caregivers, and philosophy of the institution.

    a. What is the profile of the patient/resident who requires long-term care in an institutional setting? Envision yourself working with this type of patient/resident. Is it a good fit for you?

b. The administration of medications in long-term care facilities is different than in acute care. Describe the differences and state ways to increase your comfort level with this process.

_____

_____

_____

_____

23. Your grandmother has reached a stage where your family has decided that she requires more care than the family is able to give her at home. Discuss points about choosing a nursing home.

_____

_____

_____

_____

24. Why would a nurse who works in long-term care actually need a better understanding of legal aspects, such as advance directives and power of attorney or guardianship, compared to a nurse who works in an acute care facility?

_____

_____

_____

_____

NEXT-GENERATION NCLEX™ (NGN)

25. Extended Multiple Response

Cognitive Skill: Take Action

Scenario: The Joint Commission establishes national patient safety goals and strategies to meet these goals. One of the major patient safety goals for long-term care settings is to prevent pressure injuries.

Which interventions will the nurse use to prevent pressure injuries in the long-term care setting?

Instructions: Place a check mark next to interventions that the nurse will use to prevent pressure injuries. **Check all that apply.**

_____	1.	Inspect the skin on a routine schedule according to facility policies.
_____	2.	Direct UAPs to assist ambulatory residents to walk in the hallway.
_____	3.	Keep skin clean and dry, and use moisture barriers as needed.
_____	4.	Massage dependent areas if redness or bruising is observed.
_____	5.	Use mechanical loading devices when transferring any resident.
_____	6.	Supervise UAPs for use of body mechanics to prevent injury.
_____	7.	Call for extra assistance when repositioning obese residents.
_____	8.	Encourage foods that meet individualized nutritional needs.
_____	9.	Remind UAPs that a high-Fowler's position can increase shearing forces.

Rehabilitation Nursing

Answer Key: A complete Answer Key is provided in your Additional Learning Resources on Evolve.

MULTIPLE CHOICE

Directions: Select the best answer(s) for each of the following questions.

1. Which patient is the **most** likely candidate for admission to a rehabilitation unit?
   1. Has trouble breathing with an acute exacerbation of chronic obstructive pulmonary disease (COPD)
   2. Recently treated and recovering from delirium secondary to a urinary tract infection
   3. Has moderate Alzheimer's disease and family is having increasing difficulties with home care
   4. Is recovering from a myocardial infarction (MI) and needs guidance to prevent recurrence

2. A patient had lung surgery and was recently transferred from the hospital and is now under the care of the pulmonary rehabilitation team. Which intervention is **most** likely to be assigned to the LPN/LVN?
   1. Design and teach an exercise routine.
   2. Review diet and teach nutritional modifications.
   3. Monitor use of energy conservation activities.
   4. Explain lung function and recovery prognosis.

3. An older patient who had a stroke has multiple residual symptoms. The spouse wants more therapy for her husband so he can "be like himself." What would nurse do **first**?
   1. Ask physiatrist to recertify physical therapy and increase frequency of speech therapy.
   2. Point out that some patients with stroke never fully recover to preexisting health state.
   3. Ask spouse to clarify the meaning of "be like himself" and her expectations of therapy.
   4. Ask physiatrist to review treatment goals and then compare those to the spouse's goals.

4. Which patient action is the **best** demonstration of a functional outcome?
   1. Patient states that his quality of life has improved after therapy.
   2. Patient agrees to biweekly physical therapy appointments.
   3. Patient knows signs/symptoms to report to the health care provider (HCP).
   4. Patient independently ambulates around the house.

5. Which outcome statement **best** indicates that the overall goal of rehabilitation has been successfully met?
   1. Patient telecommutes for work, regularly attends church, and joins a chess club.
   2. Patient regularly performs exercises as instructed by the occupational therapist.
   3. Patient demonstrates ability to maintain colostomy care and diet therapy.
   4. Patient completes activities of daily living (ADLs) with partial assistance.

6. The physiatrist tells the nurse that the patient with a spinal cord injury (SCI) may be developing heterotopic ossification in the right knee. How would the nurse use this information in planning care for this patient?
   1. Instruct the unlicensed assistive personnel (UAP) to handle the patient very gently.
   2. Ask the physical therapist about type and frequency of range-of-motion exercises.
   3. Frequently check the right leg for perfusion, pulse, temperature, pallor, and edema.
   4. Elevate the leg on a pillow and apply ice packs to reduce swelling and discomfort.

7. Which patient needs interventions that are based on the concept of habilitation?
   1. Man who had a transient ischemic attack
   2. Woman who had carpal tunnel surgery
   3. Older man who had knee replacement surgery
   4. Child who was born with spina bifida

8. The nurse is assisting a patient with a SCI to move to a wheelchair. Which intervention would the nurse use to prevent postural hypotension?
   1. Take the blood pressure and pulse to establish a baseline.
   2. Ask the patient if he feels dizzy or lightheaded.
   3. Make sure the patient is well hydrated and well nourished.
   4. Raise the head of the bed 15-20 minutes before moving him.

9. The nurse works at a rehabilitation unit and is assigned four patients with the following medical conditions: arthritis, SCI, stroke, and multiple sclerosis. Which basic nursing measure is common to the care of these four patients?
   1. Maintaining body alignment and position changes
   2. Assessing for pain and administering pain medication
   3. Assessing for orthostatic hypotension and dizziness
   4. Initiating bladder training and monitoring incontinence

10. Which patient is **most** likely to need cues and reminders to accomplish ADLs?
    1. Has COPD
    2. Has SCI
    3. Has traumatic brain injury (TBI)
    4. Has posttraumatic stress disorder (PTSD)

11. The patient experienced an SCI at the T1-T5 level. Which action should the patient be able to do?
    1. Independently perform most ADLs.
    2. Ambulate with the use of assistive devices.
    3. Resume normal sexual activities.
    4. Control bowel and bladder function.

12. A construction worker sustained an injury to C3 after a fall at a work site. Which problem does the nurse observe for?
    1. Use of the arms, but not the legs
    2. Control of bladder, but not bowels
    3. Potential for respiratory failure and infections
    4. Difficulty understanding and following instructions

13. The spouse reports that her husband tripped and bumped his head. He never lost consciousness but seemed confused for a few minutes after the accident. Which assessment finding does the nurse expect?
    1. Headache and vertigo
    2. Difficulty with judgment and reasoning
    3. Posttraumatic amnesia and aggressiveness
    4. Appears awake, but does not respond

14. The patient has an SCI above the level of T5. While assisting with hygienic care, the nurse notices that the patient is diaphoretic and shivering, and he reports a headache. His blood pressure is elevated. What would the nurse do **first**?
    1. Recheck blood pressure and call the HCP.
    2. Reposition to a position of comfort.
    3. Check for bladder distention.
    4. Give an antihypertensive medication.

15. The nurse anticipates that the patient with a SCI is at risk for venous thrombosis. Which interventions will be used for prevention? **Select all that apply.**
    1. Fluid restriction
    2. Passive and active range-of-motion exercises
    3. Application of heat
    4. Administration of anticoagulants
    5. Application of elastic stockings
    6. Assessment for swelling, redness, and heat in extremities

16. The nurse is assessing a patient who had a stroke and was recently admitted to the rehabilitation unit. What is the **best** method to determine how much assistance is required for hygienic care?
    1. Instruct the UAP to assist as needed.
    2. Ask the patient how much he can do for himself.
    3. Read the documentation from the transferring facility.
    4. Observe the patient performing tasks such as eating.

17. The older patient with a hip fracture has a self-care deficit related to bathing due to problems with ambulation and balance. Which action would the nurse use to foster independence while ensuring safety?
    1. Help the patient sit in the bathtub and bathe self, rather than attempt to stand and balance in the shower.
    2. Have the UAP stay with the patient during shower, but tell the UAP to let the patient wash herself.
    3. Have the patient remain in bed; bring warm, moist towels and suggest she wash her hands and face.
    4. Sit the patient on an elevated shower chair; adjust the water temperature of the handheld shower spray.

18. To maximize participation in therapy, which patient is **most** likely to need minimal distractions?
    1. Patient is depressed.
    2. Patient had an MI.
    3. Patient had a TBI.
    4. Patient has COPD.

19. A patient had cardiac surgery and has improved, but he is unable to return to work. The spouse feels that she must quit her job to take care of him. In this case, what would be considered the **best** outcome?
    1. Patient continuously works toward resuming his old job.
    2. Spouse acknowledges patient's ability to independently stay at home.
    3. Spouse quits her job, and concerns about husband's situation are alleviated.
    4. Patient acknowledges spouse's feelings and encourages her to stop worrying.

20. A young, healthy person was involved in an explosion at a chemical factory and sustained polytrauma/blast-related injury. Which types of injuries would the health care team expect to find? **Select all that apply.**
    1. Burns
    2. Fractures of extremities
    3. Chemical pneumonitis
    4. Brain injury
    5. MI
    6. Hearing loss

21. An experienced adult rehabilitation nurse is temporarily floated to the pediatric rehabilitation unit and assigned to care for a 7-year-old boy who sustained TBI. What would the nurse expect in caring for this pediatric patient?
    1. Child's cognitive function will be similar to an adult patient with TBI.
    2. Child is likely to respond and improve more rapidly than an adult.
    3. Child's treatment and interventions are similar to the adult care plan.
    4. Child's developmental age and capabilities are included in the care plan.

CRITICAL THINKING ACTIVITIES

22. The patient who sustained a TBI was admitted to an acute care facility then transferred to a rehabilitation facility. Now the patient is alert, stable, and ambulatory but he suffers residual effects from the TBI.

    a. In the rehabilitative assessment of this patient, what may the nurse expect to find? _____

    _____

    _____

    _____

    _____

    _____

    b. What type of interventions does the nurse anticipate for the patient with a TBI? _____

    _____

    _____

    _____

    _____

23. The nurse is caring for a patient who needs post-stroke care and rehabilitation. The patient has residual right-sided weakness in the arm and leg. The physical therapist and the occupational therapist are optimistic that the patient can recover some function, but return to pre-stroke status is unlikely. The patient is currently discouraged and is focused on loss and disability. He shows little interest in performing the exercises or in learning how to do self-care.

    a. What should the nurse do first? _____

    _____

    _____

    _____

    _____

    b. Identify several ways that the nurse can encourage independence. _____

    _____

    _____

    _____

    _____

    _____

NEXT-GENERATION NCLEX™ (NGN)

24. Extended Drag and Drop

Cognitive Skill: Take Action

Scenario: Rehabilitation is a complex process that requires knowledge and expertise from multiple disciplines. The rehabilitation team coordinates to deliver a comprehensive and individualized program for each patient. Team members listed below were recruited to meet the needs of a patient who had a stroke.

Instructions: In the left column are members of the rehabilitation team. Actions are listed in the right column. In the space provided, write in the letter for the team member who would perform the action. Each team member will be used only once.

Team Member	Actions
a. Clinical psychologist	_____ 1. Takes control of own life
b. Occupational therapist	_____ 2. Is team leader and coordinator of program
c. Rehabilitation RN	_____ 3. Educates patient and family concerning rehabilitation process
d. Speech-language pathologist	
e. Chaplain	_____ 4. Gives care and assists in treatment plan and implementation
f. Physiatrist	
g. Rehabilitation LPN/LVN	_____ 5. Designs exercise program
h. Vocational rehabilitation counselor	_____ 6. Recommends equipment modifications and adaptations
i. Patient	_____ 7. Helps patient regain communication skills
j. Physical therapist	_____ 8. Plans leisure activities and promotes patient's interest in activities
k. Therapeutic recreation therapist	
	_____ 9. Assesses patient's status on the mental health continuum
	_____ 10. Provides spiritual support and guidance
	_____ 11. Helps patient obtain training for new or current employment

Student Name_____ Date_____

Hospice Care

40

Answer Key: A complete Answer Key is provided in your Additional Learning Resources on Evolve.

MULTIPLE CHOICE

Directions: Select the best answer(s) for each of the following questions.

1. A long-term care facility resident is in hospice care and end of life is imminent. The primary health care provider (HCP) orders IV fluids. The hospice nurse objects and the nurses are not sure what to do. Who should mediate this situation?
   1. Director of nursing services for the facility
   2. Family member who has power of attorney
   3. Medical director of the core interdisciplinary team
   4. Supervisor of the hospice nurse

2. The family of an older adult is struggling with financing long-term care versus loss of income if someone quits work to provide full-time care. Which member of the core interdisciplinary team would be **most** helpful in advising the family?
   1. Social worker
   2. Nurse coordinator
   3. Medical director
   4. Admissions nurse

3. Which outcome statement **best** indicates that the goal of bereavement counseling has been met?
   1. Widow reports that family missed her dead husband during the holidays, but he was fondly remembered.
   2. Older widow appreciates bereavement counselor and a deep personal relationship develops.
   3. Widow calls bereavement counselor several times a month for several years after the death of spouse.
   4. Bereavement counselor sends cards and messages, but never hears from the widow of the deceased.

4. Which assessment is the nurse **most** likely to perform to evaluate efficacy of hypodermoclysis?
   1. Assess for bowel sounds and abdominal distention.
   2. Assess mucous membranes and skin turgor.
   3. Assess for relief of local pain and general discomfort.
   4. Assess for nausea and frequency of vomiting.

5. Which factors contribute to constipation in terminally ill patients? **Select all that apply.**
   1. Poor dietary intake
   2. Poor fluid intake
   3. Hyperglycemia
   4. Hyponatremia
   5. Opioids for pain control
   6. Decreased activity

Copyright © 2023, 2019, 2015, 2011, 2006, 2003, 1999, 1995, 1991 by Elsevier Inc. All rights reserved. **301**

6. In which circumstance would the nurse need to know whether a patient has agreed to Do Not Resuscitate (DNR)?
   1. Patient has terminal illness and refuses to eat.
   2. Patient is having chest pain with trouble breathing.
   3. Patient has no pulse and is not breathing.
   4. Patient is difficult to arouse with faint pulse.

7. Which patient **best** meets the criteria for admission to hospice?
   1. The patient is in poor health, homeless, and prognosis is uncertain; no family caregivers are available for support.
   2. The patient is undergoing cancer treatments, but pain and symptoms are difficult for the family to manage.
   3. The patient has less than 6 months to live and family is willing to participate in the planning of care.
   4. The patient wants around-the-clock skilled nursing care and emergency life support as needed.

8. The family of a dying patient is feeling physically and emotionally exhausted while taking around-the-clock shifts to care for their loved one. Which hospice service would be the **best** benefit for the family?
   1. Respite care service
   2. Palliative care consultation
   3. Bereavement counseling
   4. Hospice ethics committee

9. The HCP orders oral opioid medication for the terminally ill patient for pain control. What other types of medications would the nurse expect the HCP to order? **Select all that apply.**
   1. Anticholinergics
   2. Anticonvulsants
   3. Anticoagulants
   4. Antiemetics
   5. Antihypertensives
   6. Anxiolytics

10. The hospice nurse performs a pain assessment and gives different amounts of pain medication to the patient rather than the same dose each time. What is the **best** rationale for this practice?
    1. Determining the right dose of medication is difficult, so different amounts are tried to determine a safe dose.
    2. As a person is dying, the organs begin to shut down and absorption and metabolism of medication decreases.
    3. Every patient is different in how he or she responds to the medication, so it is administered by trial and error.
    4. The dosage is titrated to manage pain while keeping the patient alert enough to interact with the family.

11. Which nursing intervention would help the patient/family to meet the hospice goals?
    1. Encourage the family to consider putting the patient into long-term care.
    2. Remind the cancer patient that hoping for remission is therapeutic and beneficial.
    3. Reassure the primary caregiver that going out to a movie is not being selfish.
    4. Reinforce that eating and drinking as much as possible facilitates healing and recovery.

12. The patient and family are from a culture that differs from the nurse's. The family is performing rituals that are making the patient physically and emotionally uncomfortable. What would the nurse do **first**?
    1. Graciously respect the patient's and family's cultural beliefs and allow them to continue.
    2. Politely ask the patient if he wants to continue or if he would like the family to stop.
    3. Humbly attempt to understand the benefit of the rituals from a cultural point of view.
    4. Respectfully inquire if there is a way to modify the rituals to make them less traumatic.

13. The hospice volunteer says, "I might quit. I like the patient, but the wife expects me to do yardwork, errands, cooking, housework, and pet care. Now she wants the house painted." What would the nurse do?
    1. Talk to the wife and explain the role and responsibilities of the volunteer.
    2. Call the volunteer coordinator and ask for additional help to paint the house.
    3. Ask the patient how he has been getting along with the volunteer.
    4. Instruct the volunteer to explain the situation to the volunteer coordinator.

14. The patient and hospice aide frequently talk, joke, and have a close relationship. The nurse suspects that the patient is disclosing more concerns to the aide than he is to the rest of the staff. What is the **most** important action for the nurse to take?
    1. Praise the hospice aide for having a supportive rapport with the patient.
    2. Have frequent contact with the aide to get updates on the patient's concerns.
    3. Remind the aide about scope of practice and staff-patient boundaries.
    4. Try to spend more time with the patient to develop a better rapport and trust.

15. The patient is a large man who needs assistance to move and transfer to a wheelchair. His wife, the caregiver, is a relatively small woman. Which team member can **best** assist the wife with this issue?
    1. Physiatrist
    2. Hospice aide
    3. Physical therapist
    4. Nurse coordinator

16. The Edmonton Symptom Assessment System (ESAS) was used when the patient was first admitted into hospice. Which current assessment findings could be compared to the baseline established by ESAS?
    1. Patient's satisfaction with plan of care and recommendations for improvement
    2. Patient's subjective feeling of pain, tiredness, and overall feeling of well-being
    3. Patient's cognitive, intellectual, and perceptual status and ability to make judgments
    4. Patient's ability to perform activities of daily living (ADLs) and home maintenance

17. The patient is having significant pain, but refuses to take oral morphine. "Because it makes me feel confused and I hallucinate." What would the nurse do **first**?
    1. Encourage taking the medication for now, but promise to call the HCP.
    2. Offer a prescribed nonopioid drug and try several nonpharmacologic options.
    3. Call the pharmacist to see if alternative routes of administration cause fewer side effects.
    4. Give the patient a lower dose and observe for confusion or other side effects.

18. Patient has nausea to related anxiety and to obstruction caused by growth of a tumor. Which medication, if prescribed, would the nurse question?
    1. Promethazine: suppository 30 minutes before meals
    2. Prochlorperazine: oral dose as needed for nausea
    3. Lorazepam: oral dose as needed every 6-8 hours for anxiety
    4. Senna: oral dose two times per day

19. The patient is having nausea and vomiting, so the nurse gives the patient an antiemetic and the vomiting subsides. What would the nurse offer the patient **first**?
    1. Diluted bouillon
    2. Plain white rice
    3. Vanilla pudding
    4. Favorite food

20. The patient has not had a bowel movement. What is the **initial** nursing action?
    1. Advise to increase fiber and fluids in the diet.
    2. Assess the amount and frequency of opioid usage.
    3. Explain that decreased oral intake decreases the amount of stool.
    4. Assess discomfort, bowel sounds, and firmness of the abdomen.

21. The nurse notes that the patient is weak and emaciated and determines that stomatitis is contributing to the problem. Which intervention would be the **most** helpful?
    1. Administer an antiemetic medication 30 minutes before meals.
    2. Weigh the patient after meals and point out small improvements.
    3. Assist with oral hygiene and use water-soaked swabs before and after meals.
    4. Have family bring in meals, rather than cook at home.

22. The HCP has informed the hospice patient, family, and nurse that there is an invasive untreatable tumor that is contributing to the patient's anorexia. Which intervention is the **best** for the patient?
    1. Emotional support
    2. Artificial hydration
    3. Total parental nutrition
    4. Tube feedings

23. The nurse gets a phone call from the caregiver who reports hearing the "death rattle." Which instructions would the nurse give to the caregiver?
    1. "I will get an order for a bronchodilator medication and bring it to the house."
    2. "Apply oxygen and stay with him. I will come to the house right now."
    3. "Sit the patient upright in bed, apply oxygen, and call 911."
    4. "This is expected: mucus and fluids will pool in the back of his throat."

24. The patient is having difficulty with excessive secretions which cause coughing and choking, especially at night. He is unable to independently sit upright. Which intervention is **best**?
    1. Teach the patient to cough and deep-breathe.
    2. Obtain an order for droperidol.
    3. Teach the caregiver to perform oral-tracheal suctioning.
    4. Obtain an order for transdermal scopolamine.

25. The hospice aide was devastated when the patient died and the nurse discovers that the aide has been visiting the caregiver on daily basis for the past 12 months. What would the nurse do?
    1. Assess the caregiver's feelings about the frequent visits from the aide.
    2. Report the hospice aide's behavior to the nurse coordinator.
    3. Assess the hospice aide's feelings and motivations for behavior.
    4. Suggest that the hospice aide contact the bereavement counselor.

26. The caregiver is normally calm and eager to participate. Today she is frustrated and angrily says, "Nothing is working and I can't go on like this!" What would the nurse do **first**?
    1. Contact the interdisciplinary team so that the plan can be reevaluated.
    2. Call the nurse coordinator to come and assess the situation.
    3. Check the patient for changes in physical, emotional, or behavioral status.
    4. Use therapeutic communication and encourage the caregiver to express concerns.

27. The hospice patient has an increased risk for pressure injuries in the last stages of end of life. He is weak and spends most of the time reclining and dozing. Which instructions will the nurse give to the hospice aide? **Select all that apply.**
    1. Determine the need for heel and elbow protectors.
    2. Report redness or skin breakdown.
    3. Monitor for poor nutrition, decreased circulation, and immobility.
    4. Use mild soap for bathing and hygiene.
    5. Keep linens clean, dry, and free of food or other debris.

28. Which question would the nurse ask to evaluate the efficacy of droperidol?
    1. "When was your last bowel movement?"
    2. "On a scale of 1 to 10, what number is your pain?"
    3. "Has the medication helped to reduce the nausea?"
    4. "Did the medication help to reduce your anxiety?"

29. In which circumstance is it **most** important for the nurse to perform an abdominal assessment?
    1. Patient is having side effects after taking the prescribed dose of prochlorperazine.
    2. Patient's extremities are cool and the underside of the body becomes darker.
    3. Patient is refusing to eat or drink as much as he typically would for breakfast.
    4. Patient has no bowel movements despite drinking fluid and taking senna as prescribed.

30. Which outcome statement **best** indicates that the goal of palliative care has been met?
    1. Patient finalizes his will and empowers son to be medical power of attorney.
    2. Patient's pain is controlled, and he enjoys a visit with the grandchildren.
    3. Patient independently completes morning hygiene and dresses himself.
    4. Patient and family acknowledge that curing the illness is not possible.

CRITICAL THINKING ACTIVITIES

31. The family of a patient with terminal cancer has requested information about hospice care. The patient has severe pain and potential curative treatments have been exhausted.

    a. How would the nurse assess the patient's pain? _____

    _____

    _____

    _____

    _____

    b. Identify the types of medications that may be used to relieve or reduce pain for the following.

       i. Mild to moderate pain: _____

       _____

       ii. Severe pain: _____

       _____

       iii. Long-lasting results: _____

       _____

    c. What nonpharmacologic measures may also be implemented to relieve or reduce pain?

    _____

    _____

    _____

32. An 86-year-old man has Alzheimer's disease. His 80-year-old wife has been taking care of him at home for the past 10 years. He was recently diagnosed with an aggressive and inoperable cancer. His family agrees that he should be in hospice, but they are unable to agree on who should be the primary caregiver. The wife insists that she has been taking care of her husband for 10 years and is capable. The eldest son has been responsible for paying the bills and overseeing his parents' finances; he thinks that his sister, who is a nurse but lives in a different state, should move back and be the caregiver. The sister thinks that the grandson who is living with his grandparents and attends the university should be the

caregiver. The grandson agrees that he is at the house most often, but is reluctant to take the responsibility. Discuss how the hospice team can assist this family in the decision-making process.

_____

_____

_____

_____

_____

_____

_____

NEXT-GENERATION NCLEX™ (NGN)

33. Matrix

Cognitive Skill: Analyze Cues

Scenario: The hospice nurse is caring for a patient who is restless, picking at the bedspread, and talking to her dead husband. She sleeps most of the time and is difficult to arouse. She is refusing to eat or drink. Her hands and feet are cool and discolored. Her breathing is irregular with occasional apnea lasting 10-20 seconds. Oral secretions are collecting in the back of the throat and a coarse gurgling sound is heard. Bowel and bladder incontinence occur. Blood pressure is 80/60 mm Hg and pulse is 130 beats/min.

Which interventions are used for the patient at the end of life?

Instructions: Use an X to indicate which interventions are essential, nonessential, or contraindicated. All interventions should be categorized.

Nursing Intervention	Essential	Nonessential	Contraindicated
Talk calmly and gently reassure patient.			
Start an IV and titrate fluid to increase blood pressure.			
Provide a cool-mist humidifier.			
Perform endotracheal suctioning to remove secretions.			
Encourage caregiver to feed patient small spoonfuls.			
Reorient to the time of day and who is present.			
Cover with warm blankets.			
Advise limiting number of visitors and duration of visit time to prevent overtiring the patient.			
Instruct UAP to keep patient clean and dry and use pads or adult diapers as needed.			
Elevate the head of the bed with pillows.			

Professional Roles and Leadership

Answer Key: A complete Answer Key is provided in your Additional Learning Resources on Evolve.

SHORT ANSWER

Directions: Using your own words, answer each question in the space provided.

1. What are the key components of a cover letter?_____

    _____

    _____

2. What are the advantages of membership in professional organizations? _____

    _____

    _____

3. For the NCLEX-PN® examination, identify the following.

    a. Minimum number of questions: _____

    b. Maximum number of questions: _____

    c. Maximum time allowed:_____

    d. Goal of computerized adaptive testing: _____

    e. Average time to receive results:_____

    f. Approval for candidate to take the test given by:_____

    g. Examples of alternate-item format questions:_____

4. List possible job settings for an LPN/LVN. _____

    _____

    _____

    _____

    _____

MULTIPLE CHOICE

Directions: Select the best answer(s) for each of the following questions.

5. A nurse is participating in a phone interview for a job at a pediatric walk-in clinic. Which question would be inappropriate for the interviewer to ask?
   1. "Have you ever been arrested for a criminal activity?"
   2. "Do you have hobbies or recreational activities that involve children?"
   3. "Do you think that pediatrics is part of your long-term career goals?"
   4. "Do you think that a person of your age could work with children?"

6. A newly graduated nurse is interviewing for her first job. Which question is the **most** important for the nurse to ask?
   1. "Is the employment contract verbal, implied, or written?"
   2. "What kind of internship or residency programs do you offer?"
   3. "How would I fit into the existing organizational chart?"
   4. "Would I have to take a competency test for medication or math?"

7. The LPN/LVN desires to improve knowledge and skills in IV therapy. Which educational opportunity would be the **best** route?
   1. Associate nursing degree
   2. In-service education
   3. Refresher course
   4. Certification

8. A conscientious nursing student tearfully says, "The NCLEX-PN® questions were hard and increasingly difficult. At 85 questions, the examination stopped. I think I failed." What is the instructor's **best** response?
   1. "You seem really upset. Let's take a moment and talk about how you feel."
   2. "So, worst-case scenario, if you failed, what can do you to take the next steps?"
   3. "Difficult questions are selected by performance; this reflects a high competence level."
   4. "Don't worry; generally having the system stop at 85 questions means that you passed."

9. These nurses have recently relocated from another state and are working at a new job. Which nurse has the **greatest** need to clarify the nurse practice act before acting on the request?
   1. LPN/LVN gets a verbal order to insert a peripheral IV catheter; then push IV opioid medication.
   2. Supervising RN asks LPN/LVN to train and supervise new unlicensed assistive personnel (UAP).
   3. Patient requests that LPN/LVN explain the difference between power of attorney and living will.
   4. Another LPN/LVN asks if the nurse could switch a shift because of child-care issues.

10. Under which circumstance would it be **most** appropriate for the nurse to contact the state board of nursing, if the nurse has already tried to go up the chain of command at the place of employment?
    1. LPN/LVN feels that competency testing was unfair because of culturally biased questions.
    2. Charge nurse shows favoritism to her friends when making out the patient assignments.
    3. Patient has threatened to name LPN/LVN in a lawsuit that involves physician malpractice.
    4. Supervising RN is making assignments that fall outside the LPN/LVN's scope of practice.

11. There has been an earthquake in the area, and disaster victims are being brought into the emergency department. In this situation, which type of leadership would the nurse manager use?
    1. Democratic
    2. Autocratic
    3. Situational
    4. Laissez-faire

12. The nursing student will be able to take the NCLEX-PN® within a few months. However, the student's fiancé is likely to be transferred to another state within the next year. What would the student do?
    1. Wait until the fiancé has moved and then apply to that state board of nursing to take NCLEX-PN®.
    2. Wait until after legally married to take the NCLEX-PN® so that the license will be issued under the married name.
    3. Apply to take the NCLEX-PN® in the current state of residency and investigate reciprocity or endorsement with other states.
    4. Apply to take the NCLEX-PN® in the current state of residency and then retake the NCLEX-PN® in the permanent state of residency.

13. A new nurse is unsure of a prescription that is handwritten but believes that it is appropriate. What would the nurse do **first**?
    1. Transcribe it to the medication administration record.
    2. Report the problem to the nursing supervisor.
    3. Wait for the health care provider (HCP) to return and clarify prescription.
    4. Ask a charge nurse or senior nurse to look at the prescription.

14. The patient had surgery in the morning; at bedtime, he requests pain medication. The nurse administers a preoperative dose of opioid medication. An hour later, the patient reports unrelieved pain and the nurse recognizes the error. What would the nurse do **first**?
    1. Check the postoperative prescription and give the correct dose.
    2. Inform the patient that additional medication cannot be given at this time.
    3. Report the error to the HCP and ask for a one-time prescription for pain medication.
    4. Make out an incident report and document actions in the patient record.

15. The nurse is caring for several patients. Which tasks can be delegated to the UAP? **Select all that apply.**
    1. Taking the morning vital signs
    2. Changing the linens for isolation patients
    3. Restocking the medications and intravenous solutions
    4. Ambulating patients in the hallway
    5. Assessing skin condition while bathing
    6. Transcribing orders during the night shift

16. Which action could be considered negligence by the nurse and could potentially result in the loss of the nursing license?
    1. Fails to check patient allergies prior to administering medication, but patient suffers no harm
    2. Fails to report change of status to HCP; the patient declines and resuscitation is required
    3. Fails to give medication within the time limit established by the facility's policies and procedures
    4. Fails to come to work on time and so offgoing nurse has to stay later to cover patient care

17. The nurse overhears an RN, who is a friend, discussing patient information in the cafeteria. There are visitors nearby and they appear to be listening. What would the nurse do **first**?
    1. Take the RN aside and tell her that others are listening.
    2. Report the RN to the office of risk management.
    3. Walk over to the RN and quickly change the subject.
    4. Write an incident report and submit it anonymously.

18. The nurse is assigned to be the chairman of a patient satisfaction committee. The committee will include nurses, UAPs, and unit secretaries from other units in the hospital. Which style of leadership would be the **most** useful?
    1. Autocratic
    2. Democratic
    3. Laissez-faire
    4. Situational

19. The nurse is working in a long-term care facility and instructs the UAP to assist several patients with morning hygiene and report back if anyone is having any problems. Which delegation error has the nurse made?
    1. Has assigned the UAP too many patients
    2. Has given the UAP a task that is not within scope of practice
    3. Has given broad and generalized instructions to the UAP
    4. Has failed to give feedback on the UAP's performance

20. The new nurse is having difficulty with time management. She is frustrated and always stays late to complete her work. What would be the **first** step to improve time management?
    1. Ask for help if falling behind schedule.
    2. Stop socializing with colleagues.
    3. Reflect on how the time is being spent.
    4. Set goals every day and stick to them.

21. Which actions are considered part of the responsibilities of the nurse manager? **Select all that apply.**
    1. Submits staffing schedules for the unit
    2. Conducts regular staff meetings
    3. Role-models nursing care for a group of assigned patients
    4. Recruits, interviews, and hires new employees
    5. Conducts routine staff evaluations
    6. Establishes necessary staff and interdisciplinary committees

22. Which nurse needs a reminder about how to handle confidential information?
    1. Nurse A discusses patient information during change-of-shift report
    2. Nurse B makes notes during the shift and shreds notes before leaving the unit
    3. Nurse C discusses the patient's condition with the wife and adult children
    4. Nurse D monitors the UAPs and intervenes as needed to safeguard patients' privacy.

23. The newly graduated nurse has taken a new job, but the facility does not have a mentoring program. Which action would be the **best** for the nurse to accomplish self-mentoring?
    1. Shadow an experienced nurse for several days.
    2. Ask for an extended probationary period.
    3. Offer to work weekends or night shifts.
    4. Ask questions and observe experienced nurses.

24. Which nurses are using strategies to prevent burnout? **Select all that apply.**
    1. Nurse A asks colleagues and family if they notice signs of burnout.
    2. Nurse B strives to meet the expectations of supervisor and coworkers.
    3. Nurse C completes morning rounds before preparing routine medications.
    4. Nurse D schedules time to spend with family doing fun activities.
    5. Nurse E explores opportunities in different fields of nursing.
    6. Nurse F sympathizes with other nurses and offers to help them.

CRITICAL THINKING ACTIVITIES

25. Identify a job or a practice setting that you would like to apply for. Describe what you will need to do to increase your chances of getting your first choice of position.

    _____

    _____

    _____

26. The nurse has just started a new job, but has never worked the night shift before. Identify self-care behaviors that the nurse could use for each of the following.

    a. Staying alert at work: _____

    _____

b. Getting to sleep: _____

_____

c. Balancing life with work: _____

_____

d. While there are many disadvantages to working the night shift, the nurse is looking forward to the new job and decides to focus on some of the advantages. Identify several things that could be considered a benefit of being on this shift. (Hint: Interview several night-shift nurses to get a variety of opinions.)

_____

_____

_____

_____

27. Listen to several different nurses give change-of-shift report. Describe the strong points of the reports and describe parts of the reports that could have been improved.

_____

_____

_____

_____

_____

_____

_____

_____

28. Compare different styles of report that you have seen on clinical units (e.g., audio, rounding on patients, etc.). If you have only seen one method, interview nurses and discuss with classmates or senior students.

_____

_____

_____

_____

_____

_____

_____

_____

NEXT-GENERATION NCLEX™ (NGN)

29. Cloze

Cognitive Skill: Analyze Cues

Instructions: Choose the most likely options to complete the statements below.

The LPN/LVN has started a new job. The supervising RN uses a people-centered approach and encourages staff input for the decision-making process. There is an atmosphere of team-building and collaboration that reflects a(n) ___1___ style of leadership. There is a position open and duties include receiving and giving reports on assigned patients, making assignments, assisting with medications and treatments, and conferencing with team members about priority patients. The LPN/LVN considers working toward this opportunity of being a ___2___. When the LPN/LVN begins her first workday, she tells the UAP to take vital signs on assigned patients every 4 hours, report abnormalities, and feel free to ask questions. In reviewing the Five Rights of Delegation, the LPN/LVN recognizes that she made an error related to the ___3___.

Options for 1	Options for 2	Options for 3
autocratic	nurse manager	right person
laissez-faire	certified nurse	right task
democratic	preceptor	right circumstance
situational	team leader	right communication
team management	float nurse	right supervision